HEALTH PROMOTION IN NURSING PRACTICE

Fourth Edition

HEALTH PROMOTION IN NURSING PRACTICE

Fourth Edition

Nola J. Pender, PhD, RN, FAAN

Professor and Associate Dean for Research
University of Michigan
School of Nursing
Ann Arbor, Michigan

Carolyn L. Murdaugh, PhD, RN, FAAN

Professor and Associate Dean for Research
University of South Carolina
College of Nursing
Columbia, South Carolina

Mary Ann Parsons, PhD, RN, FAAN

Professor and Dean
University of South Carolina
College of Nursing
Columbia, South Carolina

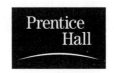

Prentice Hall

Upper Saddle River, NJ 07458

Library of Congress Cataloging-in-Publication Data

Pender, Nola J., 1941-
  Health promotion in nursing practice / Nola J.
  Pender, Carolyn L. Murdaugh, Mary Ann
  Parsons.—4th ed.
    p. ; cm.
  Includes bibliographical references and index.
  ISBN 0-13-031950-3 (paper)
  1. Health promotion. 2. Preventive health ser-
  vices. 3. Nursing. I. Murdaugh, Carolyn L.
  II. Parsons, Mary Ann. III. Title.
  [DNLM: 1. Health Promotion—Nurses'
  Instruction. 2. Nursing Care—Nurses'
  Instruction. 3. Health Behavior—Nurses'
  Instruction. 4. Health Policy—Nurses'
  Instruction. WS 350.2 G798c 2001]
RT67 .P56 2001
613—dc21   2001016328

Care has been taken to confirm the accuracy of information presented in this book. The authors, editors, and the publisher, however, cannot accept any responsibility for errors or omissions or for consequences from application of the information in this book and make no warranty, express or implied, with respect to its contents.

The authors and publisher have exerted every effort to ensure that drug selections and dosages set forth in this text are in accord with current recommendations and practice at time of publication. However, in view of ongoing research, changes in government regulations, and the constant flow of information relating to drug therapy and drug reactions, the reader is urged to check the package inserts of all drugs for any change in indications of dosage and for added warnings and precautions. This is particularly important when the recommended agent is a new and/or infrequently employed drug.

Publisher: Julie Alexander
Executive Editor: Maura Connor
Acquisitions Editor: Nancy Anselment
Production Editor: Mary Treacy
Director of Manufacturing and Production: Bruce Johnson
Managing Editor: Patrick Walsh
Manufacturing Buyer: Ilene Sanford
Editorial Assistant: Mary Ellen Ruitenberg
Cover Design: Jayne Conte
Composition: Carlisle Communications
Printing and Binding: RR Donnelley, Harrisonburg, VA

Prentice-Hall International (UK) Limited, *London*
Prentice-Hall of Australia Pty. Limited, *Sydney*
Prentice-Hall of Canada Inc., *Toronto*
Prentice-Hall Hispanoamericana, S.A., *Mexico*
Prentice-Hall of India Private Limited, *New Delhi*
Prentice-Hall of Japan, Inc., *Tokyo*
Prentice-Hall Pte., Singapore
Editora Prentice-Hall do Brasil, Ltda., *Rio de Janeiro*
Prentice-Hall, *Upper Saddle River, New Jersey*

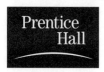

10 9 8 7 6 5 4 3 2 1
PRINTED IN THE UNITED STATES OF AMERICA

ISBN 0-13-031950-3

Contents

Preface

Over the past 30 years since I began my research and writing career in the field of health promotion, I have seen the prevention of illness and the promotion of health emerge as major objectives for the world community. The *Fifth Global Conference on Health Promotion* held in June 2000 in Mexico City, Mexico, indicates the importance that nations attribute to investing in the health of their citizens. Increasing the capacity of communities to promote health and create infrastructures for the delivery of health promotion services is a major challenge for the next decade.

In the United States, *Healthy People 2010* sets the pace for prevention and health promotion policy for the first years of the Twenty-First century. Further, the federal government has appointed two national task forces to craft guidelines for the delivery of clinical preventive services and community preventive services. The flurry of activity around the introduction of *Healthy People 2010* and its central position in national health policy bodes well for the stability of health promotion as an integral aspect of health care. Yet, much remains to be accomplished, including the systematic delivery of culturally sensitive health promotion services in primary and community care, and consistent reimbursement of health promotion and illness prevention services by public and private health care payment systems. Health promotion is here to stay. Now we must develop the appropriate multisectoral infrastructure to sustain it.

As an area of inquiry, health promotion is attracting the research talents of scholars in many fields, all of whom will contribute to a greater understanding among health professionals and consumers of what optimum health is and how it can be attained. Nurse scientists have made outstanding contributions to developing the knowledge base for the delivery of quality health promotion care to clients in varied settings. Nurses have the expertise to make major advances in designing and testing innovative health promotion interventions in schools, worksites, community health centers, as well as home-based systems using the latest scientific and technical knowledge. Now is the time for nurses to partner with community groups in designing health promotion services that meet particular population needs.

In publishing the fourth edition of this book, I have been extremely fortunate to collaborate with two superb coauthors with expertise in health promotion, nursing research, nursing education, and nursing practice. Dr. Carolyn L. Murdaugh, a well-known nursing scholar, has been funded for her research on family and individual adjustment to chronic illness and quality of life for over 20 years. Currently, she is associate dean for nursing research and also directs the Center for Health Promotion and Risk Reduction in Special Populations in the College of Nursing at the University of South Carolina. She is a fellow of the American Academy of Nursing. She previously was director of research, University of Arizona College of Nursing and Medical Center, as well as senior scientist and chief of the Laboratory for the Study of Human Responses in Health and Illness, Division of Intramural Research Programs, at the National Institute of Nursing Research, National Institutes of Health. Dr. Murdaugh has clinical experience in health screening and counseling, cardiovascular stress testing, and coronary care. She has authored over 75 publications and has been honored as one of seven national leaders who have transformed cardiovascular nursing. Dr. Mary Ann Parsons is a nationally known scholar for her work and writings in family practice and the health behaviors of adolescents. She has served as the dean of the College of Nursing at the University of South Carolina since 1988. She has been instrumental in establishing a faculty practice that includes three clinics managed by advanced practice nurse faculty who incorporate prevention and health promotion interventions into clinic services. Dr. Parsons has served as president of the State Board of Nursing for South Carolina and was instrumental in developing the current national nursing licensure examination. She has conducted federally funded research focused on comprehensive health assessment by school nurses, risk factors in high-stress jobs, and exercise behavior of middle school children. Formerly, she taught at the Medical University of South Carolina and at the University of Florida. She is a fellow of the American Academy of Nursing and a certified adult nurse practitioner with a rich background of clinical experience in adult nursing and community-based care.

The purpose of the fourth edition of this book is threefold: (1) to provide an overview of major health behavior models and theories that can guide health promotion interventions; (2) to describe strategies and tools that can be used by nursing students and nurses in practice settings to provide evidence-based health promotion care to diverse populations; and (3) to foster critical thinking about future directions for health promotion intervention research and health promotion in nursing practice. If we accomplish these goals in some measure, all of the hours that were dedicated to the preparation of this book will be worthwhile.

The content of the book is organized into five sections. Part I presents various definitions of health, a number of theories and models useful in planning health promotion services, and the health promotion model and related research. Part II addresses empowerment for self-care across the life span as well as strategies for promoting the health of vulnerable populations. Part III presents strategies for assessing health, health beliefs, and health behaviors and developing a health protection–promotion plan. Part IV describes interventions for promoting physical activity, positive nutrition practices, stress management, and social support. Part V critically analyzes a very important topic, evaluating the effectiveness of individual and community health promotion interventions. Part VI addresses forming partnerships with communities for health promotion and developing policies and programs for promoting a healthier society. At the end of each chapter, readers are encouraged to reflect on the implications of what they have read for nursing research and nursing practice. The term *client* rather than *patient* is used throughout the book to denote individuals, families, groups, and communities that are active participants in health promotion and prevention. *Health* and *wellness* are used as interchangeable terms.

Appreciation is extended to Nancy Anselment and Mary Treacy, editors, for their assistance in preparation of the book. We are also indebted to persons at our respective universities who assisted us with literature searches, preparation of tables and figures, and proofing of chapters: Karen McIlroy, administrative associate, University of Michigan Child and Adolescent Health Behavior Research Center; Amy Lanier, administrative assistant, College of Nursing, University of South Carolina; and Rebecca Baker and LiaHong Xu, graduate assistants, Office of Research, College of Nursing, University of South Carolina.

Nola J. Pender

Reviewers

Janice Donaldson Hausauer, RN, MS, FNP
College of Nursing
Montana State University
Bozeman, MT

Madeline J. Kerr, PhD
School of Nursing
University of Minnesota
Minneapolis, MN

Maryanne Lachat, RN, PhD
School of Nursing
Georgetown University
Washington, DC

Sally Lusk, PhD, RN, FAAN
School of Nursing
University of Michigan
Ann Arbor, MI

Lucia Matuk
School of Nursing
University of Windsor
Windsor, ON
Canada, N9B 3P4

Introduction

Health Promotion and Disease Prevention: The Challenges of a New Millennium

As the new millennium begins, institutionalizing health promotion and disease prevention as integral aspects of health care presents a challenge for all nations. Accumulating evidence indicates that health promotion holds promise for maintaining vigor, vitality, and productivity into the eighth and ninth decades of life for an increasing proportion of the world population. As the link between a healthy and productive population and national welfare and economic prosperity is recognized, governments of many countries are developing national health promotion plans to shape the future directions of health care. The overall goals of these plans are to help people of all ages stay healthy, to optimize health in the presence of chronic disease or disability, and to create health environments in which to live. According to the World Health Organization (WHO), health promotion includes encouraging healthy lifestyles, creating supportive environments for health, strengthening community action, reorienting health services to place primary focus on promoting health and preventing disease, and building healthy public policy. Health promotion must be geared not only to individuals but also to families and the communities in which they live. Healthy public policy can facilitate positive changes in health behavior norms as well as provide health-enhancing environments on a national and international scale.[1]

Unfortunately the gap between the generation of knowledge about health promotion and prevention and its application in practice remains problematic.[2] Although a number of theories and models to guide health promotion interventions for individuals, families, and communities have been proposed and tested, health professions education has been slow to promulgate curricula to ensure that students develop knowledge and expertise in delivering theory-based health promotion and prevention care to clients. This must change. Greater expediency is needed in moving scientific breakthroughs into evidence-based practice in order for the public to benefit in a timely manner from new knowledge. A challenge of the Twenty-First century will be to provide access to knowledge and services that promote health for all segments of an increasingly diverse population. This must be accomplished in an environment of economic constraints requiring that the resources spent on health care be balanced with other resource demands.

Another challenge is to address social problems that compromise health and well-being. Early development of positive health behaviors such as caring interpersonal relationships, community service participation, and responsible sexuality can decrease social problems such as violence, suicide, and sexually transmitted diseases that are of increasing prevalence world-wide. Youths are a valuable global asset, yet this is the population in which many social problems are most prevalent. Healthy behaviors rather than risky behaviors need to be supported by families and communities to optimize health for all in the Twenty-First century.[3] Guthrie and colleagues have suggested that gender-specific health promotion frameworks may be needed to address issues of gender socialization that impact health behaviors as well as the physical and mental health of adolescents.[4]

In an age of rapid advances in information technology, electronic media offer unprecedented opportunities to provide health-related information to the public. Innovative use of interactive computer technology and interactive television through worldwide networks is enabling health professionals and consumers to collaborate as never before in tailoring health communications to the special needs of individuals and families from diverse populations.[5,6,7] Health systems are increasing their capabilities to literally "reach around the world." Innovative use of communication networks such as the World Wide Web can provide open access to the latest health knowledge, creating a national and international resource for informed health care decision making by both providers and consumers. Care must be taken to provide access to computerized information systems for vulnerable populations. It is encouraging to note that recent research examining the acceptability of computerized assessments of smoking behavior in low-income populations indicated that 92% of the study participants found the programs either "very easy" or "easy" to use.[8]

Nurses should be at the forefront in developing interactive health education counseling programs and behavioral interventions that capitalize on emerging information technology breakthroughs. A "one size fits all" approach to health promotion programming has become outdated in the Twenty-First century. Technology offers nurses new tools for further developing the individualized health care to which they have long been committed.

Breakthroughs in understanding the human genome have the potential to markedly enhance health and prevent disease. In the next decade, molecular prevention will become a reality. Nurses will be pivotal in helping clients to combine knowledge about personal genetic makeup, genetic prevention techniques, and behavior change strategies to prevent illnesses for which they are at high risk. Nursing research agendas as well as nursing education programs should embrace evolving scientific discoveries in the health sciences, and pioneer and test innovative biopsychosocial nursing care strategies.

Toward a Global Health Agenda

All people of the world must be recognized as a global community, a health megasystem. What affects one country does not happen in isolation but affects other countries as well. Strategies suggested to achieve health for all on a global scale include the following: (1) empowering people by providing the latest health information and decision-making opportunities; (2) strengthening local systems of primary health care; (3) improving education and training programs in health promotion and prevention for health professionals; (4) applying science and technology to critical health problems; (5) using new approaches to problems such as violence that have resisted solution; (6) providing culturally appropriate assistance to the least developed countries; and (7) establishing a process for examination of the world challenges that must be addressed to make good health a reality for the masses.[9] In the next century, the health-promoting and health-damaging features of social policies, organizations, and environments will receive increased attention. As early as the mid-1980s, when WHO articulated its global commitment to health promotion as a process enabling people to make healthy personal choices within a context of social responsibility for health, the organization emphasized the necessity of going beyond the education of individuals to include organizational changes, community development, and legislation.[10] This broader approach to health promotion is well illustrated by the Healthy Cities Projects that WHO initiated in 1984 in Europe. The project stresses a municipal approach to health promotion through extensive community participation, intersectoral cooperation, and the implementation of comprehensive city plans for health promotion. The target endpoints to be evaluated are not only morbidity and mortality but also prevalence of health-promoting behaviors, quality of the physical and social environment, and extent of community empowerment and action.[11] Healthy Cities Project's focus on health as a central concern to be addressed in political, economic, and social decisions. Building healthy cities is an ecological approach that has yet to reach its full potential for improving the health of the masses. Many lessons can be learned from the WHO project that will enable cities and nations to make health a priority and improve well-being throughout the life span, especially for vulnerable populations.

The Fifth Global Conference on Health Promotion provided an international forum in which to explore approaches for strengthening the evidence base for health promotion. A challenge for scientists is to develop credible, widely recognized, high-quality standards for evaluation of the effectiveness of multisectoral health promotion interventions. This task presents a formidable challenge given the complexity of health promotion interventions ranging from changing the behavior of individuals and collectives to changing policies that set norms for behavior.[12] Use of behavioral surveillance systems will be critical to assessing progress toward health promotion objectives. Time-sensitive strategies for analyzing data and using data to make strategic decisions about "what works" will be essential to further the public health agenda for prevention and health promotion.[13]

A progressive step toward international collaboration among nurses for health promotion and prevention was the establishment of World Health Organization Collaborating Centers. Nurses from centers throughout the world share information about innovative models for delivery of health promotion and prevention services, curricula content at the undergraduate and graduate levels to prepare nursing students to deliver quality health education counseling and behavioral interventions, approaches to developing strategic national plans for health promotion, and directions for research to build scientific knowledge upon which successful health promotion and prevention nursing interventions can be based. Nurses can play a pivotal role throughout the world in mobilizing forces for change in individual, family, and organizational health behaviors. Thus, the development of nurses for leadership in health promotion is an international priority.

National Progress Toward Health

In the United States, it is estimated that unhealthy lifestyles are responsible for 55% mortality, environment for 25%, and heredity for the other 20%.[14] This is a powerful message that unless the health care system is significantly changed to influence lifestyles and environments, the nation's health profile will continue to deteriorate. Demographic changes toward an older population and a more ethnically diverse population will create new demands for health promotion and prevention services in primary care and public health.[15]

In 1979, the report *Healthy People: The Surgeon General's Report on Health Promotion and Disease Prevention* introduced a set of broad national goals for improving the health of Americans by 1990.[16] In 1980, a companion document, *Health Promotion—Disease Prevention: Objectives for the Nation,* was published and identified 226 specific health goals in three major areas: health promotion, health protection, and preventive health services.[17] The greatest gains were made in the areas of control of high blood pressure, injury prevention, smoking reduction, immunization, and dental health. Death rates for both heart attacks and strokes also decreased. Because the 1990 objectives were perceived as effective in drawing the nation's attention to the potential of disease prevention and health promotion to increase longevity and improve the quality of lives, national objectives were also set for the year 2000. In 1990, *Healthy People 2000: National Health Promotion and Disease Prevention Objectives* was published. It identified three broad goals: Increase the span of healthy life for Americans, reduce health disparities among Americans, and achieve access to preventive services for all Americans. The plan organized 300 national objectives into 22 priorities for action. These were placed in the categories of health promotion, health protection, preventive services, and surveillance and data systems.[18] Surveillance and data systems were put in place to better track achievement of national goals and greater attention was given to tracking the health status of groups by race and ethnicity. Successes included increasing immunization levels among children and older adults, reducing infant mortality, decreasing unintended pregnancies among adolescents, increasing use of seat belts, decreased driving while impaired by alcohol or drugs, and leveling off of tobacco, alcohol, and illicit drug use.[14] An excellent overview of the status of the nation on six different health behaviors is provided by a series of articles in the *American Journal of Health Promotion*.[19-25]

Healthy people in healthy communities is the vision of *Healthy People 2010*,[14] the blueprint for health services in the United States in the new millennium. The two major goals include increasing quality and years of healthy life and eliminating health disparities. It should be noted that the goal is now *eliminating health disparities* rather than *decreasing health disparities*. This is an important change for our country that indicates we will no longer tolerate the health disparities that characterize our diverse populations. The document includes 467 objectives in 28 focus areas offering an exciting array of goals to be pursued in primary care as well as by schools, work sites and other public health settings. Critical health indicators have been identified to track progress toward the overall goals. These include physical activity, overweight and obesity, tobacco use, substance abuse, responsible sexual behavior, mental health, injury and violence, environmental quality, immunization, and access to health care.[14] Of particular concern are vulnerable populations who often have inadequate health care, low-paying jobs without health insurance coverage, and chronic exposure to hazardous environments. Successful collaboration with communities to improve the health and environment of vulnerable populations is a major challenge for health care providers in the next decade. It is important that health promotion and illness prevention programs for these populations are culturally appropriate and integrated into the contexts in which they spend their daily lives.

Public support is growing for coverage of health promotion and illness prevention services by third-party payers. Increasingly, managed care organizations are interested in offering health promotion and preventive services that have been shown to be effective in promoting positive behavior change and decreasing health care costs. The federal government and private insurers should continue to evaluate the impact of providing an array of prevention and health promotion services to individuals and families including the millions of citizens in the United States who are currently uninsured or underinsured.

Health Promotion and Health Protection: Is There a Difference?

The most important difference between health promotion and health protection or illness prevention is in the underlying motivation for the behavior on the part of individuals and aggregates. *Health promotion* is behavior motivated by the desire to increase well-being and actualize human health potential. *Health protection* is behavior motivated by a desire to actively avoid illness, detect it early, or maintain functioning within the constraints of illness. The *actualizing tendency* underlying health promotion increases states of positive tension in order to promote change and growth. This increase in tension is often experienced as challenge and facilitates behaviors expressive of human potential. The *stabilizing tendency* underlying health protection is evident in the functioning of homeokinetic mechanisms and is directed toward maintaining balance and equilibrium. The stabilizing tendency is responsible for protective maneuvers, primarily maintaining the internal and external environments within a range compatible with continuing existence.

Probably the purest form of motivation for health promotion exists in childhood through young adulthood when energy, vitality, and vigor are important to attain but the threat of chronic illness seems remote. Youth may engage in health behaviors for the pure pleasure of doing so or for the improvement of physical appearance and attractiveness to others. In the adult years, when human vulnerabilities become more apparent, the two motivations for health behavior usually coexist. For example, an older adult may be motivated to jog in order to improve stamina and energy (health promotion) but also to avoid cardiovascular disease (health protection). Regulatory measures for clean air may be passed to prevent exposure to asbestos as a cancer risk factor (health protection) but also to improve the overall quality of the environment (health promotion).

The reader should note three important theoretical differences between health promotion and health protection. First, health promotion is not illness or injury specific; health protection is. Second, health promotion is "approach" motivated, whereas health protection is "avoidance" motivated. Third, health promotion seeks to expand positive potential for health, whereas health protection seeks to thwart the occurrence of insults to health and well-being. When interventions are being tailored to particular clients, a distinction between the *motivational dynamics* of health promotion and health protection (prevention) is likely to be helpful. In reality, health promotion and health protection are complementary processes. Both are critical to the quality of life at all developmental stages. More attention will be given to these two concepts throughout the rest of the book.

The Multidimensional Nature of Health Promotion

The health of individuals and families is affected markedly by the community, environment, and society in which they live. The context for living can either sustain and expand health potential or inhibit the emergence of health and well-being. It is important that nurses appreciate and consider the complexity of health promotion endeavors. Dunn in his early classic writings on high-level wellness provided the following schema for health promotion efforts:[26]

- Individual wellness
- Family wellness
- Community wellness
- Environmental wellness
- Societal wellness

Individual Wellness

Individuals play a critical role in the determination of their own health status, because self-care represents the dominant mode of health care in our society. Many personal decisions are made daily that shape lifestyle and the social and physical environments. Health promotion at the individual level improves personal decision making and health practices. Throughout this book, the frame of reference for individual prevention and health promotion activities will be the total life span from childhood to the older adult years. Every developmental stage must be considered in formulating national health policy and programs if the quality of life for people of all ages is to be significantly enhanced through health promotion efforts.

Family Wellness

Although the family plays a critical role in the development of health beliefs and health behaviors, there is very little research on the health-promoting role of the family. Almost all individuals can identify with a family group in which members influence one another's ideas and actions. Each family has a characteristic value, role, and power structure as well as unique communication patterns. In addition, families fulfill affective, socialization, health care, and coping functions in varying ways. Parenting styles and family environments can encourage healthy or unhealthy behaviors that may persist throughout the life span. Much more attention should be given to the development of strategies for promoting family wellness.

Community Wellness

According to Dunn, community wellness is achieved by a multiplicity of actions that improve the conditions of family and community life.[26] A number of benefits of community-based health promotion programs can be identified:

1. Enhanced opportunities for information exchange and social support among members of the target population
2. Reduced unit cost of programming because large groups, rather than individuals, receive health promotion services
3. Availability of interorganizational networks that can facilitate and coordinate health promotion efforts
4. Potential for widespread change in social norms regarding health and health behavior
5. Coordinated rather than piecemeal approach to the promotion of health in large populations
6. Access to a broad array of media for dissemination of health information
7. Availability of aggregate indices to be used for tracking the health status of the population
8. Use of the talents and resources of community residents resulting in a sense of commitment to health promotion programming

Community programming for prevention and health promotion can result in rapid dissemination of health information and in marked changes in cultural norms relevant to health and health behavior.

Environmental Wellness

The level of environmental wellness affects the extent to which individuals, families, and communities can achieve their optimum potential. *Environment* is a comprehensive term meaning the physical, interpersonal, and economic circumstances in which we live. The quality of the environment is dependent on the absence of toxic substances, the availability of aesthetic or restorative experiences, and the accessibility of human and economic resources needed for healthful and productive living. Socioeconomic conditions such as unemployment, poverty, crime, prejudice, and isolation can have adverse effects on health. Environmental wellness is manifest in harmony and balance between human beings and their surroundings.

Societal Wellness

The wellness of a society depends largely on the passage of laws and the establishment through social action of policies that protect the health and welfare of all age groups. A well society is one in which all members have a standard of living and way of life that allows them to meet basic human needs and engage in activities that express their human potential. Essential to a well society is the collective citizenry's willingness to accept responsibility for health and to foster a level of education commensurate with informed decision making. A well society recognizes the dignity of all human beings, adopts policies to maintain that dignity, and avoids policies and programs that are demeaning or belittling to its members. A well society empowers its members to use their talents throughout the life span without premature retirement or relegation to a status of less value with age. Societal wellness requires involvement of a number of sectors, including those of education, food production, housing, and employment as well as the health sector, in joint efforts to improve a population's health profile. Prerequisites for a well society include

1. A belief that disease and illness are not inevitable consequences of human existence
2. A vision for the population beyond that of immediate survival
3. Awareness of the close relationship between individual, family, and community health assets and the well-being and productivity of a society
4. Acceptance of high-level wellness as the goal of the society

Societal wellness provides the framework in which individual, family, community, and environmental wellness can exist. Decisions made at all levels of bureaucracy in the public and private sectors affect the range of health-promoting options available.

Coordinated interventions at all five levels are likely to be the most cost-efficient and effective approach to health promotion. Such interventions are complex but synergistic, optimizing ultimate chances of success.

The Contribution of Nurses to the Prevention and Health Promotion Team

Nurses, because of their biopsychosocial expertise and frequent, continuing contact with clients, have the unique opportunity of providing global leadership to health professionals in the promotion of better health for the world community. Nurses should serve as role models of health-promoting lifestyles and as leaders to activate communities for health promotion. Nurses, as the largest single group of health care providers, will continue to play a vital role in making health promotion and illness prevention services available to all population groups, including those who are underserved and vulnerable. Payers are increasingly willing to reimburse for health promotion and prevention services that add value to health care.[27] Many managed care organizations already provide selected prevention and health promotion services to their members. This trend will escalate in the future. It is important that primary care and community care delivery systems be reorganized to eliminate any system barriers to delivery of quality health promotion and illness prevention services. These barriers include lack of trained personnel, lack of tracking systems, absence of reminder systems for systematic follow-up, and inadequate intervention materials.[28,29] Nurses as major health care providers must continue to work toward the redistribution of health care resources so that quality health promotion and illness prevention services are available to all.

REFERENCES

1. Turner J. World Health Organization—Charter for health promotion. *Lancet*. 1986;2:1407
2. Johnson JL, Green LW, Frankish CJ, MacLean DR, Stachenko S. A dissemination research agenda to strengthen health promotion and disease prevention. *Can J Public Health*. 1996;87:S5–S10.

3. Wilson DK, Rodrigue JR, Taylor WC, eds. *Health-Promoting and Health-Compromising Behaviors Among Minority Adolescents.* Washington, DC: American Psychological Association; 1997.

4. Guthrie BJ, Caldwell CH, Hunter AG. Minority adolescent female health: Strategies for the next millennium. In: Wilson DK, Rodrigue JR, Taylor WC, eds. *Health-Promoting and Health-Compromising Behaviors Among Minority Adolescents.* Washington, DC: American Psychological Association; 1997:153–171.

5. Kreuter, M, Farrell, D, Olevitch, L, Brennan, L. *Tailoring Health Messages: Customizing Communication with Computer Technology.* Mahwah, NJ: Lawrence Erlbaum Associates, Inc.; 2000.

6. Kreuter MW, Strecher VJ, Glassman B. One size does not fit all: The case for tailoring print materials. *Annals of Behavioral Medicine.* 1999;21(4):276–283.

7. Skinner CS, Campbell MK, Rimer BK, Curry S, Prochaska JO. How effective is tailored print communication? *Annals of Behavioral Medicine.* 1999;21(4):290–298.

8. Bock B, Niaura R, Fontes A, Bock F. Acceptability of computer assessments among ethnically diverse, low-income smokers. *Am J Health Prom.* 1999;13(5):299–304.

9. World Health Organization. *From Alma-Ata to the Year 2000: Reflections at Midpoint.* Geneva, Switzerland: WHO; 1988.

10. *Report of the Working Group on Concepts and Principles of Health Promotion.* Copenhagen, Denmark: WHO; 1984.

11. Ashton J, Grey P, Barnard K. Healthy cities: WHO's new public health initiative. *Health Prom.* 1986;1:319–324.

12. McQueen D. Strengthening the evidence base for health promotion. Technical Report #1. Fifth Global Conference on Health Promotion. Sponsored by World Health Organization, Pan American Health Organization, and Ministry of Health of Mexico. Mexico City, Mexico, June 5–9, 2000.

13. McQueen D. A world behaving badly: The global challenge for behavioral surveillance. *American Journal of Public Health.* 1999;89(9):1312–1314.

14. U.S. Department of Health and Human Services. *Healthy People 2010* (Conference Edition, in two volumes). Washington, DC: U.S. Government Printing Office; January 2000.

15. U.S. Department of Health and Human Services. *Developing Objectives for Healthy People 2010.* Washington, DC: Office of Disease Prevention and Health Promotion; 1997.

16. *Healthy People: The Surgeon General's Report on Health Promotion and Disease Prevention.* Washington, DC: U.S. Public Health Service; U.S. Department of Health, Education, and Welfare publication PHS 79-55071; 1979.

17. *Promoting Health–Preventing Disease: Objectives for the Nation.* Washington, DC: U.S. Public Health Service; 1980.

18. *Health People 2000: National Health Promotion and Disease Prevention Objectives.* Washington, DC: U.S. Public Health Service; 1990.

19. Orleans CT, Gruman J, Ulmer C, Emont SL, Hollendonner JK. Rating our progress in population health promotion: Report card on six behaviors. *Am J Health Prom.* 1999;14(2):75–82.

20. Orleans CT, Cummings KM. Population-based tobacco control: Progress and prospects. *Am J Health Prom.* 1999;14(2):83–91.

21. Gutman M, Clayton R. Treatment and prevention of use and abuse of illegal drugs: Progress on intervention and future directions. *Am J Health Prom.* 1999;14(2):92–97.

22. Babor TF, Aguirre-Molina M, Marlatt GA, Clayton R. Managing alcohol problems and risky drinking. *Am J Health Prom.* 1999;14(2):98–103.

23. Carey MP. Prevention of HIV infection through changes in sexual behavior. *Am J Health Prom.* 1999;14(2):104–111.

24 Glanz K. Progress in dietary behavior change. *Am J Health Prom.*1999;14(2):112–117.

25. Marcus BH, Forsyth LH. How are we doing with physical activity? *Am J Health Prom.* 1999;14(2):118–124.

26. Dunn HL. *High-Level Wellness.* Arlington, VA: R. W. Beatty Co., 1973.

27. Atkins D, Best D, Shapiro E N. The Third U.S. Preventive Services Task Force: Background, methods, and first recommendations. *Am J Prev Med.* April 2001;20(35):1–107.

28. Solberg LI, Kottke TE, Conn SA, et al. Delivering clinical preventive services is a systems problem. *Annals of Behavioral Medicine.*1997;19(3):271–278.

29. Solberg LI, Kottke TE, Brekke ML. Will primary care clinics organize themselves to improve the delivery of preventive services? A randomized controlled trial. *Prev Med.* 1998; 27:623–631.

Part I

The Human Quest for Health

1

Toward a Definition of Health

Health, person, environment, and nursing constitute the commonly accepted metaparadigm of the discipline of nursing.[1,2] Although health is the frequently articulated goal of nursing, disagreements about the meaning of health are common. These disagreements may result from the increasingly diverse social values and norms that shape conceptualizations of health in pluralistic societies. What many health professionals once assumed was a universally accepted definition of health, the absence of diagnosable disease, is actually only one of many views of health held. All people free of disease are not equally healthy. Furthermore, health can exist without illness, but illness never exists without health as its context.[3]

The emergence of health promotion as the central global strategy for improving health has shifted the paradigm from defining health in traditional medical terms (the curative model within a biologic perspective) to a new one that considers health to be a multidimensional phenomenon with biopsychosocial, spiritual, environmental, and cultural dimensions. In the context of a multidimensional model of health, health benefits can potentially be achieved from positive changes in any of the health dimensions.[4] Such a perspective of health is empowering, as it opens up multiple options for improving health status.

During the course of human development, an expansive definition of health emerges over the life span. As children mature and move into adolescence, their definition of health becomes more inclusive and more abstract.[5] Health definitions of adolescents show a trend toward greater thematic diversity (physical, mental, social, and emotional health) and less emphasis on the absence of illness with increasing age.[6] Conceptions of health need to be studied qualitatively and quantitatively over the life span to understand developmental variations across genders, races, and cultures.

In a positive model of health, emphasis is placed on strengths, resiliencies, resources, potentials, and capabilities rather than on existing pathology. Despite a philosophic and conceptual shift in thinking about health, the nature of health as a positive life process is less understood empirically. Most measures of health continue to focus primarily on mortality or on morbidity-related indices such as dysfunction, disability, or impairment. Such "measures of health" are really "measures of illness." Defining health simply in terms of morbidity (prevalence of illness) or mortality (deaths) is inadequate for the Twenty-first century, as "conditions of life" rather than "pathologic states" compromise health for many people. Life conditions positively or negatively influence health long before morbid states are evident.

In general, few health measures in the nursing literature incorporate the holistic and expansive views of health to which nurses claim to subscribe. Instead, nurses, just as other professionals, choose empirical indicators for health that are derived from an illness or curative model.[7] New measures of health that adequately encompass the complexity of health are critically needed. They should (1) characterize health by the conditions defining its presence rather than its absence, (2) identify a spectrum of health states, and (3) reflect a life-span developmental perspective.

The fundamental mechanisms underlying human health processes are now receiving attention from nurse scientists. However, many questions remain to be addressed. How is human health expressed biologically and behaviorally? What are the gender-specific, culture-specific, and race-specific expressions of health? Are expressions of health qualitatively different at varying points of development? What is maximum human health potential? What are the interactive conditions between the person and the environment that enhance or deplete health? What dimensions are critical to assess the health of families? What dimensions are key to evaluating the health of communities? Generating knowledge relevant to these questions will advance nursing science and provide an empirical base for effective health-promoting and health-protecting interventions.

Health as an Evolving Concept

A brief review of the historical development of the concept of health will provide the context for examining definitions of health found in the professional literature. The word *health* as it is commonly used did not appear in writing until approximately AD 1000. It is derived from the Old English word *hoelth*, meaning being safe or sound and whole of body.[8(p3)] Historically, physical wholeness was of major importance for acceptance in social groups. Persons suffering from disfiguring diseases, such as leprosy, or from congenital malformations were ostracized from society. Not only was there fear of contagion of physically obvious disease, there was also repulsion at the grotesque appearance. Being healthy was construed as natural or in harmony with nature, whereas being unhealthy was thought of as unnatural or contrary to nature.[9]

The concept of mental health as we now know it did not exist until the latter part of the Nineteenth century. Individuals who exhibited unpredictable or hostile behavior were labeled "lunatics" and ostracized in much the same way as were those with disfiguring physical ailments. Being put away with little if any human care was considered their "just due," because mental illness was often ascribed to evil spirits or satanic powers. The visibility of the ill served only as a reminder of personal vulnerability and mortality, aspects of human existence that society wished to ignore.

With the advent of the scientific era and the resultant increase in the rate of medical discoveries, illness came to be regarded with less disgust, and society became concerned about assisting individuals to escape its catastrophic effects. *Health* in this context was defined as "freedom from disease." Because disease could be traced to a specific cause, often microbial, it could be diagnosed. The notion that health was a disease-free state was extremely popular into the first half of the Twentieth century and was recognized by many as *the* definition of health.[10] Health and illness were viewed as extremes on a continuum; the absence of one indicated the presence of the other. This gave rise to "ruling out disease" to assess health, an approach still prevalent in the medical community today. The underlying erroneous assumption is that a disease-free population is a healthy population.

For several decades, the importance of mental health became obscured in the rapid barrage of medical discoveries for treatment of physical disorders. However, the psychologic trauma resulting from the high-stress situations of combat during World War II expanded the scope of health as a concept to include consideration of the mental status of the individual. Mental health was manifest in the ability of an individual to withstand stresses imposed by the environment. When individuals succumbed to the rigors of life around them and could no longer carry out the functions of daily living, they were declared to be mentally ill. Despite efforts to develop a more holistic definition of health, the dichotomy between individuals suffering from physical illness and those suffering from mental illness persisted.

In 1974, the World Health Organization (WHO) proposed a definition of health that emphasized "wholeness" and the positive qualities of health: "Health is a state of complete

physical, mental, and social well-being and not merely the absence of disease and infir-
mity."[11],[12] This definition increased the number of components to take into consideration
in assessing health. However, the criteria for recognizing health as a positive human experience were difficult to deduce from the definition. The definition was revolutionary in that it
did (1) reflect concern for the individual as a total person; (2) place health in the context of
the social environment; and (3) equate health with productive and creative living.

The WHO definition called attention to the multidimensionality of health. However,
the definition has been criticized by many who state that the definition is utopian, too broad,
too abstract, and not subject to scientific application.[13] Despite these criticisms, the WHO
definition of health is the most popular and most comprehensive definition of health world-
wide. Based on the WHO definition, Ware proposed five distinct dimensions as a minimum
standard for a comprehensive health measure: physical health (functional and structural
integrity), mental health (emotional and intellectual functioning), social functioning, role
functioning, and general perceptions of well-being, which are now widely accepted measures
of health status.[14],[15] These health dimensions are reflected in *Healthy People 2010,* a 10-year
strategy for improving the nation's health, developed under the direction of the Secretary of
Health and coordinated by the Office of Disease Prevention and Promotion, United States
Department of Health and Human Services. *Healthy People 2010* is designed to serve as a
guiding instrument or roadmap for addressing obstacles to public health in America. The
document builds on health initiatives pursued over the past two decades and outlines targeted goals and objectives to achieve in the next decade. In the *Healthy People 2010* initiative, ten health indicators are identified.[16] These health indicators reflect individual
behaviors, the physical and social environment, and important health system issues that
affect health. Health is now recognized as a concept that is not only multidimensional but
also applicable to both individuals and aggregates. In the following sections, definitions of
health are discussed that focus on the individual, family, and community. In the past, defining health for individuals received more attention in nursing and other health disciplines
than did defining health for families and communities. However, it has become clear that
individual health is linked closely to both family and community health. The underlying
premise of *Healthy People 2010* is that the health of individuals is almost inseparable from the
health of the larger community, and the health of every community determines the overall
health status of the nation.[16]

Definitions of Health That Focus on Individuals

Health as Stability

For individuals, stability-based definitions of health derive primarily from the physiologic
concepts of homeostasis and adaptation. Dubos, an early advocate of the stability position,
defined health as a state or condition that enables the individual to adapt to the environment. The degree of health experienced is dependent on one's ability to adjust to the various internal and external tensions that one faces. Dubos considered optimum health to be a
mirage because in the real world individuals must face the physical and social forces that are
forever changing, frequently unpredictable, and often dangerous. According to Dubos, the

nearest approach to high-level health is a physical and mental state free of discomfort and pain that permits one to function effectively within the environment.[17]

Definitions of health based on normality can be described as stability oriented. Statistical norms for a variety of human functions are already well defined. A major problem with normative definitions of health is that they predict "what could be" based on "what is," leaving little room for incorporating growth, maturation, and evolutionary emergence into a definition of health. A norm represents average or middle-range effectiveness rather than excellence or exceptional effectiveness in human functioning.

Environmental models can also be described as stability oriented, as the essence of these models is individual adaptation to the environment—physical, social, and other environments. According to these models, health is related to the ability of an individual to maintain a balance with the environment, with relative freedom from pain, disability, or limitations, including social limitations. Health exists when one is able to work with the environment successfully and is able to grow, function, and thrive. In contrast, lack of adaptation is a gap between one's ability and the demands of the environment.[18]

Parsons' conceptualization of health is compatible with an environmental model, as he defined health in terms of social norms rather than physiologic norms more than 40 years ago. He described health as "the effective performance of valued roles and tasks for which an individual has been socialized."[19] According to Parsons, health is determined by application of normative standards of adequacy for present and future role and task performance.

Similar to Parsons' sociologic model of health, Patrick, Bush, and Chen have defined health in terms of functional norms as ". . . evidence of socially valued function levels in the performance of activities usual for a person's age and social roles with a minimum probability of change to less valued function levels."[20] The desirability of the immediate function level, as well as the probability that the current condition or state will change to a higher or lower preference function level, must be considered in assessing present health status.

A number of nurse-theorists have proposed definitions of health emphasizing stability. Levine defined health as a state in which there is balance between input and output of energy and in which structural, personal, and social integrity exist.[21] Johnson, in her behavioral system model, does not explicitly define health. A conception of health that focuses on stability can, however, be inferred from her conceptualization of internal homeostasis. Health or wellness is balance and stability among the following behavioral systems: attachment or affiliative, dependency, ingestive, eliminative, sexual, aggressive, and achievement. Behavioral system balance and stability is demonstrated by efficient and effective behavior that is purposeful, goal directed, orderly, and predictable.[22] Neuman has defined health or wellness as a condition in which all subsystems—physiologic, psychologic, and sociocultural—are in balance and in harmony with the whole of man. It is also a state of saturation, of inertness, free of disruptive needs. Disrupting forces or noxious stressors with which individuals cannot cope create disharmony, reducing the level of wellness. In a wellness state, total needs are met and more energy is generated and stored than expended. A strong, flexible line of defense is maintained, providing the individual with considerable resistance to disequilibrium.[23]

Roy also subscribes to a stability definition of health. The central concept in Roy's model is adaptation. Health is a state and process of successful adaptation that promotes being and becoming an integrated whole person. The four adaptive modes through which coping energies are expressed are physiologic, self-concept, role performance, and interdependence modes. Adaptation promotes integrity. Integrity implies soundness or an unimpaired condition that can lead to completeness and unity. The person in an adapted state is freed from ineffective coping attempts that deplete energy. Available energy can be used to enhance health.[24]

Tripp-Reimer also proposed a model for health that is stability oriented. The conceptualization of health is based on a two-dimensional perspective: an *emic* dimension (wellness–illness), which represents the subjective perception and experiences of health by an individual and social group; and an *etic* dimension (disease–nondisease), which reflects the objective interpretation of health by a health care professional. The emic–etic health grid and its two dimensions indicate either congruence or incongruence between the perspectives of client and practitioner. This definition focuses on a medical model of normality or homeostasis. The model is proposed to be useful cross-culturally when perceptions of scientifically trained personnel and clients of differing ethnic background may disagree about the concept of health or health status.[25]

Health as Actualization

When health is defined more broadly as actualization of human potential, some scholars have proposed that a different term, *wellness,* be used. The argument has been made that a new term must be employed because the definition of health has been so narrowly constrained historically that attempts to expand it will be futile. Despite this legitimate concern, *health* and *wellness* tend to be used interchangeably in the scientific literature and are used interchangeably in this text.

Halbert Dunn was one of the early advocates for definitions of health emphasizing actualization. Dunn coined the term *high-level wellness,* which he described as integrated human functioning that is oriented toward maximizing the potential of which the individual is capable. This requires that individuals maintain balance and purposeful direction within the environment where they are functioning.[26] Although the definition advanced by Dunn identifies balance as a dimension of health, major emphasis is on the realization of human potential through purposeful activity.

Dunn stated that high-level wellness, or optimum health, involves three components: (1) progress in a forward and upward direction toward a higher potential of functioning, (2) an open-ended and ever-expanding challenge to live at a fuller potential, and (3) progressive integration or maturation of the individual at increasingly higher levels throughout the life cycle.[27] Well individuals function at a high level within a constantly changing environment. Individuals need freedom to realize personal uniqueness through creative expression and thereby achieve a high level of wellness. Dunn proposes that high-level wellness can emerge only in a favorable environment. Health, according to Dunn, is not simply a "passive state of freedom from illness in which the individual is at peace with his environment,"[28(p4)] it is an emergent process characteristic of the entire life span.

Orem used health and well-being to refer to two different but related human states in her self-care theory. She defined health as a state characterized by soundness or wholeness of human structures and bodily and mental functions. Well-being was defined as a state characterized by experiences of contentment, pleasure, and happiness; by spiritual experiences; by movement toward fulfillment of one's self-ideal; and by continuing personalization. Personalization is movement toward maturation and achievement of human potential. Engaging in responsible self-care and continuing development of self-care competency are facets of the process of personalization. Individuals can experience well-being even under conditions of adversity, including disorders of human structure and function.[29]

Newman, building on the work of Martha Rogers, defined health as the totality of the life process, which is evolving toward expanded consciousness.[30] This definition emphasizes the actualizing properties of individuals throughout the life span. Four dimensions of health as a concept are identified:

1. Health is a fusion of disease and nondisease.
2. Health is the manifestation of an individual's unique pattern.
3. Health is expansion of consciousness. Time is a measure of consciousness, and movement is a reflection of consciousness.
4. Health encompasses the entire life process, which evolves toward higher and greater frequency of energy exchange.

Key life process phenomena include consciousness, movement, space, and time. Newman's model of health addresses holistic characteristics of human beings. However, empirical referents for many of the terms within the model have not been identified, which limit testing or applying the model empirically.

Parse, in describing her man-living-health theory of nursing, presents five assumptions about health that essentially define the concept from her perspective:[31]

1. Health is an open process of becoming, experienced by mankind.
2. Health is a rhythmically coconstituting process of the man–environment relationship.
3. Health is man's patterns of relating value priorities.
4. Health is an intersubjective process of transcending with the possibles.
5. Health is unitary man's negentropic (toward increasing order, complexity, and heterogeneity) unfolding.

Both Parse and Newman build on Martha Rogers' theory of unitary man. Both represent early attempts to define health in terms of the holistic human as opposed to defining health in terms of humankind's component parts. The emergent nature or actualization potential of the healthy individual and the capacity for open energy exchange with the environment are characteristics of both Parse's and Newman's definitions of health.

Actualization or wellness models have been criticized because of the difficulties in measuring subjective perceptions. In addition, perceptions of health and wellness vary according to age and cultural context.[16] Another criticism is that the expanded definitions of health in these models do not distinguish health from happiness, quality of life, and other global concepts.[32] In spite of these criticisms, the wellness models provide a focus on the whole person and promote the positive aspects of health. Also, persons who accept the wellness model of health are more likely to seek alternative sources of therapy, not because of dissatisfaction with conventional medicine, but because of their different beliefs and values about life and health.[33]

Health as Stability and Actualization

Models of health also incorporate both stability and actualization. For example, Wu has described health as a feeling of well-being, a capacity to perform to the best of one's ability, and the flexibility to adapt and adjust to varying situations created by the subsystems of humans or the suprasystems in which they exist.[34] Wu proposed that wellness and illness represent distinct entities, with a repertory of behaviors for each. Within this frame of reference, both wellness and illness can exist simultaneously. Evaluation of both wellness and illness are critical to comprehensive health assessment.

King proposed a definition of health that emphasized both stabilizing and actualizing tendencies. She defined health as a dynamic state in the life cycle of a person that implies adjustment to stressors in the internal and external environment through optimum use of resources to achieve maximum potential for daily living.[35] In King's model, a holistic health perspective relates to the way individuals handle stressors while functioning within the culture to which they were born and attempt to conform.[36] King viewed health as a functional state in the life cycle, with illness defined as interference in the cycle.

Smith proposed a model of health encompassing four dimensions, three focused on stability and one on actualization.[37] Each health dimension is defined by the extremes on the health–illness continuum identified by the dimension.

- *Clinical dimension.* Health extreme: absence of signs or symptoms of disease or disability as identified by medical science; illness extreme: conspicuous presence of these signs or symptoms
- *Role-performance dimension.* Health extreme: performance of social roles with maximum expected output; illness extreme: failure in performance of roles
- *Adaptive dimension.* Health extreme: flexible adaptation to the environment is maintained by the individual who interacts with environment with maximum advantage; illness extreme: alienation of the person from environment, failure of self-corrective responses
- *Eudaimonistic dimension.* Health extreme: exuberant well-being; illness extreme: enervation, languishing debility

Each dimension requires a distinct approach and a different mode of intervention, depending on which dimension is used as the guiding framework for care.

A definition of health needs to be applicable to everyone: to the well, to those with a treatable disease or illness, and to those with chronic disease or disability.[38] The first author of this text has proposed a definition of health that incorporates both actualizing and stabilizing tendencies. Health is defined as the actualization of inherent and acquired human potential through goal-directed behavior, competent self-care, and satisfying relationships with others, while adjustments are made as needed to maintain structural integrity and harmony with relevant environments. This broad conceptual definition has led to a classification system that describes affective and behavioral expressions of health by individuals (Table 1–1). The major culture-free dimensions of health expression include affect, attitudes, activity, aspirations, and accomplishments. The physical, mental, social, and spiritual components of health that are now cited within expanded definitions of health, including the WHO definition, are encompassed in this classification. Pender's dimensions are further divided into 15 subcategories that may be culture specific. The system is based on the assumption that health is a manifestation of person and environment interactional patterns that become increasingly complex throughout the life span. The classification system provides a framework for the comprehensive assessment of health that is consistent with a positive, unitary, humanistic view.

TABLE 1-1 Classification System for Affective and Behavioral Expressions of Health

Affect

Serenity	Harmony	Vitality	Sensitivity
Calm	Spiritual	Energetic	Aware
Relaxed	Contemplative	Vigorous	Connected
Peaceful	At one with the universe	Zestful	Intimate
Content		Alert	Loving
Comfortable		Fit	Warm
Glowing		Buoyant	
Happy		Exhilarated	
Joyous		Powerful	
Pleasant		Courageous	
Satisfied			

Attitudes

Optimism	Relevancy	Competency
Hopeful	Useful	Purposive
Enthusiastic	Contributing	Initiating
Open	Valued	Self-motivating
Reverent	Caring	Self-affirming
Trustful	Committed	Innovative
Resilient	Involved	Masterful
		Challenged

Activity

Positive Life Patterns	Meaningful Work	Invigorating Play
Eating a healthy diet	Setting realistic goals	Having meaningful hobbies
Exercising regularly	Varying activities	Engaging in satisfying leisure activities
Managing stress	Undertaking challenging tasks	
Obtaining adequate rest	Assuming responsibility for self	Planning energizing diversions
Avoiding harmful substances	Collaborating with coworkers	
Building positive relationships	Receiving intrinsic or extrinsic rewards	
Seeking and using health information		
Monitoring health		
Coping constructively		
Maintaining a health-strengthening environment		

(Continued)

TABLE 1-1 *Continued*

Aspirations

Self-Actualization	Social Contribution
Growth or emergence	Enhancement of global harmony and interdependence
Personal mastery	Preservation of the environment
Organismic efficiency	

Accomplishments

Enjoyment	Creativity	Transcendence
Pleasure from daily living	Maximum use of capacities	Freedom
Sense of achievement	Innovative contribution	Expansion of consciousness
		Optimized harmony between individual and environment

 # The Need for an Integrated View of Health

Health is a holistic experience and becomes fragmented only in the minds of health professionals. The biological model has provided for technological excellence and sophisticated medical care, but it has led to a narrow focus on disease. An expansive view of health and its dimensions has been proposed that is positive, holistic, and humanistic. The affective and behavioral expressions in the classification system for expression of health can be integrated with traditional biomedical models (disease) and public health models (mortality, morbidity, risks) of health to provide an expansive, holistic biopsychosocial view.[38,39] The biopsychosocial view eliminates the need to reject one view of health at the cost of another and enables clinicians and researchers to work with health and disease together rather than isolating the concepts.[39] Also, socioeconomic status is now recognized as a powerful determinant of health.[16,38] Therefore, understanding the relevance of a broad definition of health to individuals in all socioeconomic segments is critical to improving their health. Clinical investigations are needed that study the interrelationships of these models in the expression of health, as well as their combined contributions to health at different points in the life span in culturally diverse populations. In addition, culturally sensitive, age-appropriate objective measures need to be developed to assess the expanded definition that has been proposed in order to advance knowledge about an integrated holistic view of health.

 # Health and Illness: Distinct Entities or Opposite Ends of a Continuum?

The issue of whether health and illness are separate entities or opposite ends of a continuum continues to be debated by scientists. Are health and illness quantitatively or qualitatively different concepts? Are they bipolar?

Theorists who present health and illness as a continuum usually identify possible reference points such as (1) optimum health, (2) suboptimal health or incipient illness, (3) overt illness and disability, (4) very serious illness or approaching death.[28(p5)] Such scales have only one point representing health, whereas three points on the scale represent varying states of illness. Dunn's model of wellness maintained that the two concepts are separate and proposed construction of continua that allow the differentiation of varying levels of health as well as varying levels of illness.[27(p5)]

When health and illness are assumed to represent a single continuum, it is difficult to discuss healthy aspects of the ill individual. The presence of illness ascribes the "sick role," and the individual is expected to direct all energies toward finding the cause of the illness and engaging in behaviors that will result in a return to health as soon as possible. Health can be manifested in the presence of illness, so a case can be made for separate but parallel continua for health and illness. Poor health can exist even if disease is not present, and good health can be present in spite of disease.[40] Oelbaum stressed the interrelationship of health and illness, even though she considers the concepts to be separate entities rather than opposite ends of a continuum. She stated that apathy toward the work of wellness is the precursor of disease. The particular health behaviors or functions that are poorly performed will influence the type of disease, disorder, or damage that will follow.[41]

The authors of this book believe health and illness are qualitatively different but interrelated concepts. In Figure 1–1, multiple levels of health are depicted in interaction with the experience of illness. Illness is represented as discrete events throughout the life span and may be of short (acute) or long (chronic) duration. These illness experiences can either hinder or facilitate one's continuing quest for health. Thus, optimum health or poor health can exist with or without overt illness.

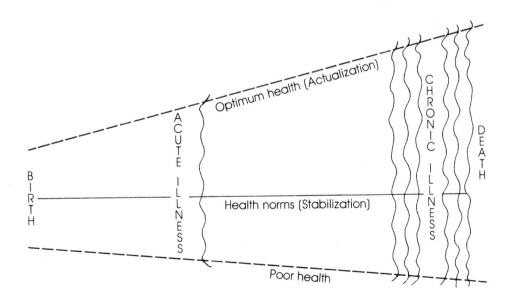

FIGURE 1-1 The health continuum throughout the life span

Definitions of Health That Focus on the Family

The complexity of the family and the diversity of family life in different ethnic and geographic settings pose a challenge for defining and promoting family health. The traditional definition of family as two or more persons living together who are related by marriage, blood, or adoption is no longer inclusive for all of American society. A definition of family that is more inclusive is two or more persons who depend on one another for emotional, physical, or financial support.[42] In this definition, family members are self-defined and may include any individuals who make a significant commitment to each other, inside or outside of marriage. It is critical that variation in family structure be taken into consideration in defining and measuring family health.

Conceptual frameworks of family health are evolving with the changing definition. Although there is no single conceptual framework, family nursing conceptual frameworks and theories are emerging from the family social science disciplines, family therapy theory, and nursing theories.[43] Nursing theories originated with the individual as a focus; and only a few, such as Rogers, Roy, King, and Neuman have expanded to include the family. Four major social science theories that have provided direction for development of nursing knowledge in family health include developmental theory, systems theory, structural functional theory, and interactional theory.

Loveland-Cherry has observed that family health is a concept often referred to as a goal of nursing but seldom defined. She defines family health as possessing the abilities and resources to accomplish the development tasks of the family. Adapting Smith's[37] models of health to families, she has proposed the following dimensions of family health.[44]

- *Clinical model:* lack of evidence of physical, mental, or social disease; deterioration; or dysfunction of family system
- *Role-performance model:* ability of family system to carry on family functions effectively and to achieve family developmental tasks
- *Adaptive model:* family patterns of interaction with the physical and social environment, characterized by flexible, effective adaptation or ability to change and grow
- *Eudaimonistic model:* ongoing provision of resources, guidance, and support for realization of family's maximum well-being and potential throughout the life span

This framework specifies the critical dimensions of family health conceptually and enables the nurse to apply them empirically.

Other approaches to family nursing have been proposed as a basis for assessment to promote health.[45] These include the family as context, family as client, family as system, and family as a component of society. All of the perspectives move the basic unit of analysis from the individual to the family system, as the interaction of the individual with other members of the family or other units in society is the focus.

A biopsychosocial definition of family health has been proposed that states it is a dynamic changing state of well-being, including biologic, psychological, sociological, spiritual, and cultural factors of the family system.[42] In this definition, an individual's health affects the functioning of the family, and in turn, family functioning affects the health of the individual. Both the family system and the individual members must be part of the health assessment.

Characteristics of healthy families have been described. These characteristics include affirmation and support for one another, shared sense of responsibility, shared leisure time, shared religious core, respect, trust, and family rituals and traditions. These qualities address stability of family functioning and balance in interaction among family members. Family typologies are being developed to identify a set of common profiles that may be linked to health in families. For example, four family types (balanced, traditional, disconnected, emotionally strained) have differentiated among health measures in two community-based samples.[46] These typologies also suggest that health promotion interventions need to be implemented in ways that are compatible with family values, beliefs, and orientations. Additional research is needed to evaluate the effects of health-related interventions based on family type.

Many factors influence how family health is defined. Social, cultural, environmental, and religious factors play a central role in determining how families view their health. Families' strengths, resources, and competencies are an integral part of a positive conceptualization of health. Family health processes are now being given increased attention by nurse researchers as well as scientists in other disciplines. Development and testing of theoretical models to describe family health will assist health professionals to identify determinants of family well-being and promote the health of families.

Definitions of Health That Focus on the Community

Communities are usually defined within one of two frameworks: geographical area or relational. Geographical definitions are based on legal or geopolitical areas such as cities, towns, or census tracts. Relational definitions are based on how people interact to achieve common goals. The World Health Organization (WHO) defines community as a social group determined by both geographical area and common values, with members who know each other and interact within a social structure.[47] Members of the community create norms, values, and social institutions for its members. The WHO definition focuses on a community's spatial, personal, and functional dimensions.

Social ecological theories of community health emphasize the interaction and interdependence of the individual with the family, community, social structure, and physical environment.[48] A social ecology model described in the Ottawa Charter for Health Promotion, a landmark policy statement, outlines the essential dimensions of community health.[49] Fundamental to community health are peace, shelter, education, food, income, a stable ecosystem, sustainable resources, social justice, and equity. Flynn, whose Healthy Cities Project is based on a social ecological view, notes that the responsibility for health is widely shared in the community with collaborative decision making about health issues.[50] Informed political action and healthy public policies are essential to a healthy community.

Three major dimensions of community health have been identified in an effort to develop a broad understanding of community health. These dimensions, which can be assessed by multiple measures, provide information that is complementary to develop a clear picture of the health of the community.[51]

1. *Status dimension:* biological, emotional, and social components, measured by morbidity, mortality, life expectancy, risk factors, consumer satisfaction, mental health, crime rates, functional levels, worker absenteeism, infant mortality
2. *Structural dimension:* community health services and resources measured by utilization patterns, treatment data, and provider–population ratios; social indicators measured by socioeconomic and racial distributions, and median education level
3. *Process dimension:* effective community functioning or problem solving that results in community competence as evidenced by commitment, self–other awareness, articulateness, effective communication, conflict containment and accommodation, participation, management of relations with larger society, and mechanisms to facilitate client interaction and decision making

Based on these dimensions, community health can be defined as meeting the collective needs of its members through identifying problems and managing interactions within the community and between the community and the larger society.[52]

Community health is more than the sum of the health states of its individual members; it encompasses the characteristics of the community as a whole. Individual, family, and community health are intimately related. The health of the community depends on whether the social, physical, and political aspects enable individuals to live healthy lives as well as on individual health. Healthy communities support healthy lifestyles. Likewise the collective attitudes, beliefs, and behaviors of individuals who live in the community influence community health.[16] *Healthy People 2010* objectives focus on determinants of health that include the effects of the individual, physical, and social community environments, and policies and interventions to promote health and access to care. All of these determinants must be assessed prior to developing strategies to create healthier communities.

The traditional focus on an individual, curative model—although successful in the care of chronic diseases—unintentionally relegated individual and community health to a position of secondary importance. However, the focus is shifting to an ecological model that goes beyond the individual to include community-level factors.[53] Although more research is needed, evidence supports an expanded view of individual health that is inseparable from the community. Effective health promotion interventions need to be based on the assessment of a community's competence and actualizing potential, as recommended by *Healthy People 2010*.

Directions for Research on the Meaning of Health

Models of health that incorporate ethnic, cultural, social, environmental, and political factors need to be developed to examine the diversity of health conceptions. Attention should be given to developing more rigorous, consistent definitions of family health and community health. Furthermore, longitudinal studies are needed to determine the developmental variations in health definitions across the life span. Multidisciplinary research teams are suggested to test theories that incorporate a clear expanded definition of health. Measures that assess the expanded conceptualizations of health can then be constructed that will provide information to guide the design of interventions to improve individual, family, and community health.

Directions for Practice in the Context of Holistic Health

The definition of health has evolved from traditional medical usage in a curative model to a multidimensional phenomenon with biopsychosocial, spiritual, environmental, and cultural dimensions. Nurses and other health care professionals need to understand the role of these multiple dimensions in their health assessments. The assessment information can then be used to target intervention strategies. For example, the traditional biological assessment may be useful in guiding genetic counseling or screening interventions. Spiritual and cultural information can provide valuable knowledge in developing health promotion interventions for diverse populations. An assessment of the social and physical environment will provide useful information about aspects of the environment that may be positively or negatively affecting the health of the individual or the community. In addition to attention to a holistic view of health, a health assessment is not complete unless it involves the individual, and the family and community in which the individual resides. Health promotion will not be successful if the person–environment interaction is not included in one's definition of health. Health also needs to be viewed from a positive perspective when conducting an assessment or designing health promotion strategies. This means that the nurse should focus on available resources, potentials, and capabilities as well as dysfunction and potential risks. When health is viewed in a positive model, strategies can be developed that concentrate on strengthening resources as well as decreasing negative risks.

SUMMARY

Varying definitions of health have been presented that provide the foundation on which health promotion efforts for individuals, families, and communities can be based. To address the promotion of health, one must know how health—the desired outcome—is defined and how achievement of health can be measured at individual, family, and community levels. The shift from rigid adherence to a biomedical model to a view of health that encompasses mental, social, and spiritual well-being, as well as a focus on family and community has begun to occur. Supporters of this shift advocate a proactive approach to health that includes building strengths, enhancing resources, and fostering resilience to enhance prospects for effective living.[53] A shift to this broader perspective of health will also facilitate development of proactive health policy to improve the nation's health (see Healthy People Website: http://www.health.gov/healthypeople).

REFERENCES

1. Faucett J. *Analysis and Evaluation of Contemporary Nursing Knowledge: Nursing Models and Theories.* Philadelphia, PA: F. A. Davis Co.; 2000.
2. American Nurses Association. *Nursing's Social Policy Statement.* Publication No. NP-197; 1995.
3. Pender NJ. Expressing health through lifestyle patterns. *Nurs Sci Q.* 1990;3(3):115–122.

4. Benson H. *Timeless Healing: The Power and Biology of Belief.* New York: Scribner; 1996.

5. Millstein SG. A view of health from the adolescent's perspective. In: Millstein SG, Petersen AC, Nightingale EO, eds. *Promoting the Health of Adolescents: New Directions for the Twenty-First Century.* New York: Oxford University Press, 1994:97–118.

6. Millstein SG, Irwin CE. Concepts of health and illness: Different constructs or variation in a theme. *Health Psychol.* 1987;6:515–524.

7. Hinshaw AS. Evolving nursing research traditions: Influencing factors. In: Hinshaw, AS, Feetham, SL, Shaver, J, eds. *Handbook of Clinical Nursing Research,* Thousand Oaks: Sage Publications; 1999;19–38.

8. Sorochan W. Health concepts as a basis for orthobiosis. In: Hart E, Sechrist W, eds. *The Dynamics of Wellness.* Belmont, CA: Wadsworth, Inc.; 1970.

9. Dolfman ML. The concept of health: An historic and analytic examination. *J School Health.* 1973;43:493.

10. Wylie CM. The definition and measurement of health and disease. *Public Health Rep.* 1970 Feb;85:100–104.

11. World Health Organization. *Alma-Alta 1978: Primary Health Care.* Geneva, Switzerland: WHO; 1986.

12. World Health Organization. *Basic Document,* ed. 36., Geneva, Switzerland: WHO; 1996.

13. Larson JS. The conceptualization of health. *Medical Care Research and Review.* 1999;56(2): 123–136.

14. Ware JE. Standards for validating health measures: Definition and content. *J Chronic Dis.* 1987;40:473–480.

15. Ware JE, Kosinski M, Gaandek B, Aaronson NK, Apolone G, Beck P, Brazier J, Bullinger M, Kaasa S, Leplege A, Prieto L, Sullivan M. The factor structure of the SF-36 Health Survey in 10 countries: Results from the IQOLA Project. International quality of life assessment. *J Clin Epidemiol.* 1998; 51(11):1159–65.

16. U.S. Department of Health and Human Services. *Healthy People 2010.* Washington, DC: U.S. Government Printing Office; January 2000.

17. Dubos R. *Man Adapting.* New Haven, CT: Yale University Press; 1965:349.

18. Verbrugge L, Jette A. The disablement process. *Social Science & Medicine.* 1994;38:1–14.

19. Parsons T. Definitions of health and illness in the light of American values and social structure. In: Jaco EG, ed. *Patients, Physicians and Illness.* New York: Free Press; 1958:176.

20. Patrick DL, Bush JW, Chen MM. Toward an operational definition of health. *J Health Soc Behav.* 1973;14:6.

21. Schaefer KM, Pond JB. *Levine's Conservation Model: A Framework for Nursing Practice.* Philadelphia PA: F. A. Davis Co.; 1991:17.

22. Loveland-Cherry C, Wilkerson SA. Dorothy Johnson's behavioral system model. In: Fitzpatrick J, Whall A, eds. *Conceptual Models of Nursing: Analysis and Application.* 2nd ed. Norwalk, CT: Appleton & Lange; 1989.

23. Neuman B. *The Neuman Systems Model: Applications to Nursing Education and Practice.* 2nd ed. Norwalk, CT: Appleton & Lange; 1995.

24. Roy C, Andrews H.A. *The Roy Adaptation Model.* Norwalk, CT: Appleton & Lange; 1999.

25. Tripp-Reimer T. Reconceptualizing the concept of health: Integrating emic and etic perspectives. *Res Nurs Health.* 1984;7:101–109.

26. Dunn HL. What high-level wellness means. *Can J Public Health.* 1959 Nov;50(11):447–457.

27. Dunn HL. Points of attack for raising the level of wellness. *J Nat Med Assoc.* 1975;49:223–235.

28. Dunn HL. *High-Level Wellness*. Thorofare, NJ: Charles B. Slack, Inc.; 1980.

29. Orem DE. *Nursing: Concepts of Practice*. 5th ed. New York: McGraw-Hill, Inc.; 1995.

30. Newman MA. Health conceptualization. In: Fitzpatrick J, Taunton RL, Jacox AK, eds. *Annual Review of Research*. New York: Springer; 1991;9:221–243.

31. Parse RR. *Man–Living–Health: A Theory of Nursing*. New York: John Wiley & Sons; 1981:25–36.

32. Saracci R. The World Health Organization needs to reconsider its definition of health. *British Medical Journal*. 1997;314:1409–1410.

33. Astin J. Why patients use alternative medicine: Results of a national study. *JAMA*. 1998;279: 1548–1553.

34. Wu R. *Behavior and Illness*. Upper Saddle River, NJ: Prentice Hall, Inc.; 1973:112.

35. King IM. *A Theory for Nursing: Systems, Concepts, Processes*. New York: Teachers College Press; 1983;31.

36. King IM. Health as the goal for nursing. *Nurs Sci Q*. 1990;3(3):123–128.

37. Smith J. *The Idea of Health: Implications for the Nursing Profession*. New York: Teachers College Press; 1983:31.

38. Institute of the Future. *Health and Healthcare 2010*. San Francisco: Jossey-Bass Publishers; 2000.

39. Engel G. From biomedical to biopsychosocial. Being scientific in the human domain. *Psychosomatics*. 1997;38(6):521–526.

40. Tamm ME. Models of health and disease. *British Journal of Medical Psychology*. 1993;66: 213–228.

41. Oelbaum CH. Hallmarks of adult wellness. *Am J Nurs*. 1974;74:1623.

42. Hanson SM, Boyd ST. *Family Healthcare Nursing: Theory, Practice and Research*. Philadelphia, PA: F. A. Davis Co.; 1996.

43. Klein DM, White JM. *Family theories: An Introduction*. Thousand Oaks: Sage Publications; 1996.

44. Loveland-Cherry CJ. Family health risks. In: Stanhope M, Lancaster J, eds. *Community and Public Health Nursing*. 5th ed. St Louis: Mosby;2000:506–525.

45. McCubbin MM. Normative family transitions and health outcomes. In: Hinshaw A, Feetham S, Shaver J, eds. *Handbook of Clinical Nursing Research*. Thousand Oaks: Sage Publications; 1999: 201–230.

46. Fisher L, Paradis G, Soubhi H, Mansai O, Gauvin L, Potvin L. Family process in health research: Extending a family typology to a new cultural context. *Health Psychol*. 1998;17(4):358–366.

47. World Health Organization. Community health nursing: Report of a WHO expert committee. *Technical Report Series No. 558*. Geneva, Switzerland: WHO; 1974.

48. Green L. Health education's contribution to public health in the Twentieth century: A glimpse through health promotion's rear-view mirror. *Annual Review of Public Health*. 1999;20:67–88.

49. World Health Organization. Ottawa Charter for Health Promotion. *Health Prom*. 1986;1(4):ii–v.

50. Flynn BC. Partnerships in healthy cities and communities: A social commitment for advanced practice nurses. *Advanced Practice Nursing Quarterly*. 1997;2(4):1–6.

51. Shuster GF, Goeppinger J. Community as client: Using the nursing process to promote health. In: Stanhope M, Lancaster J, eds. *Community and Public Health Nursing*. 5th ed. St. Louis: Mosby; 2000:306–329.

52. Hemstrom MM. Application as scholarship: A community client experience. *Public Health Nurs*. 1995;12(30):279–283.

53. Reppucci ND, Woolard JL, Fried CS. Social, community and preventive interventions. *Annual Review of Psychology*. 1999;50:387–418.

2

Motivation for Health Behavior

Services provided by health professionals in the United States are increasingly directed toward the goal of assisting individuals, families, and populations to achieve their full health potential through the adoption of healthy behaviors. Although early detection of disease, referred to as secondary prevention, is extremely important, it has produced limited health, quality-of-life, and economic benefits. Increasingly, primary prevention and health promotion have been shown to have substantial benefits in improving quality of life and longevity. Secondary prevention is based on a disease model of health care. In contrast, primary prevention (health protection) and health promotion are based on behavioral or sociopolitical models of health care consistent with an ecological perspective that recognizes the effects of multiple systems on health outcomes. The goal of improving the health of the population will best be served by placing major emphasis in the health care system on primary prevention and health promotion throughout the life span.[1-3] Progress toward this goal requires an understanding of the motivational dynamics of actions that enhance health. This chapter and the subsequent one, which focuses on the Health Promotion Model, describe models and theories useful in explaining and predicting health behaviors—those actions motivated by the desire to protect or promote health. Further, specific theory-based strategies that nurses can use to assist individuals and families in making health-behavior changes are presented. Theory-based change strategies for use with communities or larger population groups are discussed in Part VI of this book.

Health behavior may be motivated by a desire to protect health by avoiding illness or a desire to increase one's level of health in either the presence or absence of illness. The following important distinctions are made by the authors of this book. *Health protection* is directed toward decreasing the probability of experiencing health problems by active protection against pathologic stressors or detection of health problems in the asymptomatic stage. Health protection focuses on efforts to move away from or avoid the negatively valanced states of illness and injury. *Health promotion* is directed toward increasing the level of well-being and self-actualization of a given individual or group. Health promotion focuses on efforts to approach or move toward a positively valenced state of high-level health and well-being. In reality, for many health behaviors, both "approaching a positive state" and "avoiding a negative state" serve as sources of motivation for behavior. A *mixed* motivation model (approach and avoidance) may be the rule rather than the exception for most health behaviors of adults who are middle age or older. In contrast, healthy children are relatively pure examples of approach motivation because negative illness events in the distant future lack the immediacy needed to motivate behavior.

The Health Belief Model, discussed in this chapter, is targeted for application to health protection because of its dominant emphasis on avoidance of negative events. Other models presented here are not primarily "threat oriented" and thus are applicable to behaviors motivated by either health protection or health promotion or a combination of both. Because illness frequently thwarts the attainment of high-level wellness, maintaining an illness-free state through health protection is highly desirable. Freedom from illness and the resultant stresses and strains allows individuals and families to direct more energy toward the promotion of health. The terms *health-protecting behavior* and *preventive behavior* are used interchangeably in this book. For a more expansive overview of multiple models and theories for health behavior change, the reader is referred to other sources.[4,5]

Three types of health protection (prevention) have been described in a classic article.[6] *Primary prevention* provides specific protection against a disease to prevent its occurrence. Examples include mass immunization (polio, pertussis, diphtheria) to prevent acute infectious diseases; reducing risk factors (inactivity, high dietary cholesterol, high blood pressure); and control of air (passive smoke, asbestos), water (chemical pollutants), and noise (excessive loudness of machinery) pollution to prevent chronic diseases. *Secondary prevention* consists of organized, direct screening efforts or education of the public to promote early case finding of individuals with disease so that prompt intervention can be instituted to halt pathologic processes and limit disability. Public education to promote breast self-examination and testicular self-examination or use of home kits for detection of occult blood in stool specimens are examples of secondary prevention. When primary prevention is not available, secondary prevention (early diagnosis and treatment) represents the first line of defense against disease. In other situations, primary preventive measures may be available but not used, resulting in the need for secondary prevention. *Tertiary prevention* is directed toward minimizing residual disability from disease and helping the client learn to live productively with limitations. Cardiac rehabilitation programs following myocardial infarction or cardiovascular surgery are excellent examples of tertiary prevention services.

Human Potential for Change

Individuals and groups have tremendous plasticity and potential for change. Because of human beings' capacity for self-knowledge, self-regulation, decision making, and creative problem solving, self-directed change is possible. Self-change can be defined as new behaviors that clients willingly undertake to achieve self-selected goals or desired outcomes. Clients have the power and skill to change health behaviors or modify health-related lifestyles. The nurse promotes a positive climate for change, serves as a catalyst for change, assists the client with various steps of the change process, and develops the client's capacity to maintain change.

To best promote behavior change, the nurse must have positive regard for the client and sensitivity to the client's cultural and racial heritage and socioeconomic conditions. Nurses and clients should be matched, whenever possible, so that the nurse is competent in the referent culture(s) of the client. Huff and Kline identify four approaches to developing cultural competence in health promotion: (1) developing cultural awareness or becoming sensitive to differences across cultures; (2) gaining cultural knowledge through understanding the values, beliefs, and lifeways of other cultures; (3) becoming skilled in cultural assessment as a basis for designing culturally appropriate interventions; and (4) engaging in cultural encounters or immersion experiences in which cultures are directly lived and experienced with this knowledge translated into effective care strategies.[7] Cultural competence enables the nurse to better understand the particular life situation of the client and to facilitate the client's self-directed efforts to make lifestyle changes that fit with cultural beliefs and lifeways. Health behaviors with "cultural fit" are more likely to be maintained over time as an integral aspect of lifestyle. Maintenance of positive behavior change over an extended period of time is critical if clients are to gain significant health benefits from the changes made.

Use of Multiple Theories in Behavior Change

The most successful approaches to behavior change address multiple levels of influence on behavior and the synergistic interaction of influences across levels. This approach to behavior change is referred to as the *ecological approach* in which intrapersonal, interpersonal, institutional, community, and public policy factors all represent levels of influence on human health behavior.[5] An example of an intrapersonal factor that might influence behavior is exercising because of the positive feelings experienced afterward. Avoiding overeating may be influenced by the interpersonal factor of expectations of a spouse that normal weight be maintained. A powerful institutional factor influencing smoking is "smoke free" buildings. Community influence can be exerted through easy accessibility of low-cost, fat-free foods in grocery stores and restaurants. Mandatory seat belt use is an example of public policy influence on health behavior. The ecological approach to health care fits the holistic view of nurses regarding the multiple factors that influence health behavior and health. This ecological perspective is discussed in Chapters 14 and 15 and is presented in more detail elsewhere.[8,9] Activating multiple influences on health behavior requires that the nurse become familiar with and have the flexibility to knowledgably use multiple models and theories in client counseling and behavioral interventions.

The models and theories presented in this chapter range from those that focus primarily on intrapersonal influences to those that focus across intrapersonal, interpersonal, and institutional or community influences. All of the models presented in this chapter have their origins in earlier theories such as expectancy-value theory, social learning theory, and decision theory. Key concepts in these theories include cognition, motivation, behavior, and environment. Cognitive processing of information is important in all of the models because individuals' perceptions and interpretations of what they experience directly affect their behaviors. Further, the models recognize the potential of individuals to alter their environment as well as respond to it. Awareness of the elements of behavior-change theories that have been shown to influence health behavior in research studies will enable nurses and other health care providers to optimize their effectiveness in counseling and structuring behavioral interventions for clients.[10]

 # A Model of Health Protection

Understanding the determinants of health-protecting behavior is critical for the development of effective interventions that health professionals can use to assist clients in altering behaviors that increase risk for illness. The Health Belief Model is presented here as an example of a model for health protection that has been proposed and empirically tested.

The Health Belief Model

The Health Belief Model (HBM) was proposed in the 1960s as a framework for exploring why some people who are illness-free take actions to avoid illness, whereas others fail to take protective actions.[11] At the time, a major public health concern was the widespread reluctance of individuals to accept screening for tuberculosis, Pap smear for detection of cervical cancer, immunizations, and other preventive measures that were often free or p nominal charge. The model was viewed as potentially useful to predict those indivi would or would not use preventive measures and to suggest interventions th increase predisposition of resistant individuals to engage in health-protecting behaviors.

The model is derived from social psychologic theory, primarily the work of Lewin. He conceptualized the life space in which an individual exists as composed of regions, some having negative valence, some having positive valence, and others being relatively neutral.[12] Illnesses are conceived to be regions of negative valence exerting a force moving the person away from the region. Health-protecting behaviors are strategies for avoiding the negatively valenced regions of illness. The model as modified by Becker is presented in Figure 2–1. Variables proposed as directly affecting predisposition to take action are perceiving a threat to personal health and the conviction that the benefits of taking action to protect health outweigh the barriers that will be encountered. Beliefs about personal susceptibility and the seriousness of a specific illness combine to produce the degree of threat or negative valence of that illness. Perceived susceptibility reflects individuals' feelings of personal vulnerability to a specific health problem. Perceived seriousness or severity of a given health problem can be judged either by the degree of emotional arousal created by the thought of having the disease or by the medical and clinical or social difficulties (e.g., family and work life) that individuals believe a given health condition would create for them. Perceived benefits are beliefs about the effectiveness of recommended actions in preventing the health threat. Perceived barriers are perceptions concerning the potential negative aspects of taking action such as expense, danger, unpleasantness, inconvenience, and time required. Modifying factors such as demographic, sociopsychologic, and structural variables, as well as cues to action, affect action tendencies only indirectly through their relationship with perception of threat. The HBM is appropriate as a paradigm for health-protecting or disease-preventing behavior but is clearly inappropriate as a paradigm for health-promoting behavior.

Numerous studies, both retrospective and prospective, show perceived barriers to be the most powerful of the HBM dimensions in explaining or predicting various health-protective behaviors. Perceived susceptibility has also been an important predictor of preventive behaviors. Both perceived benefits of taking action and perceived severity of illness lacked power to explain or predict health-protecting behavior.[11(p49)] It is very important to note that only two component variables in the model, *perceived barriers* and *perceived susceptibility to disease,* rather than the whole model, are supported by research as relevant to designing health-protective interventions. In 1988, Rosenstock and associates proposed adding self-efficacy (judgment of person's capabilities) from social cognitive theory to the HBM as an explanatory variable and suggested that it be incorporated in interventions based on the model.[13] They indicated that when the HBM was first developed, it was intended for application to one-time behaviors such as immunization. However, application of the model to more complex behavioral risks such as smoking and unsafe sexual practices necessitates attending to individual perceptions of competence or self-efficacy to repeatedly engage in health-protective behaviors over a long period of time. Further research will reveal whether the addition of self-efficacy to the model increases its value in structuring preventive interventions. Recent applications of the model have been targeted to prediction of perceived and actual dietary quality,[14] tuberculosis screening behaviors of Mexican migrant farmworkers,[15] perceived susceptibility to breast cancer, and benefits and barriers for mammography screening.[16]

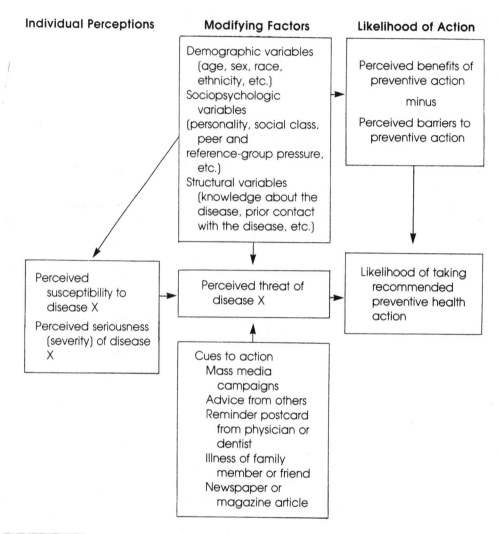

Individual Perceptions

Modifying Factors

Likelihood of Action

Demographic variables
(age, sex, race,
ethnicity, etc.)
Sociopsychologic
variables
(personality, social class,
peer and
reference-group pressure,
etc.)
Structural variables
(knowledge about the
disease, prior contact
with the disease, etc.)

Perceived benefits of
preventive action

minus

Perceived barriers to
preventive action

Perceived
susceptibility to
disease X

Perceived seriousness
(severity) of disease
X

Perceived threat of
disease X

Likelihood of taking
recommended
preventive health
action

Cues to action
Mass media
campaigns
Advice from others
Reminder postcard
from physician or
dentist
Illness of family
member or friend
Newspaper or
magazine article

FIGURE 2-1 The Health Belief Model

(From Becker MH, Haefner DP, Kasl SV, et al. Selected psychosocial models and correlates of individual health-related behaviors. *Med Care.* 1977;15:27–46, with permission.)

Models and Theories of Health Promotion and Health Protection

The models and theories discussed in this section can be used to understand both health-promoting and health-protecting behaviors. Thus, they can be applied in research and clinical settings across a wide range of health behaviors.

Theory of Reasoned Action and Theory of Planned Behavior

Ajzen and Fishbein proposed the Theory of Reasoned Action (TRA) in which attitudes and subjective norms, both intrapersonal factors, constitute the fundamental building blocks of the theory.[17] Attitudes and subjective norms influence behavioral intention, which is the immediate determinant of behavior. These relationships are depicted as follows:

$$\text{Behavior} \approx \text{Intention to Perform the Behavior}$$

$$\text{Intention} = \text{Attitude Toward Behavior} + \text{Subjective Norm for Behavior}$$

$$(\approx - \text{ is a function of})$$

The first determinant of intention, attitude toward a behavior, is a function of beliefs concerning the consequences of performing the behavior and evaluation of each of these consequences as either positive or negative. Evaluation of outcomes of a behavior as primarily desirable results in a positive attitude. Evaluation of outcomes as primarily undesirable results in a negative attitude. The second determinant of intention, subjective norms, is a function of what significant others expect a person to do—that is, what they would approve or disapprove of—and the motivation of the individual to comply with their expectations. The relative importance of attitudes and subjective norms in predicting any given behavior will vary depending on the target behavior, the context, and the population being studied.[18]

The TRA is based on the assumption that both attitudes and subjective norms are amenable to change. Thus, targets for intervention by health care professionals can be changing attitudes through addressing beliefs about outcomes and values related to the outcomes or changing subjective norms by focusing on perceptions concerning normative expectations of others and motivation to comply with what others expect. A number of research studies have tested the applicability of the TRA to various health behaviors. An overview of related research findings indicates that intentions are, for the most part, moderately to highly correlated with behavior, attitudes are moderately correlated with behavior, and subjective norms are uncorrelated to modestly correlated with behavior. Thus, attitudes and intentions have been the only components of the model clearly supported by research findings. Relationships vary by type of health behavior studied and study methods. Recent research studies have shown components of the theory of reasoned action to influence a range of health behaviors such as increasing milk consumption among women,[19] increasing physical activity,[20] and promoting the practice of HIV-preventive behaviors.[21]

The TRA assumes that behavior is under volitional control; that is, that there are no barriers to performance of the intended behavior. Ajzen, in a critique of the TRA, commented that behavior may not be completely under the control of the individual. Thus, he added a third variable of perceived behavioral control to the original Fishbein and Ajzen concepts of attitude and subjective norms, resulting in three proposed predictors of behavioral intentions. He labeled the extended theory the Theory of Planned Behavior (TPB).[22] Perceived behavioral control is measured by beliefs concerning the opportunities to engage in the behavior as well as the power of various factors to inhibit or facilitate the behavior. An example of a control belief is "How likely is it that I can get a ride to the gym tomorrow with my friend?" An inhibiting factor is illustrated by "If I cannot get a ride to the gym tomorrow, how likely am I to walk in my neighborhood?" In a study of fifth and eighth graders' intentions to participate in physical activity, perceived behavioral control predicted behavioral intentions.[23] Likewise, in a study of health care workers, perceived behavioral control predicted intention to use gloves to prevent the risk of exposure to bloodborne pathogens.[24]

Social Cognitive Theory

Social cognitive theory is a broad theoretical approach to explaining human behavior. This theory is the framework used most frequently to design behavior change interventions. Within this perspective, individuals are neither driven by inner forces nor automatically controlled by external stimuli. Human behavior is explained in terms of triadic reciprocal determinism, in which cognition, behavior, and environmental events all operate as interacting determinants of one another. That is, what we think can influence what we do as well as what we do influencing what we think (beliefs and expectations). The environment influences our thoughts and our behavior, in turn, our thoughts and behavior influence how we shape the environment in which we live. Basic human capabilities undergirding regulation of behavior include symbolization, forethought, vicarious learning, self-knowledge, self-regulation, and self-reflection. Self-efficacy, a form of self-knowledge relevant to self-regulation, is a central concept in the theory.[25,26] This concept will be the focus of the presentation here.

Perceived self-efficacy is a judgment of personal capability to successfully execute a specific behavior. Examples are a person's evaluation of their ability to select low fat foods at the grocery store or their ability to climb four flights of stairs rapidly. Efficacy expectations (judgments of personal capabilities) are distinct from outcome expectations (judgments concerning behavioral consequences). Efficacy expectations are proposed by Bandura as a primary determinant of behavior. Sources of efficacy expectations include performance attainments (mastery experiences), vicarious experiences (observing the behavior of others), verbal persuasion (being convinced by others of personal capabilities), and physiologic states during or immediately following behavior (negative arousal such as anxiety, fatigue, pain, or positive arousal such as pleasure or happiness). Individuals derive their sense of self-efficacy for a given behavior by weighing and integrating efficacy information from these diverse sources. According to social cognitive theory, the cumulative perception of efficacy determines predisposition to undertake a given behavior.[26] Nurse scientists have developed instruments to measure self-efficacy for a wide range of health behaviors including the prevention of osteoporosis[27] and successful breast-feeding.[28] The interaction of self-efficacy with other predictors of health behaviors needs to be explored further to understand the intricate nature of the motivational dynamics underlying health behavior.

Transtheoretical Model

The transtheoretical model was developed by Prochaska and DiClemente, based on their extensive research on smoking cessation among adults.[29] They propose that health-related behavior change progresses through five stages, regardless of whether the client is trying to quit a health-threatening behavior or adopt a healthy behavior. These stages are:

- *Precontemplation:* A client is not thinking about quitting or adopting a particular behavior, at least not within the next six months (not intending to make changes).
- *Contemplation:* A client is seriously thinking about quitting or adopting a particular behavior *in the next six months* (considering a change).

- *Planning or preparation:* A client who has tried to quit a negative behavior or adopt a positive behavior in the past year is seriously thinking about engaging in the contemplated change *within the next month* (making small or sporadic changes).
- *Action:* This phase covers the period of six months during which the client has made the behavior change and it has persisted (actively engaged in behavior change).
- *Maintenance:* This is the period beginning six months after action has started and continuing indefinitely. This stage involves continuation and stabilization of the change (sustaining the change over time).[29]

An attempt has been made to integrate various core concepts from other models of behavior change into the transtheoretical model. In particular, the concept of *decisional balance* from Janis and Mann's decision-making model[30] is integral to the theory. The Janis and Mann conflict model assumes sound decision making involves comparison of all potential gains and losses, which are entered into a balance sheet. The behavior should occur when the potential gains of engaging in the behavior outbalance the losses. Decisional balance has been shown to have particular patterns across behavior change stages. Cross-sectional studies of 12 health behaviors indicated that during precontemplation, the cons of changing the behavior were higher than the pros. During either contemplation or preparation, depending on the behavior, the pros' increase was followed by a decrease in the cons so that there was a crossover in decision balance. That is, for the majority of behaviors studied, the balance between the pros and cons had reversed before action occurred. During the maintenance stage, the pros of engaging in the desirable behavior or not engaging in the undesirable behavior continued to outweigh the cons.[31,32] Based on shifts in self-efficacy in a predictable way across the stages of behavior change, with clients progressively becoming more efficacious, it has been suggested that self-efficacy be integrated into the transtheoretical model.[33]

Prochaska proposes that different processes of change are appropriate at different stages of behavior change. The 10 processes of change are presented in Table 2–1. They are categorized as either experiential or behavioral processes or strategies. According to Prochaska, experiential processes are much more important than behavioral processes for understanding and predicting progress in the early stages of change. Behavioral processes are much more important for understanding and predicting transition from preparation to action and from action to maintenance. Experiential processes are to a large extent internally focused on behavior-linked emotions, values, and cognitions. Behavioral processes focus directly on behavioral change. Once an individual's stage has been assessed using the transtheoretical model, the nurse can select appropriate processes to help the client progress from stage to stage. Peterson tested the model in an intervention study to increase physical activity among working adults.[34] Participants were randomly assigned to one of three groups: stage-based information, generic information, and a no information control group. Six weeks after the intervention, there was a self-reported 13% increase in physical activity in the stage-based information group, a 1% increase in the generic information group, and an 8% decrease in the control group. Abrams describes a unique intervention model for cessation of smoking combining stepped-care and stage matching to derive personalized intervention strategies.[35] For more specific information on processes of change proposed in the transtheoretical model, the reader is referred to other sources.[36,37]

TABLE 2-1 Processes of Change

Process	Definition
Experiential Processes	
Consciousness raising	Efforts by the individual to seek new information and to gain understanding and feedback about the problem
Dramatic relief	Affective aspects of change, often involving intense emotional experiences related to the problem behavior
Environmental re-evaluation	Consideration and assessment by the individual of how the problem affects the physical and social environments
Self-reevaluation	Emotional and cognitive reappraisal of values by the individual with respect to the problem behavior
Social liberation	Awareness, availability, and acceptance by the individual of alternative lifestyles in society
Behavioral Processes	
Counterconditioning	Substitution of alternative behaviors for the problem behavior
Helping relationships	Trusting, accepting, and utilizing the support of caring others during attempts to change the problem behavior
Reinforcement management	Changing the contingencies that control or maintain the problem behavior
Self-liberation	The individual's choice and commitment to change the problem behavior, including the belief that one *can* change
Stimulus control	Control of situations and other causes that trigger the problem behavior

(From Marcus BH, Rossi JS, Selby VC, et al. The stages and processes of exercise adoption and maintenance in a worksite sample. *Health Psychol.* 1992;11:387. With permission.)

The Interaction Model of Client Health Behavior

The Interaction Model of Client Health Behavior (IMCHB) focuses on both characteristics of the client and factors external to the client to provide a comprehensive explanation of actions directed toward risk reduction and health promotion. Client background variables included in the model are demographic characteristics, social influence, previous health care experience, and environmental resources. These background variables and the intrinsic motivation, cognitive appraisal, and affective response of the client in regard to a particular behavior interface with elements of client–professional interaction (affective support, health information, decisional control, and professional–technical competencies) to affect health outcomes.[38] Based on Cognitive Evaluation Theory proposed by Deci and Ryan,[39] Cox indicates that intrinsic motivation, or doing an activity for its own sake because of interest or positive cognitive or emotional responses, is an important source of motivation for health behavior. Critical elements of health outcomes are use of health care services, clinical health status indicators, severity of health care problems, adherence to the recommended care regimen, and satisfaction with care. The model is depicted in Figure 2–2.

A Health Self-Determinism Index (HSDI) has been derived from the cognitive evaluation framework proposed by Deci and Ryan as an approach to measuring intrinsic motivation.

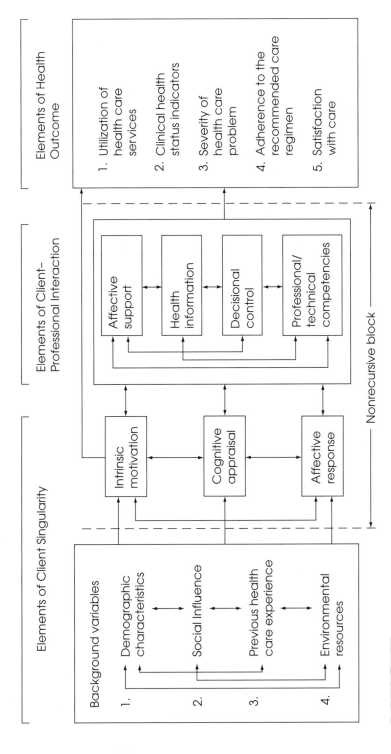

FIGURE 2-2 Interaction Model of Client Health Behavior

(From Cox [38[p47]] with permission from Aspen Publishers.)

Elements of Health Outcome

1. Utilization of health care services
2. Clinical health status indicators
3. Severity of health care problem
4. Adherence to the recommended care regimen
5. Satisfaction with care

Elements of Client-Professional Interaction

Affective support

Health information

Decisional control

Professional/technical competencies

Intrinsic motivation

Cognitive appraisal

Affective response

Nonrecursive block

Elements of Client Singularity

Background variables

1. Demographic characteristics
2. Social Influence
3. Previous health care experience
4. Environmental resources

The four subscales constituting the instrument are self-determined health judgments, self-determined health behavior, perceived competency in health matters, and internal and external cue responsiveness.[40] A Health Self-Determinism Index for Children (HSDI-C) has also been developed to measure their intrinsic motivation in health behavior. The psychometric characteristics of both instruments are reported elsewhere.[41]

A number of tests of the model have been published. Troumbley and Lenz applied the IMCHB to explaining relationships between client singularity variables (demographic characteristics, intrinsic motivation, cognitive appraisal of designating self as overweight or normal weight, and affective response of psychologic distress to weight concerns) and health outcomes (health risk and health status) among enlisted U.S. Army soldiers. Client singularity variables were explanatory of both health status and health risk.[42] The IMCHB was tested among a sample of 260 fourth-grade children and their mothers to determine its explanatory potential for a composite of 36 health behaviors. Health perception exerted the only direct effect on health behaviors, among girls as well as among boys.[43] The IMCHB merits further exploration in prospective studies to determine its explanatory potential for health behaviors.

Relapse Prevention

Marlatt and Gordon proposed a model of relapse prevention for addictive behaviors such as alcoholism, smoking, obesity, and drug dependency.[44] Because of the addictive nature of these behaviors and the high rates of recidivism, researchers have focused on understanding various factors affecting relapse to health-damaging behaviors and on designing interventions to prevent relapse.

In understanding the natural history of relapse, it is important to differentiate between lapse and relapse. A lapse is a "slip" that results in a single repeat of the addictive behavior. In relapse, the client returns to the addictive behavior often engaging in it with increased frequency. Marlatt and Gordon have indicated that by allowing room for mistakes to occur but providing clients with preparatory training (coping responses) to deal with these lapses, relapses can be prevented.[44] For example, the client in a smoking cessation program who has been abstinent and suddenly finds him- or herself smoking a cigarette, if taught appropriate coping responses, may smoke no additional cigarettes and feel efficacious or competent in being able to stop after one smoke. According to the theory, this should result in a decreased probability of experiencing relapse. In contrast, the client who lapses and has no coping responses to draw upon is likely to experience decreased self-efficacy for quitting, positive effects from return to substance use, and the abstinence violation effect (AVE) of feeling guilty and "out of control." Shiffman and colleagues provide evidence regarding the occurrence of AVE following smoking lapses.[45] The cognitive–behavioral model of the relapse process appears in Figure 2–3.

Marlatt and Gordon propose that individuals experience enhanced self-efficacy and personal control from maintaining abstinence. Perceived control will continue to strengthen but can be threatened by a high-risk situation. A high-risk situation is defined as any one that threatens self-control and can potentially trigger relapse. Three categories of events associated with high rates of relapse are negative emotional states (anger, frustration, depression, boredom); social situations (negative situations, such as interpersonal

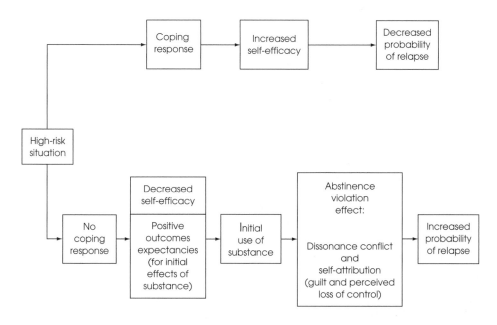

 FIGURE 2-3 A Cognitive Behavioral Model of the Relapse Process

(From Marlatt GA, and Gordon, JR,[44][p38] with permission.)

conflict or positive situations (such as partying or relaxing with friends); and physical craving (withdrawal symptoms and physical response to cues). In these situations, use of coping responses that have been learned and rehearsed as part of relapse-prevention training can prevent a lapse from becoming a relapse. Specific relapse-prevention strategies that are suggested include self-monitoring, relaxation training, and relapse rehearsal.[44,46] Investigators have suggested that combining relapse prevention strategies with strategies for enhancing self-efficacy may be promising for maintaining cessation of addictive behaviors.[47]

Interventions for Health Behavior Change

Increasing healthy behaviors and decreasing risky or health-damaging behaviors is the major challenge facing health professionals and populations globally during the next several decades. Thus, a critical question is what do major theories suggest are the critical strategies nurses should use in working with clients to make the desired changes in health-related behaviors. In this section, selected behavior-change strategies gleaned from a number of different theories will be identified in a multitheory approach to illustrate evidence-based counseling and behavioral interventions. An exhaustive coverage of all constructs from the previously presented theories is not possible so exemplars will be used.

Raising Consciousness

The transtheoretical model emphasizes the importance of consciousness raising at the point that the client is either not considering behavior change or just beginning to consider it. Through seeking and processing information, observing others, and interpreting information in light of one's personal situation, awareness of the benefits of adopting a healthy behavior or discontinuing a risky behavior can be enhanced. The client should be provided with materials that discuss the health-related issues relevant to the target behavior including the short- and long-term consequences for the individual and for significant others. Risk-appraisal and risk-reduction counseling can be used to raise consciousness concerning how changing behavior can lower risk for chronic illness. "Headliners" from national newspapers and magazines focused on the benefits of change or the negative consequences of not changing may be particularly effective in consciousness raising due to the "eye-catching" format in which the information is presented. The client should be given a list of potential information resources and encouraged to become an active participant in information gathering.[36] The materials used for consciousness raising need to be culturally specific to the client to optimize impact.

Reevaluating the Self

Self-reevaluation, a process identified in social cognitive theory, is based on the premise that change results from the arousal of an affective state of dissatisfaction within the client as a result of recognition of disturbing inconsistencies between self-standards (values, beliefs) and behaviors. The client may ask questions such as Will I like myself better if I am thinner, more physically active, or no longer smoke? When a contradiction exists between the personal values central to the self-concept and current behavior, it can most directly be resolved by engaging in behavior change. Further, the more clients perceive that they are the kind of persons that engage in a particular behavior, the more likely they are to intend to perform the behavior consistent with self-standards. Adherence to standards that we set for personal behavior enhances self-concept through feelings of pride and self-satisfaction, whereas violation of self-standards for behavior result in negative feelings of guilt and self-censure. Strong intentions to meet personal standards should lead to increasing performance of the behavior and eventually to permanent behavior change.[37]

The client can also use self-reevaluation to contrast the personal behavioral consequences of continuing a health-damaging behavior with the consequences of discontinuing the behavior. For example, the nurse can ask the client to list several activities that would be possible if smoking were discontinued, then list likely restrictions on activities if smoking behavior were not changed. Also, considering specific differences between self and "models" or important reference groups the client admires can be the impetus for clients to make personal changes in behavior consistent with a reorientation in self-standards and values.

Promoting Self-Efficacy

Self-efficacy is a central construct in social cognitive theory.[26] Self-efficacy refers to beliefs in personal capabilities to carry out a given behavior. Perceived behavioral control in the TPB and decisional control in the IMCHB are constructs highly similar to self-efficacy. Two types of self-efficacy can be identified: Task self-efficacy refers to beliefs in being able to carry out progressively more demanding levels of the behavior, and regulatory self-efficacy, sometimes referred to as barriers self-efficacy, refers to beliefs in being able to overcome barriers to engage in the behavior. Information about self-efficacy is gleaned from performance experiences, observation of others, verbal persuasion, and physiologic states associated with performance.[48]

The most powerful input to self-efficacy is successful performance of a behavior. Thus, whenever possible, the nurse should facilitate the client's performing the target behavior in the presence of the nurse and should provide positive feedback on those aspects of the behavior that were performed appropriately. For example, having the client select low-fat foods from an array of pictures or models of foods and providing immediate feedback on correct choices can enhance task self-efficacy. Praise and positive feedback along with persuasion and reassurance that the client can perform the behavior successfully are concrete ways to build self-efficacy relevant to a particular behavior. The nurse can build regulatory self-efficacy by providing the client with a set of strategies to overcome barriers to performing the target behavior as well as enhancing confidence that the client can successfully overcome the barriers encountered. Learning from the reported experiences of others or directly observing their coping behaviors can further increase clients' perceptions of self-efficacy and lower perceived barriers to successful behavior change.

Observation of others engaging in the desired behavior is important during the action phase to refine clients' performance capabilities and enhance self-efficacy. Modeling of behavior by others is especially helpful when clients are aware of their specific health goal but are uncertain about the exact behaviors that should be developed to move toward the goal. The following considerations are important in the effective use of modeling to facilitate self-efficacy and resultant behavior change:

- There must be models available with whom the client can identify (e.g., gender specific, age specific, culture specific).
- The learner must have an actual opportunity to observe the desired behavior and must attend to important aspects of the behavior.
- The client must have the requisite knowledge and skills to reproduce the behavior.
- The client must perceive benefits from imitating the target behavior.
- The learner must have the opportunity for rehearsal of the target behavior.

Enhancing the Benefits of Change

Behavioral beliefs in the TRA and the TPB as well as outcome expectations in social cognitive theory are considered to be necessary conditions for behavior change.[17,22,25] Planning for reward or reinforcement is a unique way of expanding the benefits or positive outcomes derived from behavior change. The importance of reinforcement is based on the premise that all behaviors are determined by their consequences. If positive consequences result, the probability is high that the behavior will occur again. If negative consequences occur, the probability is low for the behavior's being repeated. Positive reinforcement (reward) rather than negative reinforcement (removal of an aversive condition) or punishment (aversive experience) provide the most effective motivation for behavioral change. When self-modification is the focus of nursing intervention, clients select the behavior they will change and the rewards they will receive for change.

Behaviors that are to be reinforced must be clearly identified and a plan or contract for change negotiated either between the client and the health care provider or between the client and significant others.

If a client wishes to increase the incidence of a specific health-promoting behavior or decrease the incidence of a health-damaging behavior, it is important that an initial frequency count of the target behavior (baseline data) be obtained so that extent of progress toward the desired change can be accurately assessed. An example of a daily record of smoking behavior is presented in Figure 2–4.

Reinforcers or benefits can be classified as tangible, social, or self-generated. Tangible reinforcers for desired behavior include objects or activities, such as purchasing a new magazine or going to a movie. Social reinforcers can include telephoning a friend or visiting with a neighbor. Self-generated reinforcers include self-praise and self-compliments. The time frame for application of reinforcement is critical. Immediate and continuous reinforcement is highly desirable, particularly in the early phases of self-change as it promotes rapid learning of the desired behaviors. Intermittent reinforcement applied later stabilizes the behavior and makes it resistant to extinction.

Behavior to Be Observed:	Smoking	
Observation Categories:	Morning Afternoon Evening	
Method of Coding Behavior:		E = Smoking after or during eating and drinking S = Smoking while nervous in a social situation D = Smoking while driving the car O = Smoking at other times

Smoking Record

Date: Tuesday, August 26

Morning	Afternoon	Evening
E E D O S S E	O S S D S E E E	E O

Date: Wednesday, August 27

Morning	Afternoon	Evening
E E E D D S S E E	S S S S D D E E E E	S E O

FIGURE 2–4 Self-observation Sheet

(From Watson DL, Tharp RG. *Self-Directed Behavior: Self-Modification for Personal Adjustment.* Monterey, CA: Brooks/Cole Publishing Co.; 1972, with permission.)

Many behaviors are too complex to be acquired all at once. Gradually shaping desired behaviors is an effective approach to making permanent changes in lifestyle. An example of shaping is the following:

- Brisk walk for 15 minutes 2 days of first week
- Brisk walk for 20 minutes 3 days of second and third week
- Brisk walk for 30 minutes 3 days of fourth and fifth week
- Brisk walk for 45 minutes 4 days of sixth and seventh week
- Brisk walk for 60 minutes 5 days of eighth and ninth week

Each step toward the final behavior should be mastered before the next step is attempted.

Once the client starts engaging in a desired behavior, losing weight, feeling more relaxed, or feeling more energetic, these consequences of health behaviors have reinforcing properties. When the behavior begins to offer its own reward, the nurse can counsel the client that other sources of reward to enhance the benefits of the behavior may no longer be necessary.[49]

Controlling the Environment

Modifying the environment to support behavior change is an important tenet of social cognitive theory.[24] The locus of attention in environmental regulation is on the antecedents of a behavior, rather than on its consequences. Stimulus control includes structuring multiple environments to elicit the desired behavior. Internal prompts can be coupled with external prompts; for example, "feeling good after brisk walking" coupled with "the invitation from spouse to take a walk." Synergistically, this can provide powerful stimuli for behavior change. Table 2–2 presents an overview of possible stimulus configurations that can prompt health-protecting and -promoting behavior.

Individuals define for themselves the relevant environmental changes they should make based on past knowledge and experience. Reconfiguring environmental stimuli can augment conditions for desirable behaviors or decrease conditions for undesirable behaviors. Specific approaches to stimulus refiguration or control include *cue elimination, cue restriction,* and *cue expansion.* In *cue elimination,* environmental cues for undesired behaviors are decreased to zero. For example, a setting can be selected that is incompatible with an undesirable response (cue elimination). Examples include sitting in no-smoking areas of restaurants or eating meals only with nonsmokers if cessation of smoking is the goal. In successful cue elimination, extinction of the behavior should result.

More frequently, cues cannot be totally eliminated but can be reduced or restricted. In *cue restriction,* for example, the cues to eating may be reduced to one room in the house, the kitchen or dining room. By localizing the cues that activate behavior, arrangements can be made for limited encounter with these cues. In *cue expansion,* the number of prompts to desired behaviors is increased. For instance, whereas personal preparation of food at home in one's own kitchen may prompt small servings of meats, fruits, and vegetables, the environment of a restaurant may prompt selection of rich entrées and desserts. In cue expansion, being given a menu at a restaurant provides cues for looking only at salad and vegetable options as opposed to scanning the dessert section. By expanding the range of cues that elicit specific responses, desirable behaviors can occur more frequently and with greater regularity. Controlling

TABLE 2-2 Possible Cues for Health-Protecting and Health-Promoting Actions

Internal Cues

Bodily states; e.g., feeling good, feeling energetic, recognizing aging, fatigue, cyclical discomfort

Affective states; e.g., enthusiasm, motivation for self-preservation, high level of self-esteem, happiness, concern

External Cues

Interactions with significant others; e.g., family, friends, colleagues, nurse, and physician

Impact of communication media; e.g., motivational messages from television, radio, newspapers, advertisements, and special mailings

Visual stimuli from the environment; e.g., passing a diabetic screening clinic, billboards, attendance at a health fair, passing a gym or exercise center, or viewing others participating in target activity

antecedents of behavior through the elimination, restriction, or expansion of cues can assist clients in creating internal and external conditions supportive of positive health practices.

Dealing with Barriers to Change

Barriers to change are central constructs in the Health Belief Model. Interference with action can arise from external barriers within the environment, such as lack of facilities, materials, or social support, or from internal barriers, such as lack of knowledge, skills, or appropriate affective or motivational orientation on the part of the client. The professional nurse facilitates the preparation, action, and maintenance stages of behavior change by assisting clients in minimizing or eliminating barriers to action. It is futile to encourage clients to take actions that are highly likely to be blocked or frustrated.

Internal barriers to self-modification include:

- Unclear short-term and long-term goals
- Insufficient skill to follow through with self-modification
- Perceptions of lack of control over the environment (cues, reinforcements, time)
- Lack of motivation to pursue selected health actions

Barriers such as these often reflect insufficient attention to the preparation stage of behavior change.

The interaction of level of readiness and barriers to action is depicted in Table 2–3. Consequences for the client and appropriate nursing actions are also presented. When clients evidence a high level of readiness to engage in health-protecting–promoting behaviors and barriers are low, only a low-intensity cue is needed to activate behavior. A high-intensity cue under these conditions may actually be aversive. When readiness is high and barriers to action are also formidable, barriers need to be reduced or eliminated. When both readiness and barriers are low, readiness to act should be increased in order to initiate action. When readiness is low and barriers high, both factors should be addressed, or behavior change is unlikely to occur.

Significant others can serve as barriers to health actions. When family members or other persons or groups disagree or are neutral or apathetic toward health behaviors, the constraints created for the client depends on the following factors:

TABLE 2-3 Interrelationships Among Level of Readiness to take Health Actions, Barriers, Consequences for Clients, and Nursing Interventions

Level of Readiness	Barriers to Action	Consequences for Client	Nursing Interventions
High	Low	Action	Support and encouragement; provide low-intensity cue
High	High	Conflict	Assist client in lowering barriers to action
Low	Low	Conflict	Provide high-intensity cue
Low	High	No action	Assist client in lowering barriers to action and then provide high-intensity cue

- The relevance of disagreeing persons or groups
- Attractiveness to the client of disagreeing persons or groups
- Extent of disagreement of relevant persons or groups
- Number of persons relevant to the client who are in disagreement with behavior
- Extent to which client is self-directed rather than other-dependent

Membership in self-help or self-change groups can be critical at this point, because the group can provide input to the client on the process of change, the barriers or environmental constraints likely to be encountered in making changes, and various means of overcoming these constraints.

Tailoring Behavior Change Interventions

Increasing use of tailored print and interactive computer communications in health promotion and prevention offers exciting opportunities for nurses to engage in the development, testing, and implementation of individualized behavior-change strategies. The computer does not replace the nurse but provides the nurse–client team with more power in information gathering, information processing, collaborative goal setting, and tailoring care strategies to assist individuals and families in achieving important health goals. One-size-fits-all health education materials are rapidly becoming outdated as information technology expands the range of possibilities for using complex, interactive behavior change strategies that are relevant to clients, practical for providers, and most likely cost effective for health care systems.[50] The one-size-fits-all approach cannot address the range of details that vary from person to person and influence individuals' health-related decisions and health behaviors.[51] Kreuter and colleagues distinguished between generic materials, targeted generic materials, and tailored communications. Generic materials include the same general information for everyone and usually consist of a single communication. Targeted generic materials are aimed at reaching some specific subgroup of the population. Tailored materials are intended to reach one specific person, are based on characteristics unique to that person, are related to the outcome of interest, and have been derived from an individual assessment.[51]

Tailored materials should be theoretically based resulting in a logically related set of constructs or tailoring components for the intervention. For example, using the Theory of

Reasoned Action to construct the intervention would result in emphasis on attitudes, subjective norms, and intentions. Using social cognitive theory would result in emphasis on outcome expectations and efficacy expectations as well as relevant components of the environment. The selected theory provides the conceptual structure for designing the assessment tool, the message database, and the algorithms to match client characteristics to individually tailored interventions.[52] Tailored messages can be delivered through many channels: print, interactive computer programs, telephone, audio, video, or the Internet. Nurse researchers and practitioners should take advantage of this broad array of information technologies to develop and test innovative counseling and behavioral intervention programs to meet the needs of individuals across diverse populations.

Kreuter and Strecher evaluated the effectiveness of health risk appraisal using tailored behavior change messages in comparison to typical messages with minimal feedback or to no feedback. They found that patients receiving the tailored health risk feedback were 18% more likely to change at least one risk behavior when queried six months later than were patients receiving typical or no feedback. The most frequent changes made were obtaining cholesterol screening, decreasing dietary fat consumption, and increasing physical activity.[53] Marcus assessed the effectiveness of an individualized, motivationally tailored physical activity intervention compared to a standardized self-help intervention. The individually tailored intervention used an expert system to assess motivational readiness for physical activity adoption, self-efficacy, decisional balance between pros and cons of change, use of cognitive and behavioral processes of change, and actual physical activity participation. Feedback at three subsequent time points was tailored to progress that the individual had made since baseline measurement. Motivationally matched manuals, according to stage of behavior change, were also used. The standard intervention consisted of four self-help physical activity booklets from the American Heart Association. At the end of the intervention, 44% of the tailored group compared to 18% in the standardized group met the CDC/ACSM criteria of participating in moderate-intensity physical activity at least 5 days per week for a total of 30 minutes each day.[54]

Velicer and colleagues evaluated whether interactive, individually tailored sequential messages were more effective than simply stage-matched manuals for smoking cessation among adults in a managed care system. The interactive, tailored intervention outperformed the stage-matched manual intervention in abstinence rates at 6, 12, and 18 months. The results of this study indicate giving everyone at the same stage the same materials, may not be as effective as further individualizing the materials on multiple personal characteristics.[55] Although some studies have not found tailored materials to be superior,[56] most studies provide support for continuing to build tailoring capabilities for health counseling and intervention in health care agencies. Skinner and colleagues provide an excellent overview of intervention studies using tailored print health communications.[57] Further assessment of tailored interventions is needed to determine when they are likely to be most effective and the dose–response relationship.

Maintaining Behavior Change

The maintenance stage of health behavior raises special challenges for the client. Changes in behavior that are transient accomplish little in enhancing client health status. Not only must behavior be sustained in the environment in which it is learned, but the behavior must be generalized to other situations. Factors that affect continuation of positive health behaviors include:

- Extent of personal skill to carry out the behavior
- Number of personal beliefs and attitudes that support the target behavior, including beliefs about self-efficacy
- Extent of positive emotional response (positive affect) and cognitive commitment (intention) to perform the behavior
- Ease of incorporating behavior into lifestyle
- Absence of environmental constraints to performing the behavior
- Extent to which the behavior is intrinsically rewarding
- Extent to which decision to take action has been communicated to others and there is social support for the behavior
- Consistency of behavior with self-image
- Personal attractiveness of incompatible actions[58]

The maintenance phase of health behavior is proposed as extending from beginning stabilization of the new behavior throughout the client's life span. Habit formation facilitates maintenance of behaviors. Habits are behaviors that become automatic and are maintained on a stimulus–response level with little conscious effort. Habit formation results in stable patterns of behavior. The nurse can assist clients in habit formation by helping them plan for certain health-promoting behaviors to occur repeatedly in the same setting or context. For example, a client can exercise each noon in the company fitness center, three to five days a week. After a period of time, if habituation has occurred, exercising at noon should become a habit just like brushing teeth or showering.

Going beyond maintenance, a sixth stage of behavior change, transformation, has been elaborated in the literature. Cardinal found evidence for the transformed stage in a study of health education professionals' physical activity behavior.[59] Of the individuals studied, 16% had well-established patterns of physical activity and were 100% confident that they could maintain regular physical activity for the rest of their life. Transformation appeared to differ from maintenance. Individuals in the transformed stage were active at a higher level of intensity and had a more positive attitude toward being role models of healthy behavior than did individuals in the maintenance stage. Persons in the transformed stage appeared highly resistant to relapse. Research is needed to determine if there is a stage beyond maintenance in which habit and personal confidence ensure permanent behavior change and transformation of behavioral patterns.

Ethics of Behavior Change

Within the nursing profession, the right of autonomy and self-determinism of the client is a major tenet of professional practice in situations in which autonomous behavior is not a threat to the health and welfare of other human beings. Thus, individuals and families should select their behavioral patterns and lifestyle based on sound information from health professionals or other credible information sources. Not all members of society will choose the most healthful behaviors, and this is their right when their actions do not affect others.[60] As the nurse assists clients who have sought help in adopting health-promoting lifestyles, authoritarian and coercive strategies should be avoided. Allowing clients to assume leadership in modifying their lifestyles is an ethical, nonmanipulative approach to improving the health of individuals and families.

 # Directions for Research in Health Behavior

It is becoming evident that a multitheory approach to intervention is the most productive.[61] How to assess clients in order to select optimal behavior-change strategies and how to combine change strategies from different theories in scientifically sound ways that are culturally relevant need further exploration.

Research in the following areas is recommended:

1. Developing and testing interventions that are based on a logical integration of multiple theories
2. Determining developmental patterns in the importance of concepts from various theories for motivating a range of health behaviors
3. Developing and testing the effectiveness of multisectoral interventions that focus on removal of environmental constraints and creation of environmental supports for behavior change
4. Developing and evaluating the outcomes of policy interventions that socially anchor health-behavior change

This research will require the best thinking of scientists from multiple disciplines in collaboration with communities to design and test the effectiveness of behavior-change interventions that are culturally and developmentally sensitive to the needs of clients. For information about funding for nursing research in the areas of health promotion and prevention intervention research, view the National Institute of Nursing Research Web site at www.nih.gov/ninr.

 # Directions for Practice in Motivating Health Behavior

In this chapter, major health-behavior-change theories that the nurse can use with clients in counseling and behavioral interventions have been reviewed. A knowledge of multiple theories makes it possible for the nurse to select the theory or theories that seem most appropriate for the client and the behavior change anticipated. Further, the nurse can select critical constructs for focus that are most important to the client. For example, barriers such as discomfort, travel, or cost may be most important to address with a woman who needs to obtain mammography. In contrast, self-efficacy may be most important to address for the individual seeking to develop healthy food preparation and eating patterns. The emerging availability of interactive information technology will augment the efforts of the nurse to assist clients in assessing their health beliefs and health behaviors and in successfully changing behavior.

The strategies for behavior change discussed in this chapter are useful nursing interventions at different stages of behavior change. For example, consciousness raising has been shown to be an effective strategy in making clients aware of the benefits of behavior change. This strategy is most effective in the early stages of behavior change such as precontemplation, contemplation, or preparation. On the other hand, restructuring the environment to achieve stimulus control is most effective in the adoption and maintenance stages of behavior change when cues for behavior need to be abundant to trigger the behavior on a regular basis. Healthy family eating can be triggered by having only healthy foods such as fruits and vegetables available in the house. Avoiding tobacco can be triggered by sitting in only the smoke-free area of a restaurant. Regular walking can be cued by building walking paths in visible places in the community.

Existing theories, models, and related strategies enable the nurse to engage in evidence-based counseling and behavioral intervention for health promotion and prevention. The flexible use of this knowledge to fit each individual, family, or community will enhance the quality of health-promotive and -preventive care for diverse groups. For more information on evidence-based counseling strategies, view the Agency for Health Care Research and Quality Website at www.preventiveservices.gov.

SUMMARY

This chapter has presented an overview of a number of models and theories relevant to health behavior and health behavior change. Continuing attempts should be made to develop integrated theories that incorporate a wider range of powerful explanatory and predictive variables as a basis for highly effective interventions for health promotion and health protection. Further, a number of theory-based behavior-change strategies have also been presented. The nurse, in assisting individuals, families, and communities to modify health behaviors, not only promotes desired changes but also provides clients with skills for continuing self-change and self-actualization. Learning that has lifelong application can empower clients to engage in a wide array of behavior changes that will improve their health and well-being.

SELECTED WEB SITES RELEVANT TO HEALTH BEHAVIOR

Agency for Healthcare Research and Quality: Guide to Clinical Preventive Services—
    http://www.ahrq.gov/clinic/prevenix.htm
American Medical Association: Guidelines for Adolescent Preventive Services—
    http://www.ama-assn.org/adolhlth/recommend/monogrf1.htm
Bureau of Maternal/Child Health: Bright Futures: *http://www.brightfutures.org*
Healthy People 2010—*http://www.health.gov/healthypeople*
National Institute of Nursing Research—*http://www.nih.gov/ninr*

REFERENCES

1. Kaplan RM. Two pathways to prevention. *American Psychol.* 2000;55(4):382–396.

2. Brown AD, Garber AM. Cost effectiveness of coronary heart prevention strategies in adults. *Pharmacoeconomics.* 1998;14:27–48.

3. McKinlay JB. The promotion of health through planned sociopolitical change: Challenges for research and policy. *Social Science and Medicine.* 1993;36:109–117.

4. Glantz K, Lewis FM, Rimer BK, eds. *Health Behavior and Health Education: Theory, Research and Practice.* San Francisco: Jossey-Bass Publishers, 1997.

5. Glanz K, Rimer BK, eds. *Theory at a Glance: A Guide for Health Promotion Practice.* Bethesda, MD: National Cancer Institute, National Institutes of Health; 1997.

6. Shamansky SL, Clausen CL. Levels of prevention: Examination of the concept. *Nurs Outlook.* 1980;28:104–108.

7. Huff RM, Kline MV. Health promotion in the context of culture. In Huff RM, Kline MV, eds. *Promoting Health in Multicultural Populations: A Handbook for Practitioners.* Thousand Oaks: Sage Publications; 1999:3–22.

8. Green LW, Richard L, Potvin L. Ecological foundations for health promotion. *Am J Health Prom.* 1996;10(4):270–281.

9. Sokols D. Translating social ecological theory into guidelines for community health promotion. *Am J Health Prom.* 1996;10(4):282–298.

10. Elder JP, Ayala GX, Harris S. Theories and intervention approaches to health-behavior change in primary care. *Am J Prev Med.* 1999:17(4);275–284.

11. Strecher VJ, Rosenstock IM. The health belief model. In: Glanz K, Lewis FM, Rimer BK, eds. *Health Behavior and Health Education: Theory, Research and Practice.* San Francisco: Jossey-Bass Publishers; 1997:41–59.

12. Lewin K, Dembo T, Festinger L, et al. Level of aspiration. In: Hunt J, ed. *Personality and the Behavioral Disorders: A Handbook Based on Experimental and Clinical Research.* New York: Ronald Press; 1944:333–378.

13. Rosenstock IM, Strecher VJ, Becker MH. Social learning theory and the Health Belief Model. *Health Educ Q.* 1988;15(2):175–183.

14. Sapp SG, Jensen HH. An evaluation of the health belief model for predicting perceived and actual dietary quality. *J Appl Soc Psychol.* 1998;28(3):235–248.

15. Poss JE. Developing an instrument to study the tuberculosis screening behaviors of Mexican migrant farmworkers. *Journal of Transcultural Nursing.* 1999;10(4):306–319.

16. Champion V. Revised susceptibility, benefits and barriers scale for mammography screening. *Res Nurs Health.* 1999;22:341–348.

17. Fishbein M, Ajzen I. *Belief, Attitude, Intention and Behavior: An Introduction to Theory and Research.* Reading, MA: Addison-Wesley Publishing Co., Inc.; 1975.

18. Montano DE, Kasprzyk D, Taplin SH. The theory of reasoned action and the theory of planned behavior. In: Glanz K, Lewis FM, Rimer BK, eds. *Health Behavior and Health Education: Theory, Research and Practice.* San Francisco: Jossey-Bass Publishers; 1997:85–112.

19. Brewer JL, Blake AJ, Rankin SA. Theory of reasoned action predicts milk consumption in women. *Journal of the American Dietetic Association.* 1999;99(1):39–44.

20. Hausenblas HA, Carron AV, Mack DE. Application of the theories of reasoned action and planned behavior to exercise behavior: A meta-analysis. *J Sport Exerc Psychol.* 1997;19:36–51.

21. Jemmott JB III, Jemmott LS. HIV behavioral interventions for adolescents in community settings. In: *Handbook of HIV Prevention*. New York: Kluwer/Plenum; 2000:(xvi) 330:103–127.

22. Ajzen I. The theory of planned behavior. *Organizational Behavior and Human Decision Processes*. 1991;50:179–211.

23. Craig S, Goldberg J, Dietz WH. Psychosocial correlates of physical activity among fifth and eighth graders. *Prev Med*. 1996;25(5):506–514.

24. Levin PF. Test of the Fishbein and Ajzen models as predictors of health care workers' glove use. *Res Nurs Health*. 1999;22:295–307.

25. Schwarzer R, ed. *Self-Efficacy: Thought Control of Action*. Washington, DC: Hemisphere Publishing Corp.; 1992.

26. Bandura A. *Self-Efficacy: The Exercise of Control*. New York: W. H. Freeman; 1997.

27. Horan ML, Kim KK, Gendler P, Froman RD, Patel MD. Development and evaluation of the osteoporosis self-efficacy scale. *Res Nurs Health*. 1998;21:395–403.

28. Dennis CL, Faux S. Development and psychometric testing of the breastfeeding self-efficacy scale. *Res Nurs Health*. 1999;22:399–409.

29. Prochaska JO, DiClemente CC. *The Transtheoretical Approach: Crossing Traditional Boundaries of Change*. Homewood, IL: Dow Jones–Irwin; 1984.

30. Janis IL, Mann L. *Decision-Making: A Psychological Analysis of Conflict, Choice, and Commitment*. London, England: Cassell & Collier Macmillan; 1977.

31. Prochaska JO, Velicer WF, Rossi JS, et al. Stages of change and decisional balance for 12 problem behaviors. *Health Psychol*. 1994;13(1):39–46.

32. Prochaska JO. Strong and weak principles for progressing from precontemplation to action on the basis of twelve problem behaviors. *Health Psychol*. 1994;13(1):47–51.

33. Marcus BH, Selby VC, Niaura RS, et al. Self-efficacy and the stages of exercise behavior change. *Res Q Exerc Sport*. 1992;63(1):60–66.

34. Peterson TR, Aldana SG. Improving exercise behavior: An application of the stages of change model in a worksite setting. *Am J Health Prom*. 1999;13(4):229–232.

35. Abrams DB, Orleans CT, Niaura RS, et al. Integrating individual and public health perspectives for treatment of tobacco dependence under managed care: A combined stepped-care and matching model. *Annals of Behavioral Medicine*. 1996;18(4):290–304.

36. Prochaska JO, DiClemente CC, Norcross JC. In search of the structure of change. In: Klar Y, Fisher JD, Chinsky JM, et al., eds. *Self-Change: Social Psychological and Clinical Perspectives*. New York: Springer-Verlag; 1992:87–114.

37. Prochaska JO, Norcross JC, DiClemente CC. *Changing for Good: A Revolutionary Six-Stage Program for Overcoming Bad Habits and Moving Your Life Positively Forward*. New York: Avon; 1994.

38. Cox C. An interaction model of client health behavior: Theoretical prescription for nursing. *Adv Nurs Sci*. 1982;5:41–56.

39. Deci EL, Ryan RM. *Intrinsic Motivation and Self-Determination in Human Behavior*. New York: Plenum Press; 1985.

40. Cox C. The health self-determinism index. *Nurs Res*. 1985;34(3):177–183.

41. Cox CL, Cowell JM, Marion LN, et al. The health self-determinism index for children. *Res Nurs Health*. 1990;13(4):237–246.

42. Troumbley PF, Lenz ER. Application of Cox's interaction model of client health behavior in a weight control program for military personnel: A preintervention baseline. *Adv Nurs Sci*. 1992;14(4):65–78.

43. Farrand LL, Cox CL. Determinants of positive health behavior in middle childhood. *Nurs Res.* 1993;42(4):208–213.

44. Marlatt GA, Gordon JR. *Relapse Prevention: Maintenance Strategies in the Treatment of Addictive Behaviors.* New York: Guilford Press; 1985.

45. Shiffman S, Hickcox M, Paty J, Gnys M, Kassel J, Richards T. The abstinence violation effect following smoking lapses and temptations. *Cognitive Therapy and Research.* 1997;21:497–523.

46. Brownell KD, Marlatt GA, Lichtenstein E, et al. Understanding and preventing relapse. *Am Psychol.* 1986;41:765–782.

47. Velicer WF, DiClemente CD, Rossi JS, et al. Relapse situations and self-efficacy: An integrative model. *Addict Behav.* 1990;15:271–283.

48. McAuley E, Mihalko SL. Measuring exercise-related self-efficacy. In: Duda JL, ed. *Advances in Sport and Exercise Psychology Measurement.* Morgantown, WV: Fitness Information Technology; 1998:371–390.

49. Deci EL, Ryan RM. *Intrinsic Motivation and Self-Determination in Human Behavior.* New York: Plenum Press; 1985:113–148.

50. Kreuter, MW, Strecher VJ, Glassman, B. One size does not fit all: The case for tailoring print materials. *Annals of Behavioral Medicine.* 1999;21(4):276–283.

51. Kreuter MW, Farrell D, Olevitch L, Brennan, L. *Tailoring Health Messages: Customizing Communication Using Computer Technology.* Mahwah, NJ: Lawrence Erlbaum Associates, Inc.; 2000.

52. Rakowski, W. The potential variances of tailoring in health behavior interventions. *Annals of Behavioral Medicine.* 1999;21(4):284–289.

53. Kreuter MW, Strecher VJ. Do tailored behavior change messages enhance the effectiveness of health risk appraisal? Results from a randomized trial. *Health Educ Res.* 1996;11(1):97–105.

54. Marcus BH, Bock BC, Pinto BM, Forsyth LA, Roberts MB, Traficante RM. Efficacy of an individualized, motivationally tailored physical activity intervention. *Annals of Behavioral Medicine.* 1998;20(3):174–180.

55. Velicer WF, Prochaska JO, Fava JL, Laforge RG, Rossi JS. Interactive versus noninteractive interventions and dose–response relationships for stage-matched smoking cessation programs in a managed care setting. *Health Psychol.* 1999;18(1):21–28.

56. Brug J, Steenhuis I, VanAssema P, DeVries H. The impact of a computer-tailored nutrition intervention. *Prev Med.* 1996;25:236–242.

57. Skinner CS, Campbell MK, Rimer BK, Curry S, Prochaska JO. How effective is tailored print communication? *Annals of Behavioral Medicine.* 1999;21(4):290–298.

58. Fishbein M, Bandura A, Triandis HC, et al. Factors influencing behavior and behavior change: Final report of a theorists' workshop on AIDS-related behaviors. National Institute of Mental Health, National Institutes of Health, Washington, DC; October 3–5, 1991.

59. Cardinal BJ. Extended stage model of physical activity behavior. *J Human Movement Studies.* 1999;37:37–54.

60. O'Connell JK, Price JH. Ethical theories for promoting health through behavior change. *J School Health.* 1983:53:476–479.

61. Weinstein ND. Testing four competing theories of health-protective behavior. *Health Psychol.* 1993;12:324–333.

3

The Health Promotion Model

In the early 1980s, the initial version of the Health Promotion Model (HPM) first appeared in nursing literature. It was proposed as a framework for integrating nursing and behavioral science perspectives on factors influencing health behaviors. The framework was offered as a guide for exploration of the complex biopsychosocial processes that motivate individuals to engage in behaviors directed toward the enhancement of health.[1] The term *health behavior* was being used with increasing frequency in health literature, and there was renewed interest in earlier work by Dunn[2,3] on high-level wellness and behavior that was motivated by a desire to promote personal health and well-being.

The initial HPM stimulated a number of studies to determine the power of its seven cognitive–perceptual factors and five modifying factors to explain and predict health behaviors. The cognitive–perceptual factors were importance of health, perceived control of health, definition of health, perceived health status, perceived self-efficacy, perceived bene-

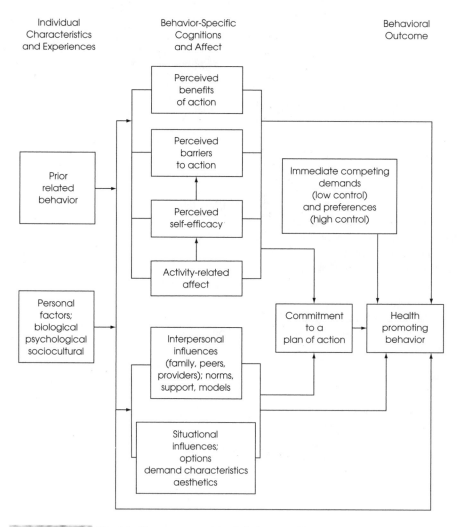

FIGURE 3-1 Health Promotion Model (revised)

fits, and perceived barriers. The modifying factors were demographic and biologic characteristics, interpersonal influences, situational influences, and behavioral factors. The initial model[4,5] has since been replaced by the Health Promotion Model (revised) as depicted in Figure 3–1. Researchers are encouraged to direct their investigative efforts toward testing the revised model using the initial model only for historic reference. The initial version of the model appears in Appendix A.

The HPM is a competence- or approach-oriented model. Unlike the Health Belief Model described in the previous chapter, the HPM does not include "fear" or "threat" as a source of motivation for health behavior. Although immediate threats to health have been shown to motivate action, threats in the distant future lack the same motivational strength. Thus, avoidance-oriented models of health behavior are of limited usefulness in motivating overall healthy lifestyles particularly in children, youths, and young adults, who often for varying reasons perceive themselves to be invulnerable to illness. Because the HPM does not rely on personal threat as a primary source of health motivation, it is a model with potential applicability across the life span. In reality, the sources of health behavior motivation for any given individual have unique combinational properties, from predominantly health promotion or approach-oriented motives, through mixed motives of both approach *and* avoidance, to predominantly avoidance-oriented or protective motives. The HPM is applicable to any health behavior in which threat is not proposed as a major source of motivation for the behavior.

The Theoretical Basis for the Health Promotion Model

The HPM is an attempt to depict the multidimensional nature of persons interacting with their interpersonal and physical environments as they pursue health. The model integrates a number of constructs from expectancy-value theory and social learning theory (now renamed social cognitive theory), within a nursing perspective of holistic human functioning. Expectancy-value theory and social cognitive theory will be briefly described here.

Expectancy-Value Theory

Many conceptions of goal-directed behavior, including social cognitive theory, are based on the expectancy-value model of human motivation described by Feather.[6] According to the expectancy-value model, behavior is rational and economical. Specifically, a person will engage in a given action and will persist in it (1) to the extent that the outcome of taking action is of positive personal value, and (2) to the degree that based on available information, taking this course of action is likely to bring about the desired outcome. Thus, individuals will not invest their effort and personal resources in working toward goals that are of little or no value to them. Furthermore, most individuals will not invest their efforts in goals that, despite their attractiveness, are perceived as impossible to achieve. Personal change can best be understood within this theoretical framework by considering the subjective value of the change and the subjective expectancy of achieving it. The motivational significance of the *subjective value of change* is based on the supposition that the more a person is dissatisfied with his or her present situation in a particular domain, the greater will be the rewards or benefits associated with favorable change. This subjective value of change can be viewed as comparable to the perceived benefits of engaging in a given health behavior. The motivational significance of the *subjective expectancy of successfully obtaining the change* or outcome is based on prior knowledge of personal successes or the successes of others in attaining the outcome and the personal confidence that one's success will be the same or even superior to others.[7] This concept is similar to the concept of self-efficacy in social cognitive theory.

Social Cognitive Theory

Social cognitive theory presents an interactional model of causation in which environmental events, personal factors, and behavior act as reciprocal determinants of each other. The theory places major emphasis on self-direction, self-regulation, and perceptions of self-efficacy. Social cognitive theory proposes that human beings possess the following basic capabilities:[8]

1. *Symbolization:* processing and transforming transient experiences into internal models that serve as guides for future action
2. *Forethought:* anticipating likely consequences of prospective actions and planning future courses of action to achieve valued goals
3. *Vicarious learning:* acquiring rules for the generation and regulation of behavior through observation of others without the need to engage in extensive trial and error
4. *Self-regulation:* using internal standards and self-evaluative reactions as a means to motivate and regulate behavior; arranging the external environment to create incentives for action
5. *Self-reflection:* thinking about one's own thought processes and actively modifying them

Given these basic capabilities, behavior is neither solely driven by inner forces nor automatically shaped by external stimuli. Instead, cognitions and other personal factors, behavior, and environmental events are interactive. Behavior can modify cognitions and other personal factors as well as change the environment. On the other hand, the environment can augment or constrain behavior. This dynamic interactional causality provides a rich array of human possibilities.[9]

According to social cognitive theory, self-beliefs formed through self-observation and self-reflective thought powerfully influence human functioning. These self-beliefs include self-attribution, self-evaluation, and self-efficacy. Beliefs concerning self-efficacy are particularly important. Perceived self-efficacy is a judgment of one's ability to carry out a particular course of action. Perceptions of self-efficacy develop through mastery experiences, vicarious learning, verbal persuasion, and somatic responses to particular situations. Marked overestimation of competencies can result in failure and marked underestimation can result in lack of challenge and resultant growth. Efficacy judgments that appear to be most functional are those that slightly exceed present capabilities. Such judgments facilitate undertaking realistically demanding tasks that build competencies and confidence. The greater the perceived efficacy, the more vigorous and persistent individuals will be to engage in a behavior, even in the face of obstacles and aversive experiences.[10] Self-efficacy is a central construct in the HPM. For a comprehensive description of social cognitive theory, the reader is referred to the book *Social Foundations of Thought and Action* by Albert Bandura.[8(pp 393–401)] For an in-depth discussion of self-efficacy, the reader is referred to the book *Self-Efficacy: The Exercise of Control* by Albert Bandura.[10]

Assumptions of the Health Promotion Model

The HPM is based on the following assumptions, which reflect both nursing and behavioral science perspectives:

1. Persons seek to create conditions of living through which they can express their unique human health potential.
2. Persons have the capacity for reflective self-awareness, including assessment of their own competencies.
3. Persons value growth in directions viewed as positive and attempt to achieve a personally acceptable balance between change and stability.
4. Individuals seek to actively regulate their own behavior.
5. Individuals in all their biopsychosocial complexity interact with the environment, progressively transforming the environment and being transformed over time.
6. Health professionals constitute a part of the interpersonal environment, which exerts influence on persons throughout their life span.
7. Self-initiated reconfiguration of person–environment interactive patterns is essential to behavior change.

These assumptions emphasize the *active role* of the client in shaping and maintaining health behaviors and in modifying the environmental context for health behaviors.

Theoretical Propositions of the Health Promotion Model

Theoretical statements derived from the model provide a basis for investigative work in regard to health behaviors. The Health Promotion Model is based on the following 15 theoretical propositions:

1. Prior behavior and inherited and acquired characteristics influence beliefs, affect, and enactment of health-promoting behavior.
2. Persons commit to engaging in behaviors from which they anticipate deriving personally valued benefits.
3. Perceived barriers can constrain commitment to action, a mediator of behavior, as well as actual behavior.
4. Perceived competence or self-efficacy to execute a given behavior increases the likelihood of commitment to action and actual performance of the behavior.
5. Greater perceived self-efficacy results in fewer perceived barriers to a specific health behavior.
6. Positive affect toward a behavior results in greater perceived self-efficacy, which can, in turn, result in increased positive affect.
7. When positive emotions or affect are associated with a behavior, the probability of commitment and action are increased.

are more likely to commit to and engage in health-promoting behaviors gnificant others model the behavior, expect the behavior to occur, and pro- stance and support to enable the behavior.

9. Families, peers, and health care providers are important sources of interpersonal influence that can increase or decrease commitment to and engagement in health-promoting behavior.

10. Situational influences in the external environment can increase or decrease commitment to or participation in health-promoting behavior.

11. The greater the commitment to a specific plan of action, the more likely health-promoting behaviors are to be maintained over time.

12. Commitment to a plan of action is less likely to result in the desired behavior when competing demands over which persons have little control require immediate attention.

13. Commitment to a plan of action is less likely to result in the desired behavior when other actions are more attractive and thus preferred over the target behavior.

14. Persons can modify cognitions, affect, and the interpersonal and physical environments to create incentives for health actions.

Tests of the Health Promotion Model

To date, the initial HPM has been used as a framework for studies aimed at testing its predictive capabilities for overall health-promoting lifestyle as well as specific behaviors, such as exercise, nutrition practices, and use of hearing protection. An overview of results of 38 explanatory or predictive studies is presented in Table 3–1.[11–40] In some of the studies, the majority of variables in the model were tested. In other studies, a small set of variables was selected from the model to test as predictors of health-promoting lifestyle or a specific health behavior.

A summary of the supporting evidence for various constructs in the HPM is presented in Table 3–2. In addition, the disposition of each construct is indicated in terms of retention or deletion in configuring the revised HPM. Importance of health, perceived control of health, and definition of health were deleted from the revised model due to lack of sufficient empirical evidence of explanatory or predictive power, particularly in studies of specific health behaviors. Demographic and biologic characteristics and perceived health status were retained as potential personal factors to be incorporated selectively in studies as appropriate to a particular behavior. Biologic characteristics were not predictive of health behavior in any of the seven studies in which they were tested; however, better measures of these characteristics are needed before a decision can be made regarding their usefulness in predicting health-promoting behaviors. The category of personal factors can be tailored as needed for each study with only those factors included that are hypothesized to be most salient to the behavior being considered.

Cues to action are transient and difficult to assess. No studies were found that tested this construct in relation to health-promoting behavior. Thus, this variable was deleted from the model. Recently, Jones, Fowler, and Hubbard[41] report developing and refining a tool to measure cues to action. The instrument, if refined further, may prove useful in operationalizing these transient but potentially important predictors of health-promoting behaviors.

The variables in the revised HPM that were significant in the highest percentage of previous studies were perceived self-efficacy, perceived barriers, and prior behavior. Demographic

TABLE 3-1 Summary of Findings From Studies Using the Health Promotion Model

Author	Population	Dependent Variable	Variables Studied	Variance Explained
Health-Specific Outcome Measures				
Weitzel[11]	Blue-collar workers	Health-promoting lifestyle	1,6, 7, 8,10	20%
Pender et al[13]	White-collar workers	Health-promoting lifestyle	1,5, 6, 7, 8, 9, 10	31%
Walker[12]	Community-dwelling older adults	Health-promoting lifestyle	1, 6, 7, 9, 10	28%
Sechrist[12]	Cardiac rehabilitation participants	Health-promoting lifestyle	1, 3, 5, 6, 7, 9, 10	21%
Frank-Stromborg et al[14]	Ambulatory cancer patients	Health-promoting lifestyle	1, 6, 7, 9, 10	24%
Johnson et al[15]	National data sample	Health-promoting lifestyle	1, 2, 7, 8, 10 (proxy items used)	Not reported for HPLP total score
Suwonnaroop[16]	Black and white older adults	Health-promoting lifestyle	1, 3, 10	31%
Bolio[17]	Incarcerated males	Health-promoting lifestyle	1, 3, 8	9–20% for subscales
Millard[18]	Older adults (Seventh-day Adventists)	Health-promoting lifestyle	1, 7, 10	19%
Nikulich-Barrett[19]	Rural, older black and white females	Health-promoting lifestyle	8, 10	22%—Blacks 33%—Whites
Hutchinson[20]	Black university students	Health-promoting lifestyle	1, 6, 7, 8, 9, 10	34%
Warren[21]	Adult males in cardiac rehabilitation	Health-promoting lifestyle	8, 10	38%
Gillis[22]	Adolescent females	Health-promoting lifestyle	1, 3, 8, 9, 10	41%
Harrison[23]	HIV seropositive males	Health-promoting lifestyle	10	12%
Moore[24]	Older adults	Health-promoting lifestyle	1, 8, 10	—
Wilson[25]	Married and unmarried mothers	Health-promoting lifestyle	1, 10, 11, 12	—
Barnett[26]	Adolescents	Health-promoting lifestyle	6, 8, 9, 10	—
Fehir[27]	Adult males	Health-promoting lifestyle	1, 8, 10	42%
Behavior-Specific Outcome Measures				
Pender[12]	White-collar workers	Exercise (acquisition stage)	1, 2, 3, 4, 5[a], 6, 7, 8, 9, 10, 11, 12	22%
Pender[12]	White-collar workers	Exercise (maintenance stage)	1, 2, 3, 4, 5[a], 6, 7, 8, 9, 10, 11, 12	21%
Pender[12]	White-collar workers	Exercise (total group with stages combined)	1, 2, 3, 4, 5[b], 6, 7, 8, 9, 10, 11, 12	59%

continued

	Population	Dependent Variable	Variables Studied	Variance Explained

...vior-specific Outcome Measures

	Population	Dependent Variable	Variables Studied	Variance Explained
Walker[12]	Community-dwelling older adults	Exercise	<u>1</u>, 2, 5, 6, <u>7</u>, <u>9</u>, 10, 11, <u>12</u>	24%
Sechrist[12]	Cardiac rehabilitation patients	Exercise	1, 2, 3, <u>5</u>, <u>6</u>, 7, <u>8</u>, 9, 10, 11, <u>12</u>	23%
Frank-Stromborg[12]	Ambulatory cancer patients	Exercise	1, 6, 7, 9, <u>10</u> <u>11</u>, <u>12</u>	42%
Garcia et al.[28]	Preadolescents and adolescents	Exercise	<u>1</u>, 3, <u>4</u>, 5, 8, 10, <u>11</u>, <u>12</u>	19%
Lusk et al.[29]	Factory workers (skilled trades)	Use of hearing protection	<u>1</u>, <u>4</u>, 7, <u>8</u>, 9, 10, <u>11</u>, <u>12</u>	49%
			(modifying factors allowed to have direct paths to use)	53%
Lusk et al.[30]	Blue-collar workers (manufacturing plant)	Use of hearing protection	<u>6</u>, 7, <u>8</u>, 9, 10, <u>11</u>, <u>12</u>	42%
Lusk et al.[31]	Construction workers	Use of hearing protection	1, <u>3</u>, <u>4</u>, 7, <u>8</u>, 9, 10, 11, <u>12</u>	46%
Kerr[32]	Mexican American industrial workers	Use of hearing protection	3, 4, 7, <u>8</u>, <u>9</u>, <u>10</u>, <u>11</u>, <u>12</u>	25%
			(modifying factors allowed to have direct paths to use)	55%
McCullagh[33]	Farmers	Use of hearing protection	1, <u>3</u>, <u>4</u>, 8, <u>12</u>	—
Wu[34]	Taiwanese adolescents	Exercise	<u>3</u>, <u>8</u>, <u>11</u>, 12	30%
Stutts[35]	Adult males and females	Exercise	1, <u>8</u>, 11, 12	10%
Chen[36]	Taiwanese elderly	Physical activity	<u>1</u>, <u>6</u>, <u>8</u>, <u>10</u>, <u>11</u>, <u>12</u>	46%
Jeffries[37]	Expatriots in Indonesia	Exercise	<u>1</u>, 6, 7, <u>8</u>, 9, <u>10</u>, <u>11</u>, <u>12</u>	—
Oesterle[38]	Women in structured exercise programs	Exercise	<u>3</u>, <u>11</u>, <u>12</u>	—
Jeffries[37]	Expatriates in Indonesia	Nutrition	<u>1</u>, 6, 7, <u>8</u>, 9, 10, <u>11</u>, <u>12</u>	—
Martinelli[39]	Young adults	Environmental tobacco smoke exposure	1, 2, <u>4</u>, 7, <u>8</u>	34%
Tober[40]	Obese adults	Weight loss	7, 8	—

KEY 1 = Demographic characteristics   7 = Perceived control of health
     2 = Biologic characteristics   8 = Perceived self-efficacy
     3 = Interpersonal influences   9 = Definition of health
     4 = Situational influences   10 = Perceived health status
     5 = Behavioral factors (prior behavior) 11 = Perceived benefits
     6 = Importance of health   12 = Perceived barriers

Underlined number indicates significant predictor of dependent variable

[a]Prior exercise measured by self-report on a single item

[b]Prior exericise measured by fitness center exercise records from previous month

TABLE 3-2 Summary of Empirical Support for Constructs in the Health Promotion Model

Construct	#Studies/#Significant	Percent	Disposition of Construct
Demographic characteristics	29/17	59%	Retained in HPM (personal factors)
Biologic characteristics	7/0	0%	Retained in HPM (personal factors) for further testing
Behavioral factors (prior behavior)	8/6	75%	Retained in HPM
Perceived benefits	18/11	61%	Retained in HPM
Perceived barriers	19/15	79%	Retained in HPM
Perceived self-efficacy	28/24	86%	Retained in HPM
Interpersonal influences	14/8	57%	Retained in HPM
Situational influences	9/5	56%	Retained in HPM
Perceived health status	31/16	52%	Retained in HPM (personal factors)
Importance of health	17/6	35%	Deleted from HPM
Perceived control of health	22/9	41%	Deleted from HPM
Definition of health	19/9	47%	Deleted from HPM

Note: #Studies = Number of studies testing the construct for explanation or prediction
#Significant = Number of studies in which construct was found to be significantly related to health-promoting behavior

characteristics, perceived benefits, interpersonal and situational influences, as well as perceived health status (personal factor) were significant in the majority of studies conducted. Improved measures of interpersonal and situational influences are needed to provide a more rigorous test of their explanatory and predictive value for health-promoting behavior.

Intervention Studies Using the Health Promotion Model

Intervention studies need to be conducted that test the usefulness of HPM-based programs in changing health behaviors. A number of constructs in the model have been shown to be predictive and explanatory of health behaviors. These constructs provide a rich source of intervention content and strategies. Lusk and colleagues[42] report the first test of an HPM-based intervention. The purpose of the intervention study was to measure the effectiveness of a training program developed to increase the use of hearing protection devices among construction workers for whom the most common work hazard is noise-induced hearing loss. The program of research progressed systematically from examining associations between HPM variables and use of hearing protection to focusing on significant predictors in developing the behavioral intervention program. Significant predictors of construction workers' use of hearing protection identified in prior studies included interpersonal influences, situational influences, perceived self-efficacy, and perceived barriers. These constructs were used as the core elements of the intervention program.

A total of 837 construction workers were recruited to participate in the study. The training program consisted of a 20-minute video including guided practice in inserting the hearing protection devices. Role models using hearing protection (interpersonal influences), mastery experiences in actual use (perceived self-efficacy), discussion of environmental factors affecting use (situational influences), and role models successfully coping with impediments to use (perceived barriers) were all addressed in the video.

Assessment of use of hearing protection 10 to 12 months later revealed that reported use of protection increased by 20% from baseline as a result of this single intervention. This was a statistically significant increase. Lusk and her colleagues are now testing the effectiveness of a computerized interactive intervention that is tailored on HPM constructs to individual workers. Results from this study are not yet available. The systematic research program of Lusk and her colleagues serves as a model for other researchers interested in developing interventions based on the Health Promotion Model.

The Health Promotion Model (Revised)

The revised HPM that first appeared in the third edition of *Health Promotion in Nursing Practice*[5] appears in Figure 3–1. The variables in the revised HPM and their interrelationships are described below. Three new variables appear in the revised model: activity-related affect, commitment to a plan of action, and immediate competing demands and preferences. It is beyond the scope of this chapter to describe approaches to measuring each variable in the model, but information regarding measurement of variables that is not already reported in the literature can be obtained from the first author.

Individual Characteristics and Experiences

Each person has unique personal characteristics and experiences that affect subsequent actions. The importance of their effect will depend on the target behavior being considered. The individual characteristics or aspects of past experience selected for measurement provide flexibility in the HPM to capture variables that may be highly relevant to a particular health behavior but not to all health behaviors or in a particular target population but not in all populations.

PRIOR RELATED BEHAVIOR
Behavioral factors have been retained in the HPM as "prior related behavior." Of the HPM studies that were reviewed, 75% supported its importance in determining subsequent behavior. Empirical studies indicate that often the best predictor of behavior is the frequency of the same or a similar behavior in the past. Prior behavior is proposed as having both direct and indirect effects on the likelihood of engaging in health-promoting behaviors. The direct effect of past behavior on current health-promoting behavior may be due to habit formation, predisposing one to engage in the behavior automatically, with little attention to the specific details of its execution. Habit strength accrues each time the behavior occurs and is particularly augmented by concentrated, repetitive practice of the behavior.

Consistent with social cognitive theory, prior behavior is proposed as also having an indirect influence on health-promoting behavior through perceptions of self-efficacy, benefits, barriers, and activity-related affect. According to Bandura,[8] actual enactment of a behavior and its associated feedback is a major source of efficacy or "skill" information. Anticipated or experienced benefits from engaging in the behavior are referred to by Bandura as outcome expectations. If desired short-term benefits are experienced early in the course of the behavior, the behavior is more likely to be repeated. Barriers to a given behavior are experienced and stored in memory as "hurdles" that need to be overcome to engage successfully in the behavior. Every incident of a behavior is also accompanied by emotions or affect. Positive or negative affect either before, during, or following the behavior is encoded into memory as information that is retrieved when engaging in the behavior is contemplated at a later point in time. Prior behavior is proposed as shaping all of these behavior-specific cognitions and affect. The nurse can help the client shape a positive behavioral history for the future by focusing on the benefits of a behavior, teaching clients how to overcome hurdles to carrying out the behavior, and engendering high levels of efficacy and positive affect through successful performance experience and positive feedback.

PERSONAL FACTORS

The relevant personal factors predictive of a given behavior are shaped by the nature of the target behavior being considered. In the revised HPM, personal factors have been categorized as biologic, psychologic, and sociocultural. Biologic factors include but are not limited to variables such as age, body mass index, pubertal status, menopausal status, aerobic capacity, strength, agility, or balance. Psychologic factors can include variables such as self-esteem, self-motivation, and perceived health status. Sociocultural factors include variables such as race, ethnicity, acculturation, education, and socioeconomic status. Because numerous personal factors exist, those factors to be included in any given study should be limited to the few that are theoretically relevant to explanation or prediction of a given target behavior. The difference in behavioral relevance of these factors is illustrated by the fact that aerobic capacity may directly influence participation in vigorous exercise but is unlikely to influence eating a nutritious diet directly. Although personal factors may influence cognitions, affect, and health behaviors, some personal factors cannot be changed; thus, they cannot be incorporated as variables to be modified in nursing interventions.

Behavior-Specific Cognitions and Affect

This set of variables within the HPM is considered to be of major motivational significance. Thus, these variables constitute a critical "core" for intervention, because they are subject to modification through nursing actions. Measuring change in these variables is essential to determine if such changes actually result from the intervention and, in turn, influence changes in commitment or in the occurrence of health-promoting behaviors.

PERCEIVED BENEFITS OF ACTION

Of the studies reviewed that tested the HPM, 61% reported empirical support for the importance of perceived benefits in influencing health behaviors. This provides moderate support for the construct. One's plan to engage in a particular behavior is proposed as hinging on the anticipated benefits or outcomes that will occur. In the HPM, perceived benefits are proposed as directly motivating behavior as well as indirectly motivating behavior through determining the extent of commitment to a plan of action to engage in the behaviors from which the anticipated benefits will result. Anticipated benefits of action are mental representations of the positive or reinforcing consequences of a behavior. According to expectancy-value theory, the motivational importance of anticipated benefits is based on personal outcomes from prior direct experience with the behavior or vicarious experience through observational learning from others engaging in the behavior. Individuals tend to invest time and resources in activities with a high likelihood of increasing their experience of positive outcomes. Benefits from performance of the behavior may be intrinsic or extrinsic. Examples of intrinsic benefits include increased alertness and decreased feelings of fatigue. Extrinsic benefits include monetary rewards or social interactions possible as a result of engaging in the behavior. Initially, extrinsic benefits of health behaviors may be of high motivational significance, whereas intrinsic benefits may be more powerful in motivating continuation of health behaviors. The expected magnitude of benefits and the temporal relation of benefits to action impact the potency of anticipated benefits as a determinant of health behavior. Beliefs in benefits or positive outcome expectations have generally been shown to be a necessary although not sufficient condition for engagement in a specific health behavior.

PERCEIVED BARRIERS TO ACTION

Anticipated barriers have been repeatedly shown in empirical studies to affect intentions to engage in a particular behavior and the actual execution of the behavior. Of the studies testing the HPM, 79% provided empirical support for the importance of barriers as a determinant of health-promoting behavior. In relation to health-promoting behaviors, barriers may be imagined or real. They consist of perceptions concerning the unavailability, inconvenience, expense, difficulty, or time-consuming nature of a particular action. Barriers are often viewed as the blocks, hurdles, and personal costs of undertaking a given behavior. Loss of satisfaction from giving up health-damaging behaviors such as smoking or eating high-fat foods to adopt a healthier lifestyle can also constitute a barrier. Barriers usually arouse motives of avoidance in relation to a given behavior.

When readiness to act is low and barriers are high, action is unlikely to occur. When readiness to act is high and barriers are low, the probability of action is much greater. Perceived barriers to action as depicted in the revised HPM affect health-promoting behavior directly by serving as blocks to action as well as indirectly through decreasing commitment to a plan of action.

PERCEIVED SELF-EFFICACY

Self-efficacy, as defined by Bandura,[10] is the judgment of personal capability to organize and execute a particular course of action. It is concerned not with the skill one has but with judgments of what one can do with whatever skills one possesses. Judgments of personal efficacy are distinguished from outcome expectations. Perceived self-efficacy is a judgment of one's abilities to accomplish a certain level of performance, whereas an outcome expectation is a judgment of the likely consequences (e.g., benefits, costs) such behavior will produce. Perceptions of skill and competence in a particular domain motivate individuals to engage in those behaviors that they excel in. Feeling efficacious and skilled in one's performance is likely to encourage one to engage in the target behavior more frequently than is feeling inept and unskilled. Of the HPM studies reviewed, 86% provided support for the importance of self-efficacy as a determinant of health-promoting behavior.

Personal knowledge about one's self-efficacy is based on four types of information: (1) performance attainments from actually engaging in the behavior and evaluating performance in relation to some self-standard or external feedback given by others, (2) vicarious experiences of observing the performance of others and their related self-evaluation and feedback, (3) verbal persuasion on the part of others that one does possess the ability to carry out a particular course of action, and (4) physiologic states (e.g., anxiety, fear, calm, tranquility) from which people judge their competencies.[10] In the HPM, perceived self-efficacy is proposed as being influenced by activity-related affect. The more positive the affect, the greater the perceptions of efficacy. However, in reality this relationship is reciprocal with greater perceptions of efficacy, in turn, increasing positive affect. Self-efficacy is proposed as influencing perceived barriers to action, with higher efficacy resulting in lowered perception of barriers to the performance of the target behavior. Self-efficacy motivates health-promoting behavior directly by efficacy expectations and indirectly by affecting perceived barriers and determining level of commitment or persistence in pursuing a plan of action.

ACTIVITY-RELATED AFFECT

Subjective feeling states occur prior to, during, and following an activity, based on the stimulus properties associated with the behavioral event. These affective responses may be mild, moderate, or strong and are cognitively labeled, stored in memory, and associated with subsequent thoughts of the behavior. Activity-related affect consists of three components: emotional arousal to the act itself (act related), the self acting (self related), or the environment in which the action takes place (context related). The resultant feeling state is likely to affect whether an individual will repeat the behavior again or maintain the behavior long term.[43] Behavior-contingent feeling states have been explored as determinants of health behaviors in recent studies.[43–47] The affect associated with the behavior reflects a direct emotional reaction or gut-level response to the thought of the behavior, which can be positive or negative—is it fun, delightful, enjoyable, disgusting, or unpleasant? Behaviors associated with positive affect are likely to be repeated, whereas those associated with negative affect are likely to be avoided. For some behaviors, both positive and negative feeling states will be induced. Thus, the relative balance between positive and negative affect prior to, during, and following the behavior is important to ascertain. Activity-related affect is different from the evaluative dimension of attitude as proposed by Fishbein and Ajzen.[48] The evaluative dimension of attitude reflects affective evaluation of the specific outcomes of a behavior rather than the response to the stimulus properties of the behavioral event itself.

For any given behavior, the full range of negative and positive feelings states in relation to the act, self as actor, and context for action should be elaborated so that they are adequately measured. In many instruments proposed to measure affect, negative feelings are elaborated more extensively than are positive feelings. This is not surprising because anxiety, fear, and depression have been studied much more than have joy, elation, and calm. Based on social cognitive theory, there is a relationship between self-efficacy and activity-related affect. McAuley and Courneya[44] found that positive affective response during exercise was a significant predictor of postexercise efficacy. This is consistent with Bandura's proposal that emotional responses and their induced physiologic states during a behavior serve as sources of efficacy information.[10] Thus, activity-related affect is proposed as influencing health behavior directly as well as indirectly through self-efficacy and commitment to a plan of action.

Because of the recent addition of activity-related affect to the HPM, few studies have explored the contribution of this construct to the explanatory and predictive power of the model. Further studies are needed to determine the importance of activity-related affect in regard to various health behaviors.

INTERPERSONAL INFLUENCES

According to the HPM, interpersonal influences are cognitions concerning the behaviors, beliefs, or attitudes of others. These cognitions may or may not correspond with reality. Primary sources of interpersonal influence on health-promoting behaviors are family (parents or siblings), peers, and health care providers. Interpersonal influences include norms (expectations of significant others), social support (instrumental and emotional encouragement), and modeling (vicarious learning through observing others engaged in a particular behavior). These three interpersonal processes have been shown to affect individuals' predisposition to engage in health-promoting behaviors in a number of studies.

Social norms set standards for performance that individuals can adopt or reject. Social support for a behavior taps the sustaining resources offered by others. Modeling portrays the sequential components of a health behavior and is an important strategy for behavior change in social cognitive theory. In the HPM, interpersonal influences are proposed as affecting health-promoting behavior directly as well as indirectly through social pressures or encouragement to commit to a plan of action. Individuals vary in the extent to which they are sensitive to the wishes, examples, and praise of others. However, given sufficient motivation to behave in a way consistent with interpersonal influences, individuals are likely to undertake behaviors for which they will be admired and socially reinforced. In order for interpersonal influences to have an effect, individuals must attend to the behaviors, wishes, and inputs of others; comprehend them; and assimilate them into cognitive representations related to given behaviors. Susceptibility to the influence of others may vary developmentally and be particularly evident in adolescence. Some cultures may place more emphasis on interpersonal influences than do others. For example, *familismo* among Hispanic populations may encourage individuals to engage in a particular behavior for the good of the family rather than for personal gain.

In studies based on the HPM, 57% provided empirical support for the importance of interpersonal influences as determinants of health-promoting behavior. This indicates moderate support for the construct. Further efforts are needed to develop more rigorous measures of interpersonal influences so that the differential usefulness of the construct can be determined across diverse populations.

SITUATIONAL INFLUENCES

Personal perceptions and cognitions of any situation or context can facilitate or impede behavior. Situational influences on health-promoting behavior include perceptions of options available, demand characteristics, and aesthetic features of the environment in which a given behavior is proposed to take place. Kaplan and Kaplan,[49] in their work on restorative natural environments, have heightened awareness of how environments or situational contexts can impact health and health-related behaviors. Individuals are drawn to and perform more competently in situations or environmental contexts in which they feel compatible rather than incompatible, related rather than alienated, safe and reassured rather than unsafe and threatened. Environments that are fascinating and interesting are also desirable contexts for the performance of health behaviors.

In the revised HPM, situational influences have been reconceptualized as direct and as indirect influences on health behavior. Situations may directly affect behaviors by presenting an environment "loaded" with cues that trigger action. For example, a "no smoking" environment creates demand characteristics for nonsmoking behavior. Company regulations for hearing protection to be worn create demand characteristics that employees comply with regulations. Both situations enforce commitment to health actions.

Situational influences have received moderate empirical support as determinants of health behavior. Of the HPM studies reviewed, 56% reported situational influences as significant predictors of health-promoting behavior. Efforts should be directed at developing more rigorous approaches to measurement before the extent of influence of this construct can be determined. Considering the emerging ecological perspective on determinants of health behavior, the environment needs to receive more systematic study as a behavioral determinant. Situational influences may be an important key to developing new and more effective strategies for facilitating the acquisition and maintenance of health-promoting behaviors in diverse populations.

Commitment to a Plan of Action

Commitment to a plan of action initiates a behavioral event. This commitment will propel the individual into and through the behavior unless a competing demand that the individual cannot avoid or a competing preference that the individual does not resist intervenes. Human beings generally engage in organized rather than disorganized behavior. According to Ajzen and Fishbein, intentionality is a major determinant of volitional behavior.[50] *Commitment to a plan of action* in the revised HPM implies the underlying cognitive processes: (1) commitment to carry out a specific action at a given time and place and with specified persons or alone, irrespective of competing preferences; and (2) identification of definitive strategies for eliciting, carrying out, and reinforcing the behavior. The requirement of identification of specific strategies to be used at different points in the behavioral sequence goes beyond intentionality to further the likelihood that the plan of action developed by nurse and client will be successfully implemented. For example, the strategy of contracting consists of a mutually agreed-upon set of actions to which one party commits with the understanding that the other party will provide some tangible reward or reinforcement if the commitment is sustained. Strategies can be selected by clients to energize and reinforce health behaviors according to their own preferences and their stage of change. Commitment alone without associated strategies often results in "good intentions" but failure to perform a valued health behavior.

Immediate Competing Demands and Preferences

Immediate competing demands or preferences refer to alternative behaviors that intrude into consciousness as possible courses of action immediately prior to the intended occurrence of a planned health-promoting behavior. Competing demands are viewed as those alternative behaviors over which individuals have a relatively low level of control because of environmental contingencies such as work or family care responsibilities. Failure to respond to a demand may have untoward effects for the self or for significant others. Competing preferences are viewed as alternative behaviors with powerful reinforcing properties over which individuals exert a relatively high level of control. They can derail a health-promoting behavior in favor of the competing behavior.[51] The extent to which an individual is able to resist competing preferences depends on his or her ability to be self-regulating. Examples of "giving in" to competing preferences are selecting a food high in fat rather than low in fat because of taste or flavor preferences; driving past the recreation center where one usually exercises to stop at the mall (a preference for browsing or shopping rather than physical activity). Both competing demands and preferences can derail a plan of action to which one has committed. Competing demands can be differentiated from barriers in that the individual must carry out an alternative behavior based on unanticipated external demand, or untoward results are likely to occur. Competing preferences can be differentiated from barriers such as lack of time, because competing preferences are last-minute urges based on one's preference hierarchy that derail a plan for positive health action.

Individuals vary in their ability to sustain attention and avoid disruption of health behaviors. Some individuals may be predisposed developmentally or biologically to be more easily swayed from a course of action than are others. Inhibiting competing preferences requires the exercise of self-regulation and control capabilities. Strong commitment to a plan of action may sustain dedication to complete a behavior in light of competing demands or preferences. In the HPM, immediate competing demands and preferences are proposed as directly affecting the probability of occurrence of health behavior as well as moderating the effects of commitment. Only one study to date has tested "competing demands" as a predictor of health-promoting behavior. Wu[34] developed a tool to test the effects of competing demands on physical activity behavior among Taiwanese adolescents. The variable did not reach statistical significance in the data analysis. More sensitive measures of this variable in regard to various health behaviors need to be developed prior to its use in subsequent studies.

Behavioral Outcome

HEALTH-PROMOTING BEHAVIOR

This variable in the model has been addressed extensively throughout the book so needs little further discussion here. Health-promoting behavior is the endpoint or action outcome in the HPM. However, it should be noted that health-promoting behavior is ultimately directed toward *attaining positive health outcomes* for the client. Health-promoting behaviors, particularly when integrated into a healthy lifestyle that pervades all aspects of living, should result in improved health, enhanced functional ability, and better quality of life at all stages of development.

Directions for Research to Test the Health Promotion Model

The revised HPM presented in this chapter incorporates the outcome expectancies of expectancy-value theory and self-efficacy expectancies of social cognitive theory. Further, other personal factors delineated in social learning theory, as well as interpersonal, situational, and behavioral factors, are integral to the HPM. Thus, the model is theoretically consistent with these frameworks. The revised model needs to be tested empirically with particular attention to new constructs. However, some empirical evidence already exists that supports their predictive value for health behavior. Before testing the model with any specific health behavior, it is suggested that rigorous measures of behavior-specific variables be developed if they do not already exist. This may involve qualitative research to elicit appropriate content for the instruments prior to their design.

Where there is already considerable evidence supporting the predictive validity of variables in the HPM, health promotion intervention studies should be designed incorporating these variables. The extent to which the revised HPM is useful in guiding interventions that alter health behaviors will be determined through intervention studies.

Directions for Practice Using the Health Promotion Model

Evidence-based care is essential to quality care. Nurses can use the Health Promotion Model to provide a coherent and organized framework for intervening with clients to increase health-promoting behaviors. For example, nurses can develop interventions that address perceived self-efficacy, perceived barriers, perceived benefits, interpersonal influences, and situational influences relevant to a particular health behavior for any given individual. Assessment of prior behavior, demographic characteristics, and perceived health status although not components of an intervention, can shed light on how to tailor interventions to best meet the needs of diverse clients.

Information technology and computer capabilities challenge nurse researchers to creatively individualize and personalize health care. The HPM provides a framework for understanding the dimensions on which health promotion interventions can be tailored. The next decade will provide many opportunities for nurses to lead other health professionals in developing effective counseling and behavioral intervention strategies with a particular focus on eliminating health disparities. Nurses are encouraged to use the Health Promotion Model for this purpose.

SUMMARY

Assumptions and theoretical assertions of the HPM have been presented in this chapter as well as descriptions of the variables and the results of approximately 40 studies testing the HPM. The model provides an integrated perspective for nurses that depicts the range of behavioral influences to be addressed in nursing interventions in order to increase health-promoting behaviors. The extent of empirical evidence for the HPM supports its use in research and practice.

REFERENCES

1. Pender NJ. *Health Promotion in Nursing Practice*. Norwalk, CT.: Appleton-Century-Crofts; 1982.
2. Dunn HL. What high-level wellness means. *Can J Public Health*. November 1959;50(11):447–457.
3. Dunn HL. High-level wellness for men and society. *Am J Public Health*. 1959;49(6):786–792.

4. Pender NJ. *Health Promotion in Nursing Practice.* 2nd ed. Norwalk, CT: Appleton & Lange; 1987.

5. Pender NJ. *Health Promotion in Nursing Practice.* 3nd ed. Stamford, CT: Appleton & Lange; 1996.

6. Feather NT, ed. *Expectations and Actions: Expectancy-Value Models in Psychology.* Hillsdale, NJ: Lawrence Erlbaum Associates, Inc.; 1982.

7. Klar Y, Nader A, Mallor TE. Opting to change: Student's informal self-change endeavors. In: Klar Y, Fisher JD, Chinsky JM, et al., eds. *Self-Change: Social and Psychological Perspectives.* New York: Springer-Verlag; 1992:63–83.

8. Bandura A. *Social Foundations of Thought and Action: A Social Cognitive Theory.* Upper Saddle River, NJ: Prentice Hall, Inc.; 1986.

9. Bandura A. Self Efficacy: Toward a unifying theory of behavioral change. *Psychol Rev.* 1977;84:191–215.

10. Bandura, A. *Self-Efficacy: The Exercise of Control.* New York: W. H. Freeman; 1997.

11. Weitzel MH. A test of the Health Promotion Model with blue collar workers. *Nurs Res.* 1989;38(2):99–104.

12. Pender NJ, Walker SN, Frank-Stromborg M, Sechrist KR, et al. *The Health Promotion Model: Refinement and Validation.* Final Report to the National Center for Nursing Research, National Institutes of Health (Grant no. NR01121). Dekalb, IL: Northern Illinois University Press; 1990.

13. Pender NJ, Walker SN, Sechrist KR, et al. Predicting health-promoting lifestyles in the workplace. *Nurs Res.* 1990;39(6):326–332.

14. Frank-Stromborg M, Pender NJ, Walker SN. Determinants of health-promoting lifestyles in ambulatory cancer patients. *Soc Sci Med.* 1990;31:1159–1168.

15. Johnson JL, Ratner PA, Bottorff JL, et al. An exploration of Pender's Health Promotion Model using LISREL. *Nurs Res.* 1993;42(3):132–138.

16. Suwonnaroop, N. Health-promoting behaviors in older adults: The effect of social support, perceived health status, and personal factors. Case Western Reserve; 1999. *Dissertation Abstracts International* (1999). University Microfilms No. AAG9941265.

17. Bolio SM. Reported health-promoting behaviors of incarcerated males (prisoner health, family support). University of Massachusetts; 1999. *Dissertation Abstracts International* (1999). University Microfilms No. AAG9920586.

18. Millard SR. Factors related to health-promoting behaviors in Seventh-day Adventist older adults (quality of life). University of Texas at Austin; 1998. *Dissertation Abstracts International* (1998). University Microfilms No. AAG9838052.

19. Nikulich-Barrett MJ. Impact of perceived general health status, physical functioning, and self-efficacy on health promoting lifestyles of rural older black and white women (women elderly). State University of New York at Buffalo; 1997. *Dissertation Abstracts International* (1997). University Microfilms No. AAG9807369.

20. Hutchinson KC. Factors that predict health-promoting lifestyle behaviors among African-American university students. Northern Illinois University; 1996. *Dissertation Abstracts International* (1996). University Microfilms No. AAG9639920.

21. Warren MT. The relationships of self-motivation and perceived personal competence to engaging in a health-promoting lifestyle for men in cardiac rehabilitation programs. New York University; 1993. *Dissertation Abstracts International* (1993). University Microfilms No. AAG9333943.

22. Gillis AJ. The relationship of definition of health, perceived health status, self-efficacy, parental health-promoting lifestyle, and selected demographics to health-promoting lifestyle in adolescent

females. University of Texas at Austin; 1993. *Dissertation Abstracts International* (1993). University Microfilms No. AAG9323405.

23. Harrison RL. The relationship among hope, perceived health status and health-promoting lifestyle among HIV seropositive mean (immune deficiency). New York University; 1993. *Dissertation Abstracts International* (1993). University Microfilms No. AAG9317666.

24. Moore EJ. The relationship among self-efficacy, health knowledge, self-rated health status, and selected demographics as determinants of health-promoting behavior in older adults. University of Akron; 1992. *Dissertation Abstracts International* (1992). University Microfilms No. AAG9225233.

25. Wilson AH. Health-promoting behaviors among married and unmarried mothers. University of Alabama at Birmingham; 1991. *Dissertation Abstracts International* (1991). University Microfilms No. AAG9134245.

26. Barnett FC. The relationship of selected cognitive-perceptual factors to health-promoting behaviors of adolescents. University of Texas at Austin; 1989. *Dissertation Abstracts International* (1989). University Microfilms No. AAG8920656.

27. Fehir JS. Self-rated health status, self-efficacy, motivation, and selected demographics as determinants of health-promoting lifestyle behavior in men 35 to 64 years old: A nursing investigation. University of Texas at Austin; 1988. *Dissertation Abstracts International* (1988). University Microfilms No. AAG8909657.

28. Garcia A, Norton-Broda MA, Frenn M, et al. Gender and developmental differences in exercise beliefs among youth and prediction of their exercise behavior. *J School Health.* 1995;65(6):213–219.

29. Lusk SL, Ronis D, Kerr MJ, et al. Test of the Health Promotion Model as a causal model of workers' use of hearing protection. *Nurs Res.* 1994;43(3):151–157.

30. Lusk SL, Ronis DL, Kerr ML. Predictors of hearing protection use among workers: Implications for training programs. *Human Factors.* 1995;37(3):635–640.

31. Lusk SL, Kerr MJ, Ronis DL, Eakin BL. Applying the Health Promotion Model to development of a worksite intervention. *Am J Health Prom.* 1999;13(4): 219–226.

32. Kerr MJ. Factors related to Mexican-American Workers' use of hearing protection. Ann Arbor, MI: University of Michigan; 1994. *Dissertation Abstracts International* (1994). University Microfilms No. 9501083.

33. McCullagh MC. Factors affecting hearing protector use among farmers. *Dissertation Abstracts International* (1999). 61(02), University Microfilms No. AAT9959819.

34. Wu T. Determinants of physical activity among Taiwanese adolescents: An application of the Health-Promotion Model. University of Michigan; 1999. *Dissertation Abstracts International* (1999). University Microfilms No. AAG9938572.

35. Stutts WC. Use of the Health Promotion Model to predict physical activity in adults (weight control, self-efficacy). University of North Carolina at Chapel Hill; 1997. *Dissertation Abstracts International* (1997). University Microfilms No. AAG9730610.

36. Chen CH. Physical exercise and sense of well-being among Chinese elderly in Taiwan. University of Texas at Austin; 1995. *Dissertation Abstracts International* (1995). University Microfilms No. AAI9603814.

37. Jeffries PR. Predictor variables of exercise and nutrition for expatriates in Indonesia utilizing Pender's Health Promotion Model. Indiana University School of Nursing; 1996. *Dissertation Abstracts International* (1996). University Microfilms No. AAG9639877.

38. Oesterle MS. Adherence of women to structured exercise programs: The effect of cognitive-perceptual variables and social support. Northern Illinois University; 1988. *Dissertation Abstracts International* (1988). University Microfilms No. AAG8822374.

39. Martinelli AM. A study of health locus of control, self-efficacy, health promotion behaviors, and environmental factors related to the self-report of the avoidance of environmental tobacco smoke in young adults. University of Michigan; 1996. *Dissertation Abstracts International* (1996). University Microfilms No. AAG9633458.

40. Tober JA. Investigation of predictors of successful weight loss in a morbidly obese population (optifast). University of Waterloo (Canada); 1996. *Dissertation Abstracts International* (1996). University Microfilms No. AAGNN15346.

41. Jones T, Fowler MC, Hubbard D. Refining a tool to measure cues to action in encouraging health promoting behavior—The CHAQ. *Am J Health Prom.* 2000;14(3):170–173.

42. Lusk SL, Hong OS, Ronis DL, Eakin BL, Kerr MJ, Early MR. Effectiveness of an intervention to increase construction workers' use of hearing protection. *Human Factors.* 1999;41(3):487–494.

43. Gauvin L, Rejeski WJ. The exercise-induced feeling inventory: Development and initial validation. *J Sport Exerc Psychol.* 1993;15:403–423.

44. McAuley E, Courneya KS. Self-efficacy relationships with affective and exertion responses to exercise. *J Appl Soc Psychol.* 1992;22:312–326.

45. Hardy CJ, Rejeski WJ. Not what, but how one feels: The measurement of affect during exercise. *J Sport Exerc Psychol.* 1989;11:304–317.

46. Godin G. Importance of the emotional aspect of attitude to predict intention. *Psychol Rep.* 1987; 61:719–723.

47. Rejeski WJ, Gauvin L, Hobson ML, et al. Effects of baseline responses, in-task feelings, and duration of activity on exercise-induced feeling states in women. *Health Psychol.* 1995;14:350–359.

48. Fishbein M, Ajzen I. *Belief, Attitude, Intention and Behavior: An Introduction to Theory and Research.* Boston, MA: Addison-Wesley Publishing Co., Inc.; 1975.

49. Kaplan R, Kaplan S. *The Experience of Nature: A Psychological Perspective.* Cambridge, England: Cambridge University Press; 1989.

50. Ajzen I, Fishbein M. *Understanding Attitudes and Predicting Social Behavior.* Upper Saddle River, NJ: Prentice Hall, Inc.; 1980.

51. Vara LS, Epstein L. Laboratory assessment of choice between exercise or sedentary behaviors. *Res Q Exerc Sport.* 1995;64:356–360.

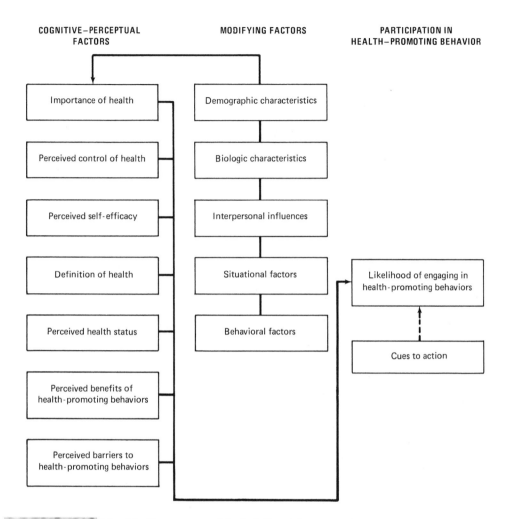

APPENDIX A Health Promotion Model (Initial version)

Part II

Health Promotion in Diverse Populations

4

Empowering for Self-Care Across the Life Span

- The Role of the Professional Nurse
- Self-Care Throughout the Life Span
  - A. Self-Care for Children and Adolescents
  - B. Self-Care for Young and Middle-Aged Adults
  - C. Self-Care for Older Adults
- Goals of Health Education for Self-Care
- The Process of Empowering for Self-Care
  - A. Mutually Assessing Self-Care Competencies and Needs
  - B. Determining Learning Priorities
  - C. Identifying Long-Term and Short-Term Objectives
  - D. Facilitating Self-Paced Learning
  - E. Using Positive Reinforcement to Empower Competence and Motivation for Learning
  - F. Creating a Supportive Environment for Learning
  - G. Decreasing Barriers to Learning
  - H. Evaluating Client Progress Toward Health Goals
- Other Considerations in Self-Care Empowerment
- The Role of the Internet in Self-Care
- Directions for Research on Self-Care
- Directions for Practice in Self-Care
- Summary

The self-care movement has become a big business targeted at consumers as a result of changes in health care financing and the proliferation of managed care. Self-responsibility and self-care are major themes in health policy.[1] In addition, the consumer movement has resulted in individuals, families, and communities expending greater energy in self-care activities to promote and maintain health. Self-care, a universal requirement for sustaining and enhancing life and health, is an area of competence to be developed. Self-care directed toward health protection and health promotion can be defined as the practice of activities initiated or performed by an individual, family, or community to achieve, maintain, or promote maximum health and well-being.[2] Participation in self-care empowers individuals, families, and communities, as self-care activities enable them to gain control of their lives and communities to improve health. Care of self and others to maximize health includes actions directed toward minimizing threats to personal health, self-nurturance, self-improvement, and continuing personal growth. Active involvement in self-care is widely acknowledged as an important strategy for achieving national health goals. *Healthy People 2010* recognizes that one of the greatest opportunities to achieve its goals is in *empowering* individuals to make informed health care decisions and to become active participants in improving their health.[3]

Self-care within chronic illness is defined as the practice of activities to manage the illness, such as self-management of side effects of treatments or symptoms of the disease.[4] In chronic illness, self-care activities may include taking medication, eating special foods, or taking direct action such as making a doctor's appointment. Self-care for health promotion goes beyond illness self-care and requires that clients gain knowledge and competencies that can be used to *maintain* and *enhance* health. In both health promotion and health protection, self-care is primary, with professional care—in the form of active protection (immunization) against disease, education, or guidance—secondary. Self-care approaches are now being extended beyond traditional strategies in medicine, nursing, and other health professions to approaches that have previously been considered complementary or alternative. Such approaches constitute a grassroots approach to enhancing self-care and will lead to new understandings of the boundaries and strengths of self-care throughout the life span.

The Role of the Professional Nurse

Professional nurses have a major responsibility for empowering clients for self-care throughout their life span. Nurses have long recognized the right of individuals and families to be informed and active participants in their own care.

In Orem's Self-Care Nursing Model, three types of self-care requisites are described: universal, developmental, and health deviation requirements.[2] Universal self-care requirements include sufficient air, water, food, elimination, a balance between activity and rest, a balance between solitude and social interaction, protection from hazards, and protection of human functioning and development. Developmental self-care requirements fall within two categories:

1. Maintenance of living conditions that support life processes, promote development, or encourage human progress toward higher levels of organization of human structure and maturation

2. Provision of care either to prevent the occurrence of deleterious effects of conditions that can affect human development or to mitigate or overcome these effects from various conditions

The nurse is primarily concerned with the universal and developmental requirements, although health deviation requirements, such as knowledge and skills needed for self-care in illness, must be attended to if they arise.

In Orem's model, individuals perform self-care to meet needs and demands consistent with their age, maturation, experience, resources, and sociocultural background. In the model, three systems are described within professional nursing practice: a compensatory system, a partially compensatory system, and an educative-developmental system. In compensatory care, the nurse provides total care for the client. Such care is most common in acute-care settings, such as hospitals during acute illness episodes. Partially compensatory care is implemented when the nurse and the client share the responsibility for care. Care during rehabilitation from illness or in advanced chronic illness is partially compensatory. In contrast, the *educative-developmental* nursing system gives the client primary responsibility for personal health, with the nurse functioning in a consultative capacity. This third nursing system is most appropriate for self-care in health protection and health promotion.

With increasing emphasis on primary care in the United States and throughout the world, the educative-developmental component of nursing practice is viewed with renewed interest as a reimbursable service by health payers, including managed care organizations. Major areas of educative-developmental nursing for self-care include enhancing clients' capacities for exercise and physical fitness, nutrition and weight control, stress management, risk reduction, maintenance of family and other social support systems, avoidance of injurious and violent behaviors and substance abuse; and environmental modifications in homes, schools, work sites, and the community to reduce hazards to health and strengthen health-enhancing features. Education, counseling, and environmental interventions directed to these ends are a shared responsibility that includes the federal government, state and local governments, policy makers, health care providers, community leaders, and individuals.

Broad-based efforts directed at activating the general public for self-care should be spearheaded by nurses in collaboration with other health professionals and community members. Empowerment of health care consumers to "take charge" of their health is based on the assumptions that they should be:

1. Actively involved in health problem solving
2. Making rational and informed choices about health and health care
3. Developing competencies and skills that foster creativity and adaptation amid changing life circumstances
4. Striving for greater mastery of environmental conditions that influence health and well-being
5. Promoting public policy making to build healthy lifestyles in diverse communities
6. Advocating for the development of health financing plans that provides payment for a range of self-care education services for all people

Individuals, families, and communities need to be empowered for health promotion. Advances will be achieved when all groups work in concert to make health promotion a coherent social movement that significantly influences the quality and cost of health care delivery. Successful programs should be integrated throughout the educational and health care sectors nationally, with tailoring to fit local needs.

Self-Care Throughout the Life Span

Self-Care for Children and Adolescents

Children represent the potential for a healthy society.[5] Currently about 60 million children are younger than 15 years in the United States and this number is expected to remain stable until 2020. This population poses multiple challenges, as almost one-third have a chronic health problem by the time they reach adolescence.[5] Childhood is a critical period in the adoption of healthy behaviors and a health-promoting lifestyle. Behaviors are developed and learned based on developmental level, social and physical environment, and personal experiences.

Childhood is a developmental period during which social and cognitive skills for autonomous decision making and health behaviors are developed. As with adults, health behaviors can be linked to family support and socioeconomic variables and socialization through family, schools, and media. Socioeconomic status plays a significant role in health behaviors, as increased socioeconomic status enables the family to provide resources, such as a more affluent school system, nutritional food choices, and access to multiple activities.[6] The family environment is thought to play a significant role in self-care for health promotion through positive, stable childhood experiences.[7] A supportive family environment shapes the child's behavior through the use of rewards and punishment in behavior choices. Family support in participating in self-care behaviors has also been shown to facilitate the development of healthy behaviors such as physical activity.

Schools have traditionally concentrated on the role of peer pressure in the adoption of self-care behaviors, rather than focusing on health in the curriculum, beginning in the early school years. Most children are exposed to television and electronic media, two health information sources that will continue to grow. For example, children participated in an Internet-based nutrition program, called the 5-a-Day Virtual Classroom, which encouraged them to eat more fruits and vegetables.[8] Children were asked their ideas about how to get other children across the country to eat 5-a-day. The suggestions cited were use of mass media, economic incentives, and social influence. The most frequently mentioned suggestion was to reward children for eating fruits and vegetables. Internet-based programs, such as this one, will be effective in providing information to promote self-care as well as information from the consumer on which to develop effective self-care interventions.

Adolescence is a critical period of physical, cognitive, emotional, and social development in a dynamic and uncertain interval between childhood and adulthood.[9] Developmentally, it is a time characterized by change and transitions.[10] The primary biological transition is puberty. Cognitively, adolescents begin to think more abstractly. However, as children, they lack the ability to apply their cognitive skills to solving problems in stressful situations. This has implications for behavioral choices under stress. Socially, the family remains an important source of support. Parents can play a positive role in providing emotional support and encouragement and can promote healthy peer interactions, as peers also serve as important role models. Schools exert an influence on the acquisition of self-care behaviors in adolescents.

Approaches to enhancing health-promoting behaviors of children and adolescents must focus on both families and peer groups. This dual approach is critical, because values, attitudes, beliefs, and behaviors of families and peers influence children's and adolescents' lifestyles. Parents serve as powerful role models of health and health-related behaviors. They depict family health care functions and various approaches to linking with the broader health care resources in the community. The rapid developmental changes that occur for children and adolescents and the emerging, yet malleable, behavioral patterns that will carry into adulthood make the preschool and school-age years an ideal time to enhance skills for health-promoting and health protecting behaviors. Peer groups play a critical role in molding lifestyles for school-age children, particularly adolescents. When peers reinforce the active health consumer role, peer pressure becomes a positive force.

An increasing number of school health programs are giving considerable attention to lifestyle education that increases children's health and resilience and teaches skills for modifying peer group affiliations and resisting the pressure of peers who encourage health-damaging behaviors. School-based health promotion research has provided valuable information about effective interventions that promote the adoption of healthy self-care behaviors in children and adolescents. The Child and Adolescent Trial for Cardiovascular Health (CATCH), the largest school-based trial ever sponsored by the National Institutes of Health,[11] was implemented into 56 schools in 4 states. The interventions consisted of an Eat Smart food service program, a physical education program, classroom curricula, and parental involvement programs. The third- to fifth-grade curricula focused on choosing healthy foods, physical activity, and intentions to smoke tobacco. Two and one-half years after implementing the interventions in the schools, significant changes were still evident in the food service program and physical education classes, and the children in the intervention schools had made significant changes in eating and physical activity self-care behaviors.[12] At three-year follow-up, significant differences still existed for physical activity and dietary knowledge and intentions.[13] In addition, differences in fat intake were evident in the fifth- and eighth-grade groups. The finding of sustained physical activity is especially significant in light of accumulating evidence of a decline in physical activity among youth because of television and computer games, which require minimal physical exertion.[14] Findings from this large study indicate that self-care behaviors can be initiated and sustained with school-based interventions that include institutional changes, personal changes, and family support and involvement.

Several nurse researchers are conducting programs of research to promote self-care in adopting health behaviors in children and adolescents. Harrell and her colleagues at the University of North Carolina have conducted research to promote cardiovascular health in third and fourth graders.[15] The intervention in the Cardiovascular Health in Children (CHIC) study consisted of an eight-week knowledge and attitude program and a physical education program. One year following the intervention, significant improvements were noted in both knowledge and cholesterol levels in those who received the intervention. A four-year follow-up is underway to see if self-care behaviors will be sustained to maintain these changes. McClowery has undertaken a school-based intervention for minority children in the first and second grade in inner-city schools.[16] Results of the ten-week program that targets parents, teachers, and the children are not yet available. Felton and Parsons have also had a sustained program of research that targets children and adolescent health behaviors. Results of their research indicate that families and the community must be included in the intervention with the child.[17,18] Participation in community sports has been shown to be a self-care activity important for the development of regular physical activity. "Best" friends have also been found to have a significant influence on adoption of risky behaviors, pointing to the importance of peers in development of healthy and unhealthy behaviors.[19] Hendricks has found that level of hope and self-efficacy are critical concepts in developing interventions to empower adolescents to make healthy behavior lifestyle choices.[20] Loveland-Cherry has investigated the role of the family in use and misuse of alcohol in fourth-grade children.[21] Her results indicate that self-efficacy, parent–child interactions, and family and peer adjustment are correlated with alcohol use–misuse. Results of a family-based intervention to study the effects of altering parental norms and behavior on adolescent alcohol use resulted in a decrease in initiation of alcohol use and subsequent misuse for adolescents who had reported no use of alcohol prior to the intervention. Loveland-Cherry's research highlights the role of family in the development of health self-care behaviors.[22]

Children and youth who have dropped out of school or are homeless need special attention in developing self-care behaviors for health promotion. Education sessions for these children may have to take place in parks, food kitchens, or homeless shelters. Children of one-parent families as well as "latchkey youth" of two working parents may also require special attention.[23] Special sensitivity to the lack of resources for daily living, lack of parental influence and supervision, and low levels of motivation because of life conditions is critical for promoting a healthy lifestyle.

Self-Care for Young and Middle-Age Adults

Young and middle-age adulthood is the time in the life cycle when many persons are intensely involved in careers and child rearing. The momentum of everyday life and the demands of dependent others may leave little time to focus on health in the absence of an illness crisis. The strengthening of intrafamilial support for self-care is particularly important at this time when adults need to accept responsibility for modeling and teaching younger and older children competent self-care, increasing family knowledge and expertise with health promotion skills, and learning how and when to use health care resources for the family. Adult learners bring many strengths to self-care education, including a background of life experiences, self-direction in learning, problem- or interest-centered (as opposed to subject-centered) learning needs, and interest in immediate rather than delayed application. Self-care empowerment education for adults consists of the following components:[24,25]

1. Provide time to express feelings.
2. Express a supportive attitude.
3. Reinforce client self-esteem.
4. Provide access to health information.
5. Practice self-care skills that can be applied immediately.
6. Present alternative views on health issues.

7. Offer multiple views related to complementary self-care therapies.
8. Provide timely feedback and reinforcement.
9. Provide flexible learning pathways.

Adults tuned in to their own needs for self-care may be effective in reducing the stress inherent in multiple societal roles, including familial and work responsibilities that many young and middle-age adults fulfill. Systematically planning health promotion activities into daily routines at work or with family members can both enhance health in a busy lifestyle and model healthy lifestyles to family members. Adequate attention to self-care during the young and middle-age years promotes optimal productivity and life satisfaction and lays the groundwork for a healthy and productive retirement and old age rather than one fraught with discomfort, disability, and compromised quality of life.

Self-Care for Older Adults

Self-care for older adults focuses on maximizing independence, vigor, and life satisfaction. Health promotion in this population is vital to prevent complications and decrease risks that affect life quality.[26] Adequate self-care education must take into account the physical, sensory, mobility, sexual, and psychosocial changes that currently characterize the aging process. Physical activity and smoking have been shown to make a significant difference in morbidity and mortality in older persons.[27] Research has indicated that exercise can enhance the self-esteem of older adults and in some cases decrease depression and anxiety. In persons age 65 and older, maintaining independence and activity has been shown to enhance their well-being, pointing to the need for ongoing health promotion self-care to maintain a regular physical activity program.[28]

Personality and coping styles do not appear to change significantly with age. Thus, persons who develop positive coping skills early in life can meet social demands in later years, find meaning in life, and direct ample energy to appropriate self-care activities. Older individuals who have been characterized as information seekers have been found to have greater health-promoting behaviors.[27] Information seeking included reading articles about health, listening to television or radio programs, talking with friends, and performing self-examinations. Other patterns linked with health-promoting behaviors and well-being include positive perceptions of one's health and aging, involvement in groups and organizations, and contact with family members.[29] Although research related to these variables has many methodological issues that have only recently begun to be addressed, the results provide helpful information on psychosocial factors that are important in healthy aging.

Retirement is a significant life event that presents a major challenge for the older population financially, socially, and emotionally. Appropriate self-care in the form of anticipatory planning is associated with successful adaptation.[30] Gioiella's[31] self-care actions that facilitate healthy retirement are still timely:

1. Planning ahead to insure adequate income
2. Developing friends not associated with work
3. Decreasing time at work in the last years before retirement by taking longer vacations, working shorter days, or working part time

4. Developing routines, including adequate physical activity, to replace the structure of the workday

5. Relying on other people and groups in addition to spouse to fill leisure time

6. Developing leisure time activities before retirement that are realistic in energy and monetary cost

7. Anticipating that exhilaration will be followed by ambivalence before satisfaction with one's retirement lifestyle develops

8. Assessing living arrangements and, if relocation is necessary, expending time in developing new social networks

9. Expecting job role loss will have a short-term effect on self-esteem and one's marital relationship

Older adults often have more time available for pursuit of personal wellness than do younger adults. They should be challenged to use this time productively and counseled about resources available within the community to facilitate such efforts.

The fastest-growing segment of the population in the United States is the group age 85 and over. These elderly individuals need safe, health-enhancing communities as well as support services to assist them in continuing health promotion activities that focus on quality versus quantity of life. With adequate support from families and health professionals and access to resources, most older adults choose to remain in their own homes throughout their old age. The nation must address the scope of health protection and health promotion services the elderly need to support their self-care capabilities. The Program of All-Inclusive Care for the Elderly (PACE) is one innovative approach to providing services for frail elders in adult day care community settings and case management by interdisciplinary teams.[32] Programs such as this one can facilitate healthy behaviors and provide the support to enable elders to remain independent as long as possible. Cost-effective and -efficient methods for developing these services using available technologies, such as Web-based communication to augment personal contact, are being tested. Major attention is beginning to be given to promoting the health and well-being of older adults, a rapidly growing segment of the U.S. citizenry.

Health and well-being in old age depend on freedom from disease, functional status, and adequate social and environmental supports.[33] Promotion of self-care activities to maintain and improve functional status includes strategies for safe mobility and prevention of falls and activities to promote social functioning and integration. All evidence to date indicates that elderly can become physically fit. However, it is much easier to remain physically active if this self-care behavior has been developed earlier in life.

Self-care for health promotion in older women needs attention because of different experiences of aging and old age in women. Women live longer than men and are more likely to live their later years alone with substantially lower incomes, more vulnerability to poverty, and more chronic health conditions than are men in the same age group.[34] Barriers to participation in health promotion activities in older women include transportation, scheduling, and cost factors.[35] However, low-cost interventions such as walking groups can be implemented in communities. Many challenges and opportunities are presented for women as they age in America. Nurses and the health care system must respond to the issues that prevent elderly women from being able to participate in healthy behaviors. Frameworks of women's health may be useful in guiding self-care interventions for women. These frameworks take into account the social context in which women experience their lives as well as their perceptions of their health and well-being, factors that must be incorporated into all health promotion activities.[36]

Goals of Health Education for Self-Care

Although education of the public for self-care is an integral part of a number of federal documents and policies, including *Healthy People 2010*,[3] it has just begun to be a viable and visible focus for federal health expenditures. Only a small percentage of the federal budget is actually spent on health education activities. Within the federal government, the Office of Disease Prevention and Health Promotion (ODPHP), the Office on Smoking and Health (OSH), the Office of Women's Health, the Office of Minority Health, and the Centers for Disease Control and Prevention are examples of major agencies that focus on meeting the health education needs of the public. National goals for health education for self-care are not well articulated in a single document but exist in numerous documents that address various self-care issues, such as those related to cardiovascular health, mental health, child development, nutrition, and elimination of health disparities. Recommended goals in the public and private sectors for self-care education directed toward health protection and health promotion include the following:

1. Raise the consciousness of the public about major threats to health that are preventable and provide the individual, group, and environmental means to do so.
2. Change the dominant definition of health to include not only the absence of illness but also high-level wellness among individuals, families, and communities.
3. Create conditions and resources to empower communities for self-care to address the social and environmental ills that prevent the community and its individuals from achieving well-being.
4. Create financial and other incentives to foster active health information seeking and positive health practices.
5. Assist people in developing the requisite knowledge and skills to successfully implement health-protecting and health-promoting behaviors.
6. Design and implement culturally and socioeconomically appropriate health-enhancing programs and techniques to diverse populations.
7. Implement curricula to provide the educational base in preschool, elementary, and secondary schools to develop behaviors for healthy living throughout the life span.

To achieve these goals, health policy makers and health professionals must be particularly sensitive to the extent to which problems of literacy and poverty present barriers to health education. Approaches to self-care education that use community workers and communication media such as radio that do not require reading but are accessible to a vast majority of the population are important in educating low-literacy populations about self-care needs and strategies. Competent self-care must also be economically plausible to individuals and families living in poverty. This requires coordination of public, private, and volunteer services to provide coherent self-care education and options to facilitate responsible yet low-cost health promotion programs and services.

The Process of Empowering for Self-Care

Responses of individuals and groups to the process of health education for self-care are multidimensional and complex. The client brings to the learning situation a unique personality and learning style, established social interaction patterns, numerous group affiliations, cultural norms and values, proximal and distal environmental influences, and a given level of readiness to adopt self-care behaviors. The nurse also comes with innate personality characteristics, values, attitudes, and social circumstances that affect the nature of the interaction. The self-care empowerment process as a collaborative endeavor between client and nurse is depicted in Figure 4–1. The interaction for self-care education brings the professional expertise of nurses and other health care professionals together with the health care knowledge and goals of the client, either individual or group. Mutual assessment of health care competencies and strengths as well as needs by the client and nurse will determine learning priorities, the pace of learning (long-term and short-term objectives), and the interpersonal and environmental support needed for learning. Barriers to learning and implementing self-care behaviors need to be identified and directly addressed with clients. Failure to identify

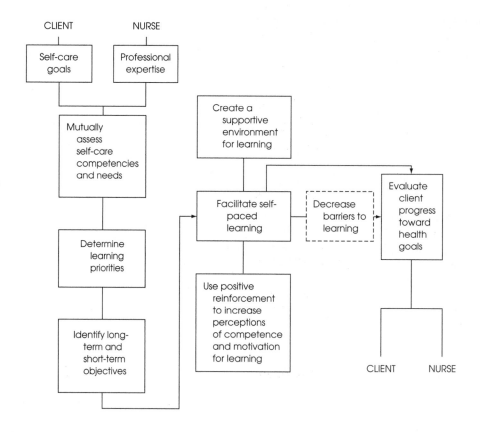

FIGURE 4-1 The self-care empowerment process

and realistically manage barriers can result in frustration and a lack of satisfaction for clients when they evaluate progress toward their self-care goals. Specific components of the self-care education empowerment process are described below.

Mutually Assessing Self-Care Competencies and Needs

The client often comes to the encounter with health care professionals with certain self-care goals in mind. Competencies related to these goals can be assessed through informal discussion, health skills checklists (Figure 4–2), or structured tests of knowledge in specific content areas. The first approach is recommended for low-literacy clients or those uncomfortable with paper-and-pencil tasks. Observation of actual behavior can also provide useful insights, if this is possible.

In the list below, please check those behaviors that you are comfortable in performing for yourself without assistance from others.

_____ Counting my pulse at the wrist for 1 minute

_____ Counting my pulse at the neck for 1 minute

_____ Selecting comfortable and appropriate shoes for brisk walking or jogging

_____ Selecting appropriate clothing for walking or jogging activities

_____ Planning a progressive schedule of exercise to meet my personal needs

_____ Indicating the ideal weight range for my height

_____ Calculating my maximal heart rate during exercise

_____ Planning time for exercise that is convenient and possible

_____ Selecting warm-up exercises that I could do before brisk walking or running

_____ Selecting procedures for cooling down after vigorous exercise

_____ Exercising at least five times a week for 30 minutes

_____ Integrating physical-fitness activities with my recreational interests

_____ Maintaining a record of my progress in physical activity over a period of several months

_____ Eating appropriately before or after vigorous exercise

_____ Avoiding injuries during exercise

FIGURE 4-2 Health-skills checklist for exercise participation

The motivated client seeks health information that will assist in self-care. The existence of apathy, lack of interest, and inattention should alert the nurse to a lack of motivation on the part of the client. Reasons for lack of interest should be explored so that the nurse can knowledgeably intervene to increase motivation.

Determining Learning Priorities

Deciding where to begin is often a dilemma for the nurse when the client needs information about multiple health topics. Clients have definite ideas about what they wish to know and what is important to them. Sometimes interest may not lie in the area that poses the greatest threat to personal health. For example, a client may smoke but be more interested in starting to exercise than in quitting smoking. Although the nurse may believe that smoking constitutes a more serious threat to the health of the client than does a sedentary lifestyle, it is obviously better to be a physically active smoker than an inactive smoker, because risks are synergistic. If the nurse assists the client to develop an exercise program, the client may also develop a heightened awareness of the negative impact of smoking on lung capacity and physical endurance. At that point, the client may exhibit readiness to discuss approaches to smoking cessation based on concrete experiences with the health- and activity-compromising effects of smoking.

Identifying Long-Term and Short-Term Objectives

Identification of both long- and short-term objectives is important in self-care education. Long-term objectives guide large segments of learning. Short-term objectives fit under a specific long-term objective and identify the particular content or activities that must be progressively mastered. The objectives should be realistic, neither too easy, resulting in boredom, nor too hard, resulting in discouragement. An example of a goal and objectives identification form is presented in Figure 4–3. Use of the form enables the client to check off each objective as it is attained and maintain awareness of the desired behavioral and health outcomes. Both the nurse and the client should retain a copy for continuing reference and update.

Facilitating Self-Paced Learning

The pace at which a client will learn depends on personal motivation, assertiveness, perseverance, skill, and learning style. The pace of learning may also vary with age, health status, and educational level. Self-pacing is important to enable the client to be self-directed and maintain control over the learning process. The pace at which the client meets each short-term objective will vary, and expectations of both the client and the health professional should be adjusted accordingly. The important factor is not how rapidly knowledge or skill is attained but the extent of mastery.

The nurse must be realistic about teaching and learning and accept both successful and unsuccessful outcomes in clients of all ages. Sometimes the nurse and client will be elated with the results, sometimes discouraged. When efforts are less rewarding than anticipated, the pace of learning should be reviewed carefully. It is possible that expanding the time frame for learning will result in increased success for the client. This is especially true for young children and adolescents, who have less experience in the learning process than do adults.

Health Goal: Increased Physical Fitness	
Long-Term Objective: To take a brisk walk for 30 minutes five times a week	
Related Short-Term Learning Objectives	**Objectives Attained**
1. Demonstrate how to check my pulse at the neck by counting beats for 10 seconds and multiplying by six. 2. State heart rate that I should achieve during exercise. 3. Demonstrate two warm-up exercises to use before walking. 4. Demonstrate two cool-down exercises to use after brisk walking. 5. Construct a weekly schedule for brisk walking. 6. Map out three different and interesting routes to take when walking.	

FIGURE 4-3 Goal and objectives identification form

Using Positive Reinforcement to Empower Competence and Motivation for Learning

In education for self-care, the client, the nurse, and the family of the client all play important roles in reinforcement. The nurse should be attuned to small steps in client progress and use positive reinforcement such as praise and compliments frequently to enhance the client's feelings of success in developing competence in self-care. Cues should be used to facilitate successful responses and immediate feedback provided to correct errors in performance. When cues and error feedback are intermingled with positive reinforcement, they are helpful, nonthreatening, and enhance intrinsic motivation of the client. Immediate and consistent reinforcement facilitates rapid learning and assists the client in deriving satisfaction from learning. Once learning has occurred, intermittent reinforcement of the desired response strengthens the behavior, making it more resistant to extinction.

Family members need to learn to serve as sources of support for one another in developing health behaviors. For example, achievement of a specific goal may be rewarded by a family outing in the park or by the family spending time together in a favorite activity at home. It is important for the family to maintain a balance between support and pressure, which will be negatively perceived. By providing mutual support, a sense of healthy interdependence rather than crippling dependence is created within the family.

Clients should be made aware of the importance of self-reward or self-reinforcement in the health education process. It is important that they learn to reward their own efforts and achievements, because much of the time, contingent reinforcement for self-care cannot be supplied by others. A schedule of rewards can be tailored by the client to personal preferences. However, use of unhealthy snack foods for reinforcement should be discouraged. It is important that the client also learn to use internal self-reinforcement such as self-praise and self-compliment. Learning to use internal self-reward in an appropriate manner permits the client to be less dependent on the availability of tangible objects to facilitate the learning process.

Creating a Supportive Environment for Learning

The environment in which health education for self-care is provided is vitally important to the success of educational efforts. If a clinic is used for health education, the rooms in which self-care is taught should be warm, comfortable, and informal. A desk should not be placed in the room; instead, tables and chairs or sofa and chairs should be placed in a conversational setting. Walls should be pleasant in color with pictures and textured materials used to create a homelike, supportive, and nonthreatening climate. Visual aids in flip-chart form on an easel at a comfortable height for the nurse to use while seated in a chair are ideal. If very young children are present during the self-care education sessions, an area with attractive toys and books may need to be provided for their use. This will minimize distraction of the parents. If children are old enough to be included in the sessions, they should be actively involved. Often, use of bright colors and interesting figures or designs on flip charts will amuse children and maintain their interest. Children can play an important role in reinforcing learning or in reminding parents and other family members to engage in the recommended behaviors.

To the extent possible, actual materials available in the home should be used in teaching. If a client is expected to use a booklet on low-cholesterol foods at home in preparing meals, the booklet to be used should be the basis for instruction. If the client is learning relaxation techniques, audiotapes and videos for practice must be usable in the client's home. They should be demonstrated in the classroom or clinic and questions answered about their use. Well-illustrated materials should be supplied liberally to the client to take home to provide reinforcement of knowledge and skills gained during health-education sessions.

Because the minimal time needed for most health instruction is 15 to 20 minutes, the nurse must decide whether to use individual or small-group teaching methods. If health education is provided to groups, the groups should be kept small to facilitate interaction and attention to the specific needs of group members. A combination of group and individual instruction may also be helpful. This combined approach allows for efficient use of professional time yet meets the unique educative–developmental needs of clients.

Decreasing Barriers to Learning

Barriers to learning can result from various sources: personal values, beliefs, and attitudes; lack of motivation; poor self-concept; or inadequate cognitive or psychomotor skills. Whatever the source, if the client exhibits lack of progress, barriers within the individual as well as within the family, relevant social groups, and the environment should be explored. Barriers must often be identified and attenuated or eliminated before progress can continue.

Approaches to managing obstacles to healthy behavior should be an integral part of the health education plan. In this way, problems are addressed systematically, and progress can be periodically assessed. The client may be unaware of what is inhibiting progress or reluctant to share such information with the nurse. A climate of trust will facilitate communication between the client and the nurse concerning obstacles to learning and performance.

Evaluating Client Progress Toward Health Goals

Evaluation is a process by which the nurse and client in collaboration judge to what degree long- and short-term objectives and health goals have been attained. All evaluation involves direct or indirect observation of behavior. The major source of error in direct measurement is inadequate sampling of the target behaviors during brief clinic or home visits. A source of error in indirect measurement is that self-observation skills of clients may be inadequately developed, or clients may ascribe a "halo effect" to themselves, seeing performance of health behaviors as more frequent or more intensive than they actually are.

A combination of methods should be used in evaluating client progress. These may include checklists of objectives (see Figure 4–3), client progress notes, laboratory measurements, paper-and-pencil tests, verbal questioning, and direct observation. The primary purpose of evaluation is to provide an accurate picture for clients of where they stand in attaining their health goals. The desired outcome from self-care education is a sustained effect of the self-care education intervention that permanently changes lifestyle or behavior.

Other Considerations in Self-Care Empowerment

Each client's desire for efficacy or competence in self-care must be assessed by the nurse. The fact cannot be ignored that some individuals do not want to be responsible for their own self-care but instead wish to function within society in a highly dependent role. Their desire for competence may have been frustrated by health care experiences that have made them feel infantile and helpless. It is critical that the nurse assess very early in interactions with clients the extent to which they desire to become empowered for their own care once they are given the requisite knowledge and skills to do so.

Clients' conceptualization of health will also determine the content that they view as meaningful in self-care education. When health is defined as maintaining stability or avoiding overt illness, health-protecting behaviors such as immunization, self-examination for signs of cancer, and periodic multiphasic screening may be most important to the client. When health is defined as self-actualization or exuberant well-being, the emphasis of health education may be placed on relaxation techniques, enhancing self-awareness, environmental appreciation during outdoor physical activity, or developing aspects of self that represent untapped potential. Culture is also a powerful influence on self-care for health promotion shaping specific health behaviors.

The Role of the Internet in Self-Care

The growth and improvement in the technology of the Internet are expected to change the way health education and health care are provided if they are incorporated as part of a multidimensional health promotion environment.[37,38] Areas such as telemedicine and communication between clients and health care professionals are expected to rapidly increase. Such communication is expected to create partnerships between clients and health care professionals. Consumers now have access to quality information that has not traditionally been obtainable. Such information has the potential to enhance personal health and quality of life. At San Diego State University, the student health center has developed a computer-based resource with hypertext links to specific health promotion information.[39] The center encourages the dissemination of health information as broadly as possible, extending the effectiveness of the college health clinics.

A positive aspect of the Internet for self-care is that information is accessible that may be difficult to obtain elsewhere. This information can be shared at any time in almost any geographic location. This has important implications for persons living in rural or inaccessible areas, persons who are homebound, and persons who work. A negative feature is lack of quality control. Information is just beginning to be made available to enable lay individuals to evaluate the quality of the information provided. The Internet is inaccessible to many who do not have adequate financial resources or who lack computer skills or an appropriate literacy level. The "digital divide" between those who have access and those who do not has received attention in the *Healthy People 2010* objectives to emphasize the need for access to information for all segments of the population to eliminate the knowledge gap.[3]

Self-help and support groups that meet on-line are called Internet newsgroups, Usenet newsgroups, and Usenet support groups.[40] Self-help groups are usually led by a layperson, whereas support groups are usually led by a health care professional. These electronic networks enable persons with similar health interests or health problems to converse electronically, gather information, and provide mutual information and support. Nurses need to share knowledge of effective programs and Internet sites that will strengthen the client's role in their self-care.

Mass education available through advanced technology is changing the way the public relates to health care professionals.[41] As consumers become more knowledgeable, they will be empowered to take a greater role in health promotion and health care. Nurses should work to insure that the information revolution is used to empower individuals and communities and is accessible to those who do not currently benefit because of poverty or other social, environmental, and cultural conditions.

Directions for Research on Self-Care

Although self-care has been practiced for centuries, it has become the focus of research for health professionals only within the last two decades. Theoretical work by Orem has been the primary driving force in nursing for empirical work on the various dimensions of self-care and related nursing care systems. Directions for research in self-care to broaden our understanding of this widely occurring but little understood phenomenon include the following:

1. Identify developmental changes in self-care across the life span.
2. Determine how peers affect self-care practices of preadolescents and adolescents.
3. Critically evaluate the health outcomes of self-care.
4. Explore self-care practices outside the domains of traditional health care.
5. Test culturally appropriate interventions to enhance self-care among individuals and families.

Further work is needed both in developing measures of self-care and in designing intervention studies to test the usefulness of empirically based self-care strategies.

Directions for Practice in Self-Care

The nurse–client relationship in self-care is reflected in the many changes in the health care system. The nurse's role as facilitator, resource, and teacher has become more important than ever before, as clients are asked to assume more responsibility for their health. In today's cost-containment environment, development of health-protecting and health-promoting behaviors at a young age and maintenance of these behaviors throughout the life span is critical. A multidisciplinary team approach should be used to implement health promotion programs in the schools, at work sites, as well as in community locations that are easily accessible. These programs should target the individual, the family, and the social and environmental factors that may facilitate or inhibit adoption of self-care behaviors. Strategies that strengthen family communication and support need to be implemented to promote adoption of healthy behaviors in children and adolescents. The nurse should encourage school systems to include instruction for healthy nutrition, allow for regular physical education, and create after-school opportunities for sports and other activities. Partnerships with churches and community organizations are needed to guide children and adolescents as well as the elderly in healthy activities. Self-care education is complex. However, use of new technologies and active involvement of individuals and their family members in the educational process can help ensure the adoption of healthy behaviors.

SUMMARY

In empowerment for self-care, it is important to emphasize the competencies of clients for self-direction and self-responsibility in planning and managing self-care activities. In addition, environmental constraints impairing self-care must be identified and resolved to optimize client success. The client should control the content and pace of learning experiences. The nurse's primary role is that of consultant. Educative–supportive care provided by the nurse should enable clients to achieve those health goals that they have set for themselves. The nurse, in functioning as a resource person, enhances the success of clients in acquiring knowledge and skills in self-care. Further research on the dimensions of self-care within the context of health protection and health promotion will provide important information for facilitating optimum self-care across diverse populations.

REFERENCES

1. Koop JE. At time of diagnosis. *Time Life Medical Video Series.* New York: Patient Education Media, Inc.; 1996.
2. Orem, DE. *Nursing: Concepts of Practice.* 5th ed. New York: McGraw-Hill, Inc.; 1995.
3. U.S. Department of Health and Human Services. *Healthy People 2010* (Conference Edition in Two Volumes). Washington, DC: U.S. Government Printing Office; January 2000.
4. Dodd MJ. Self-care: Ready or not! *Oncology Nursing Forum.* 1997; 24(6):983–990.

5. Schneider D, Northridge ME. Editorial: Promoting the health and well-being of future generations. *Am J Public Health*. 1999;89(2):155–157.

6. Marmot M, Ryff CD, Bumpass LL, Shipley M, Marks NF. Social inequalities in health: Next questions and converging evidence. *Social Science and Medicine*. 1997;44(6):901–910.

7. Hertzman C. The case for child development as a determinant of health. *Can J Public Health*. 1998;89(suppl 1):S14–19.

8. DiSorgra L, Glanz K. The 5 a day virtual classroom: An on-line strategy to promote healthful eating. *J Am Diet Assoc*. 2000;100(3):349–356.

9. Edelrman CL, Mandle CL. *Health Promotion Throughout the Lifespan*. 4th ed. St. Louis: Mosby;1998.

10. Cowell JM, Marks BA. Health behavior in adolescents. In: *Handbook of Health Behavior Research*, III. New York: Plenum Press; 1997:73–96.

11. Perry CL, Sellers DE, Johnson C, Pedersen S, Bachman KJ, Parcel GS, Stone EJ, Luepker RV, Wu M, Nader PR, Cook K. The child and adolescent trial for cardiovascular health (CATCH): Intervention, implementation, and feasibility for elementary schools in the United States. *Health Education and Behavior*. 1997 Dec;24(6):716–735.

12. Webber LS, Osganian SK, Feldman HA, Wu M, McKenzie TL, Nichaman M, Lytle LA, Edmundson E, Cutler J, Nader PR, Luepker RV. Cardiovascular risk factors among children after a 2 1/2 year intervention—The CATCH Study. *Prev Med*. 1996, Jul–Aug;25(4):432–441.

13. Nader PR, Stone EJ, Lytle LA, Perry CL, Osganian SK, Kelder S, Webber LS, Elder JP, Montgomery D, Feldman HA, Wu M, Johnson C, Parcel GS, Luepker RV. Three-year maintenance of improved diet and physical activity: The CATCH cohort. Child and adolescent trial for cardiovascular health. *Arch Pediatr Adolesc Med*. 1999, Jul;153(7):695–704.

14. Luepker RV. How physically active are American children and what can we do about it? *Int J Obes Related Metab Disord*. 1999 Mar;23(suppl 2):S12–S7.

15. Harrell JS, Gansky SA, McMurray RG, Bangdiwala SI, Frauman AC, Bradley CB. School-based interventions improve heart health in children with multiple cardiovascular disease risk factors. *Pediatrics*. 1998 Aug;102(2 Pt 1):371–380.

16. McClowry SG, School based intervention for inner city children. ROINRO4781, Abstract, CRISP, National Institutes of Health, Funding Period 1998–2003.

17. Felton GM, Parsons MA, Pate RR, Ward D, Saunders R, Valois R, Dowda M, Trost S. Predictors of alcohol use among rural adolescents. *J Rural Health*. 1996, fall;12(5):378–385.

18. Felton G, Parsons MA, Ward DS, Pate RR, Saunders RP, Dowda M, Trost S. Tracking of avoidance of alcohol use and smoking behavior in a fifth grade cohort over three years. *Public Health Nurs*. 1999, Feb;16(1):32–40.

19. Felton GM, Pate RR, Parsons MA, Ward DS, Saunders RP, Trost S, Dowda M. Health risk behaviors of rural sixth graders. *Res Nurs Health*. 1998, Dec;21(6):475–485.

20. Hendricks CS. The influence of race and gender on health promoting behavior determinants of southern "at-risk" adolescents. *The Association of Black Nursing Faculty Journal* 1998 Jan–Feb;9(1):4–10.

21. Loveland-Cherry CJ, Leech S, Laetz VB, Dielman TE. Correlates of alcohol use and misuse in fourth-grade children: Psychosocial, peer, parental, and family factors. *Health Educ Q*. 1996 Nov;23(4):497–511.

22. Loveland-Cherry CJ, Ross LT, Kaufman SR. Effects of a home-based family intervention on adolescent alcohol use and misuse. *J Stud Alcohol Suppl*. 1999 Mar;13:94–102.

23. Mott JA, Crowe PA, Richardson J, Flay B. After-school supervision and adolescent cigarette smoking: Contributions of the setting and intensity of after-school self-care. *Journal of Behavioral Medicine.* 1999;22(1):35–59.

24. Chapman JD, Aspin DN. *The School, the Community, and Lifelong Learning.* Washington, DC: Cassell; 1997.

25. Anderson D, Brown S, Race P. *Tips for Further and Continuing Education Lecturers.* London: Kogan Page; 1998.

26. Slaninka SC, Galbraith AM. Healthy endings. A collaborative health promotion project for the elderly. *J Gerontol Nurs.* 1998 Sep;24(9):35–42.

27. Rakowski W. Health behavior in the elderly. In: *Handbook of Health Behavior Research,* III. New York: Plenum Press; 1997: 97–114.

28. Kendig H, Browning CJ, Young AE. Impacts of illness and disability on the well-being of older people. *Disabil Rehabil.* 2000 Jan;22(1–2):15–22.

29. Benjamini Y, Idler EL, Levanthal H, Levanthal EA. Positive affect and function as influences on self-assessments of health: Expanding our view beyond illness and disability. *J Gerontol B Psychol Soc Sci.* 2000;55(2);107–116.

30. Lo R, Brown R. Stress and adaptation: Preparation for successful retirement. *Aust N Z J Mental Health.* 1999;8(1):30–38.

31. Giociella EC. Healthy aging through knowledge and self care. *Aging Prev.* 1983;3(1):39–51.

32. U.S. Department of Health and Human Services. *Progress Review Older Adults.* Washington, DC: U.S. Government Printing Office; 1996.

33. Kennie DC, Dinan S, Young A. Health promotion and physical activity. In: Tallis R, Fillit H, Brocklehurst JC, eds. *Brocklehurst's Textbook of Geriatric Medicine and Gerontology.* 5th ed. New York: Churchill Livingston; 1998:1461–1473.

34. Yee DL, Capitman JA. Health care access, health promotion, and older woman of color. *J Health Care Poor Underserved.* 1996;7(3):252–272.

35. Bertera EM. Assessing perceived health promotion needs and interests of low-income older women. *J Women's Health Gend Based Med.* 1999;8(10):1323.

36. Cohen M. Towards a framework for women's health. *Patient Education and Counseling.* 1998;33:187–196.

37. Lewis D. The Internet as a resource for healthcare information. *Diabetes Educ.* 1998;24(5):627–630.

38. Briggs JS, Early GH. Internet developments and their significance for healthcare. *Med Inform Internet Med.* 1999;24(3):149–164.

39. Fulop MP, Varzandeh NN. The role of computer-based resources in health promotion and disease prevention: Implications for college health. *J Am Coll Health.* 1996;45(1):11–17.

40. LaPerrière B, Edwards P, Romeder J, Maxwell-Young, L. Using the internet to support self-care. *The Canadian Nurse.* 1998 May;47–48.

41. Neuberger J. The educated patient: New challenges for the medical profession. *J Intern Med.* 2000;247(1):6–10.

5

Health Promotion in Vulnerable Populations

- Health Status of Vulnerable Populations
- Eliminating Health Disparities
- Planning Culturally Competent Health Promotion Interventions
- Essential Characteristics to Consider
- Directions for Research in Vulnerable Populations
- Directions for Practice in Vulnerable Populations

As the twenty-first century unfolds, nurses and all health care professionals will be increasingly expected to provide health care to individuals who are poor, socially marginal, or culturally different from the traditional mainstream of society. The values, attitudes, culture, and life circumstances of these individuals and the communities in which they reside must be taken into consideration when planning health protection and health promotion activities. Taking into account the factors that reflect the diversity of these populations is a key to successful behavior change.

In spite of the improvements in health in the United States during the last century, disparities continue to exist in some segments of the populations. A report by the Department of Health and Human Services has documented these disparities for certain racial and ethnic groups.[1] Major reasons for the disparities include poverty, lack of access to care, environmental hazards, and lack of community-tailored health promotion programs. Eliminating health disparities will require greater health promotion and prevention efforts than ever before. For this reason, elimination of health disparities is one of the two major themes of the *Healthy People 2010* objectives.[2] Although many of the causes of these disparities need the input of society and government, development of health promotion programs tailored for diverse communities is a realistic goal for nursing.

Health Status of Vulnerable Populations

Vulnerable populations are diverse groups of individuals who are at greatest risk of poor physical, psychological, or social health outcomes.[3] Vulnerable populations are more likely to develop health problems, usually experience worse health outcomes, and have fewer resources to improve their conditions. Various terms have been used to describe vulnerable populations including *underserved populations, special populations, medically disadvantaged, poverty-strickened populations,* and *American underclasses.*[4] Vulnerable groups include persons who experience discrimination, stigma, intolerance, and subordination and those who are politically marginized, disenfranchised, and often denied their human rights.[5] Vulnerable populations may include people of color, the poor, non-English-speaking persons, recent immigrants and refugees, homeless persons, mentally ill and disabled persons, gay men and lesbians, and substance abusers.

Societal and environmental factors play major roles in characterizing vulnerable populations.[1,6] Specifically, low socioeconomic status has been documented to be the most consistent predictor of disease and premature deaths in this country. Class-related inequities in mortality rates for three-fourths of all deaths are observed across the life span in almost every country in the world.[7] Those at greatest risk for increased morbidity and mortality are ethnic and racial minorities, two highly vulnerable groups.[8] Although there is great diversity among minority populations, overall, minorities have substantially lower incomes than whites. Income is a powerful variable that explains health status. Higher incomes facilitate access to care, better housing in safer neighborhoods, and increased opportunities for healthy food purchases as well as health promotion programs. The poverty rate continues to be almost three times greater for blacks and Hispanics than for whites.[9] Educational attainment is also lower in minority groups. High-risk behaviors have been inversely correlated with lower educational levels.[1] Higher educational levels enable persons to access and understand health-related information.

Socioeconomic status (SES) accounts for much of the observed disparities in health, as a socioeconomic gradient exists for almost every health indicator for every racial and ethnic group.[1] The socioeconomic differences are apparent in risk factors such as smoking, obesity, elevated blood pressure, and sedentary lifestyle as well as insurance coverage, physician visits, and avoidable hospitalizations. However, racial differences persist at equivalent levels of SES.[10] It has been suggested that socioeconomic status in minority populations may involve a time component.[11,12,13] Nichols suggests that populations who have been poor over several generations, suffering ongoing discrimination and frustration without substantial upward movement, may feel powerless and perceive their conditions differently from recent immigrants who are poor but hopeful about their future. Evidence for this hypothesis comes from studies related to birth outcomes and infant mortality. Black–white differences in low infant birth weight and infant mortality have existed for decades and in blacks is twice that of whites.[2] The differences persist even when the effects of social class, prenatal care, and living conditions are controlled, or when only middle-class populations with access to care are studied. When black–white differences in infant mortality were examined in 38 standard metropolitan statistical areas, they were found to differ by a factor of almost seven. The most significant predictor was an index of housing segregation, independent of black–white differences in median family income or the prevalence of poverty.[14] Thus, racism can affect health status directly as well as indirectly in the stress of experiences of discrimination and the societal stigma of inferiority.[10,15]

The health status of Hispanics has declined among immigrants as their stay in the United States increases and with succeeding generations.[16] Rates of infant mortality, adolescent pregnancy, cigarette, alcohol, and illicit drug use all increase with acculturation. For example, it has also been reported that Hispanic women in southern California have poorer birth outcomes as they become more acculturated.[17] Acculturation may increase risk factors for birth outcomes. Acculturation involves abandonment of one's cultural beliefs and assimilation of the values of the dominant society, which also involve assimilating the negative perceptions of what it means to be a person of color in the United States.

Access to care can be measured by the proportion of a population that has health insurance. Racial and ethnic minorities are much more likely to be underinsured or lack health insurance.[4] When they do have insurance, it is likely to be public insurance, primarily Medicaid. Health insurance contributes to the amount and type of health services obtained. Lack of health insurance has important implications for health protection and promotion efforts, such as screening and access to programs. Insurance status has been correlated with reported health status. Those who rated their health as fair or poor were more likely to be uninsured than those who rated their health as good or excellent.[4] Racial and ethnic minorities also experience greater barriers in accessing their usual source of care, have more difficulty getting an appointment, and wait longer during appointments. These factors are compounded by the fact that most minority communities mistrust the government and government-controlled programs. Thus financial and nonfinancial barriers to access to care exist for vulnerable populations. These barriers need to be eliminated to ensure access to quality health care.

Eliminating Health Disparities

Health disparities refer to the incidence, prevalence, mortality, and burden of diseases and other adverse health conditions that exist among certain groups or populations in the United States.[8] A vulnerable population model that focuses on the major personal and environmental resources needed to achieve and maintain health, thereby eliminating health disparities, is shown in Figure 5–1.

This model is adapted from Flaskerud and Winslow and Healthy People 2010.[2,5] The model incorporates social capital, socioeconomic status, cultural context, access to and quality of care, risk factors for disease, and health outcomes. Social capital, socioeconomic status, cultural context, and access to–quality of care are factors that affect individuals, either positively or negatively, and are indicators of the availability of resources. *Social capital* refers to features of social relationships, including levels of interpersonal trust and norms of reciprocity and mutual assistance.[18] Social capital reflects the quantity and quality of interactions with family, friends, coworkers, and others in the community. In vulnerable populations, many of these ties may be absent. *Socioeconomic status,* including income, employment, and education, are considered human factors that influence vulnerability. A higher education level correlates with greater decision making, a better economic situation, and a higher awareness about the benefits and risks to health. However, education cannot achieve its potential if young people do not attend school because of poverty and other social conditions. In addition children cannot learn effectively if they are hungry or suffer from undue stress. The *cultural context* refers to the cultural beliefs, values, and customs, including cultural explanations of illness, language, religious or spiritual beliefs, and personal lifestyle and experiences that play a role in health outcomes. *Access to care* depends on health insurance, transportation, and under-

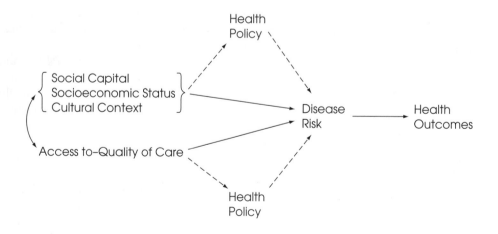

FIGURE 5-1 Vulnerable Populations Model

Adapted from Flaskerud J. Winslow B. Conceptualizing vulnerable populations health-related research. *Nursing Research.* 1998;47(2):69–78.

standing of the health care system. *Quality of care* is also related to health outcomes. For example, those who receive a lower quality of care, including poor access, often have poorer health outcomes. *Risk for disease* refers to factors that increase one's susceptibility for disease. Risk factors may be personal or present in the physical environment. Vulnerable groups have higher risk behaviors related to dietary intake, weight, activity level, cigarette smoking, and alcohol and illicit drug intake.[17] The relationship between availability of resources (social capital, socioeconomic status, cultural context) and disease risk proposes that fewer resources increase one's risks. This relationship has consistently been documented in adolescents and adults.[1] Second, disease risks are related to *health outcomes.* Birth and death rates, life expectancy, morbidity from specific diseases, accessibility of health care, and many other factors can measure health outcomes. The relationship between risks for disease and morbidity and mortality has been observed in all populations. Risk factors are higher in those who live in poverty and lack resources. As risk factors increase, morbidity also increases. The relationship between resources, risk factors, and mortality has also been documented. Health policy is proposed to mediate the relationships between social capital, socioeconomic status, cultural context, and disease risks and between access to–quality of care and disease risks. *Health policy* can promote individual and community health through health promotion campaigns, mandates, and accessible services. The role of policy in influencing both risks and health outcomes points to the need for a community and societal perspective. Aday[3] also proposes that a community perspective offers the most promise to reshape policy to eliminate the health disparities in vulnerable populations.

The Office of Minority Health, and the Office of Research on Minority Health (ORMH), U.S. Department of Health and Human Services (USDHHS), were established to focus on the president's national initiative to close the gap in health disparities.[19] The ORMH supports research to uncover knowledge to eliminate the disproportionate burden of ill health among minority Americans. African Americans, Asian and Pacific Islanders, Hispanic and Latino, and Native American and American Indians are recognized as groups that suffer from health disparities. No simple solutions are easily available to eliminate health disparities in this country or the world, for that matter. However, nurses, as frontline providers with a person–environment perspective, can implement culturally competent individual-family-and community-based programs to begin to tackle this major problem.

Planning Culturally Competent Health Promotion Interventions

Expertise in cultural competence is a needed skill, considering the diversity of vulnerable populations and the number of interacting factors operating to create health disparities. Cultural competence is defined as appropriate and effective communication that requires one to be willing to listen and learn from members of diverse populations, and the provision of information and services in appropriate languages, at appropriate comprehension and literacy levels, and in the context of the individual's health beliefs and practices.[20] In a culturally competent health promotion program, the beliefs, interpersonal style, attitudes, and behaviors of individuals and families are respected and incorporated into program planning, implementation, and evaluation activities. Nurses and other health care professionals need to be aware of their own cultural values and beliefs and recognize how these influence their attitudes and behaviors toward another group.

Bushy has described cultural–linguistic competence as a continuum of interpersonal skills ranging from *ethnocentrism* on one end of the continuum to *enculturation* at the other end of the spectrum.[21] *Ethnocentrism,* one anchoring point on the continuum, refers to prejudicial beliefs that one's own group decides the standards by which to judge all cultural groups. Thus, the beliefs of other cultural groups are devalued or treated with suspicion or hostility. *Cultural awareness,* the next stage on the continuum, refers to an appreciation of and sensitivity to another person's values, beliefs, and practices. Next, *cultural knowledge* refers to insights learned about the other culture. The continuum progresses to cultural change and then cultural competence, the level at which the health care provider is aware of, sensitive to, and knowledgeable about the other culture, and has the skills to employ appropriate health promotion activities. *Enculturation,* the opposite anchoring point on the continuum, refers to fully internalizing the values of the other culture. Enculturation is evident when the health care provider develops culturally sensitive health promotion programs in collaboration with individuals in the cultural group and incorporates members of the culture to deliver the intervention.

Developing cultural competence is not a linear process. Progress depends on life experiences, exposures to other cultures, and receptivity to learning about new cultures. Acquisition of cultural competence skills is an ongoing process to insure the delivery of health promotion interventions that are appropriate, acceptable, and meaningful for persons of diverse backgrounds. Diversity is embedded in cultural competence, but it is just one component. Accepting and understanding differences in customs and patterns of thinking are ways in which diversity is valued.

Essential Characteristics to Consider

Characteristics of vulnerable populations that must be taken into account to provide effective health promotion activities include communication patterns, family relationships, time orientation, and access to and acceptance of health promotion programs.[21,22] Culturally relevant interventions related to these characteristics are described in Table 5–1. Communications style is probably the most salient difference among diverse groups, so knowledge of cultural differences in communication is a key feature in the delivery of wellness programs. Verbal and nonverbal communication, body language, and word meanings vary across cultures. In low-literacy groups, abstract concepts may not be understood, and traditional written communication may not be appropriate. Health promotion programs are more successful when they are delivered in the same language of the participants. Therefore, persons who represent the target culture and speak the same language should be involved in development and implementation of interventions. In addition, culturally specific newspapers, radio stations, and televisions stations can be targeted to deliver health messages in the meaningful language.

TABLE 5-1 Culturally Relevant Intervention Strategies for Vulnerable Populations

Characteristic	Strategy
Communication patterns	- Assess primary language spoken, knowledge of English, literacy level - Use same language as target culture - Understand cultural meanings of health terms - Explore cultural explanations of health - Use culturally specific media to deliver messages - Involve community in developmental activities
Family relationships	- Understand role of family, extended, and nontraditional family in health - Involve family in health promotion activities - Assess religion and its role in family - Acknowledge role of church and incorporate church network
Time orientation	- Explore time orientation of target culture - Tailor message to dominant time orientation (i.e., present, past, future) - Assess meaning of "clock" time
Access to and acceptance of health promotion programs	- Assess barriers to accessibility of health promotion programs - Assess environmental resources of community - Use existing community sites to deliver programs, such as churches, schools - Incorporate health promotion activities into ongoing community activities - Explore cultural values about participating in health promotion activities such as exercise

Adapted from Keller C, Stevens K. Cultural considerations in promoting wellness. *Journal of Cardiovascular Nursing.* 1997;11(3):15–25.

Many people will hide their illiteracy due to the stigma attached, so it should never be assumed that someone can read or follow written or complex verbal instructions. Functional literacy is the ability to read at a fifth-grade level. In the United States, almost half of the population are either functionally illiterate or possess marginal literacy skills.[23] This has many implications for choice of communication channels to deliver wellness interventions.

Family relationships and the concept of family differ in many cultures. In some cultural groups, for example, it is common for the family to include more than the immediate family. The needs of the individual may be considered subordinate to the needs of the family in some cultures, such as Asians and Hispanics. In these groups, support from family members is more important than external support, which is an important factor to consider in promoting behavior change. Family members need to be intimately involved to support the individual in lifestyle change or wellness interventions. Family-oriented approaches using the family and extended family networks, rather than individual ones, are more successful in behavior change in African American and Hispanic cultures.[24] In cultures wherein the woman's role is subordinate, it may be important to emphasize the value of behavior change of the woman for the entire family.[22] Family networks may also include church relationships in certain cultures, because of the social support and communication networks offered. In these cultures, the church may be an effective place to implement health promotion programs. In addition, knowledge of and respect for religious customs is important to promote desired outcomes. Educational strategies should capitalize on the powerful effects of family and church networks to promote behavior change.

Time orientation refers to how the perception of time varies among cultures. Kluckhohn and Strodtbeck[25] identified three major time orientations that exist in every society: past, present, and future. A past orientation is based on the importance of tradition and is noted in traditional Asian groups and American Indians. For example, in these cultures, deceased relatives are considered part of the extended family, so the perspective of a deceased family member may be incorporated into the family's health practices. In the present orientation, the focus is on the here and now. A present orientation is common in persons living in poverty, as the focus is on surviving today, and the future may have no meaning. Persons with a present orientation have more difficulty changing behaviors, because the current activity is the priority. The future orientation emphasizes planning for time extending from the present. For example, middle-class Americans are considered to be more future oriented, because they work and plan for retirement, often delaying present gratification. Health promotion programs may appeal to future-oriented persons who want to be healthy in their retirement. On the other hand, these people may be so busy working for the future, health and wellness may not be a priority. Knowledge of a client's dominant time orientation as well as adherence to "clock" time will eliminate misunderstanding of response to appointments. For example, an individual who does not place a priority on "clock time" may have difficulty being punctual for appointments. Nurses need to understand how the individual prioritizes time to plan for successful attendance at programs and screening services as well as to assist individuals to learn to keep appointments.

Access to health promotion programs is a cultural competence issue because of existing cultural barriers in accessing systems of care.[20] Vulnerable populations have more problems accessing care and accepting therapeutic interventions, because of costs, distance, transportation, language, or perceived lack of acceptance by health care providers.[22] Missed appointments or program sessions may not mean the individual is not interested in health promotion. Transportation or child care may not be available, or bilingual support may not be adequate. Acceptance of interventions depends on multiple factors, including interactions with health care providers and incorporation of cultural values and lifestyle of the community. Culturally sensitive approaches based on individual and family values and lifestyles enhance access and acceptance of health interventions. Conducting focus groups with individuals in the target community to learn culturally relevant information on which to base interventions has become a successful strategy.[26] Community priorities, problems, and resources need to be identified and resources allocated to promote successful health promotion efforts. Churches or other sites within the community should be used whenever possible to facilitate easy access as well as a comfortable environment. Mobile clinics that go door to door to screen and provide information are another option.

The Office of Minority Health[27] has developed standards for culturally and linguistically appropriate health care services. Many of these standards are also relevant for the delivery of health promotion programs and are summarized in Table 5–2. Health care providers have accepted the need for culturally competent programs. Now standards need to be developed to monitor and evaluate the outcomes of culturally competent programs. Programs that improve the quality of life of individuals in the community will lead to the development of competent communities, in which members can identify and begin to solve their own issues.[20]

Giger and Davidhizar[28] propose that health promotion needs vary across groups based on six cultural phenomena. These phenomena, which may be used to assess clients prior to any health promotion activities, include *communication, space, social organization, time, environmental control, and biological variations*.[29] Communication and time are described similarly to the communication and time characteristics previously discussed. Space refers to personal space or the area surrounding a person's body that determines personal boundaries. Individuals in various cultures differ in their need for personal space. For example, in some cultures touching, such as a pat on the back or hug, is unacceptable. Social organization refers to patterns of social behavior that provide explanations for behavior related to life events such as a birth, an illness, and death. Environmental control refers to the ability to direct activities that influence the natural environment. For example, one may need to assess the sanitation conditions in the home or neighborhood and availability of resources to improve them. Last, biological variations refer to physiologic differences that may exist within a racial group. For example, American Indians are at high risk for type II diabetes mellitus. Assessment of the six cultural phenomena enables nurses and other health care providers to respond to the needs of vulnerable populations with appropriate interventions. Research is needed on the significance of these phenomena in promoting behavior change in diverse populations.

TABLE 5-2 Recommended Standards for Culturally Appropriate Health Promotion Programs

1. Acquire the attitudes, behaviors, knowledge, and skills needed to work respectfully and effectively with individuals in a culturally diverse environment.
2. Use formal mechanisms to involve communities in the design and implementation of health promotion programs.
3. Develop strategies to recruit and retain culturally competent staff who are qualified to address the health promotion needs of the diverse communities.
4. Provide ongoing education and training in culturally and linguistically competent program delivery.
5. Provide all participants with limited English proficiency programs conducted in their primary language.
6. Translate and make available signage and commonly-used written educational material.
7. Ensure that the participants' birthplace, religion, cultural dietary patterns, and self-identified race–ethnicity are documented.
8. Undertake assessments of cultural competence, integrating measures of satisfaction, quality, and outcomes of health promotions programs.

Adapted from Chin D. Culturally competent health care. *Public Health Reports.* 2000;115: 25–33.

Directions for Research in Vulnerable Populations

Although evidence indicates that health disparities exist for vulnerable populations, little research has been conducted to identify the most effective methods to eliminate these disparities successfully. In addition, the relative absence of basic information about health behaviors in diverse populations limits the development of culturally appropriate health promotion and disease prevention interventions. The effects of changing social capital, socioeconomic status, and access to and quality of care on health outcomes need rigorous investigation. Interventions that target subpopulations such as adolescents and women also need to be designed and tested, because these subgroups have received even less attention.

All types of interdisciplinary research are needed. Qualitative research must be conducted to better understand the influence of cultural beliefs and practices on health behaviors. In addition to studies that focus on individuals and families, community intervention models are needed to effectively evaluate the contribution of communities in improving and promoting health. Research needs to translate and adapt measurements that have been standardized in the dominant white population for the target culture to insure sensitive measures of the variables under study. Health service research is another area of opportunity because the effects of organizational change in providing culturally competent health promotion and prevention programs also need to be evaluated. The research questions are endless, and the issues are complex. Vulnerable groups have traditionally been underrepresented in research for many reasons, including ineffective recruitment and retention strategies, lack of attention to culturally sensitive instruments and literacy levels, and lack of trust. However, the significance of the questions that need to be asked and the complex issues that must be addressed offer many opportunities for research collaboration among nurse scientists, other health care researchers, and vulnerable populations.

Directions for Practice in Vulnerable Populations

Nurses have multiple opportunities and challenges with vulnerable populations because of the diversity, poverty, and increased risks factors for disease. Prior to working with diverse populations, nurses must become culturally competent by first examining their own attitudes and values and how these may either facilitate or impede culturally appropriate health promotion efforts. Next they should make a commitment to become culturally competent as they work with a minority group or subgroup. This may mean becoming immersed in the culture prior to any health promotion efforts. Prior to planning health promotion activities, characteristics mentioned in this chapter need to be assessed in order to develop successful strategies for lifestyle change. Lifestyle change in vulnerable populations is complex due to potential language difficulties, educational level, poverty, potentially unsafe housing or neighborhoods, and many other social, environmental, and cultural factors. This means that the cultural relevance of health behavior models that may guide one's practice needs to be examined. New dimensions, such as health care system factors and ecological factors, need to be added to insure that the models are comprehensive to guide practice interventions in vulnerable populations. In addition, understanding of potential intervening barriers is needed to plan creative primary, secondary, and tertiary interventions that encourage and facilitate healthy lifestyles.

SUMMARY

In the last century, tremendous progress was made in the health of the American people, due to such improvements as safe drinking water, advances in sanitation, more nutritious food, and advances in medical care. However, the health status of the poor and minority populations has lagged behind the health of white Americans. Disparities are noted in infant mortality, cardio-vascular disease, cerebrovascular disease, diabetes, kidney disease, AIDS, prostate cancer, and other health problems. Vulnerable populations have diverse threats to health that require atten-tion from clinicians, researchers, and policy makers. Although the contributing factors are mul-tiple and complex, many health behaviors are due to personal habits as well as social and environmental factors and are amenable to nursing interventions. Nurses, as holistic care providers, are well positioned to take a critical leadership role in designing and implementing culturally competent health promotion interventions for behavior change.

SELECTED WEB SITES RELEVANT TO VULNERABLE POPULATIONS AND MINORITY HEALTH

Race and Health Home Page of U.S. Government, *http://www.raceandhealth.hhs.gov*
Office of Minority Health, *http://www.omhrc.gov*
Office of Research on Minority Health, *http://www.nih.gov/ormh*
Resources for Cross Cultural Health Care, *http://diversityrx.org*
Healthy People 2010, http://www.health.gov/healthypeople

REFERENCES

1. U.S. Department of Health and Human Services. *Health, United States, 1998 with Socioeconomic Status and Health Chartbook.* DHHS publication number (PHS)98-1232; 1998.
2. U.S. Department of Health and Human Services. *Healthy People 2010* (Conference Edition in Two Volumes). Washington DC: U.S. Government Printing Service; January 2000.
3. Aday LA. Vulnerable populations: A community-oriented perspective. In: Sebastian JG, Bushy A. *Special Populations in the Community: Advances in Reducing Health Disparities.* MD: Aspen Publishers, Inc.; 1999;313–330.
4. Shi L. Vulnerable populations and health insurance. *Medical Care Research and Review.* 2000;57(1):110–134.
5. Flaskerud JH, Winslow BJ. Conceptualizing vulnerable populations in health-related research. *Nurs Res.* 1998;47(2):69–78.

6. Sebastian JG. Definition and theory underlying vulnerability. In: Sebastian JG, Bushy A. *Special Populations in the Community: Advances in Reducing Health Disparities.* MD: Aspen Publishers, Inc., 1999;3–9.

7. Najman JM, Smith GD. The embodiment of class-related and health inequalities: Australian policies. *Aust N Z J Public Health.* 1997;21(4 Spec No).

8. Office of Research on Minority Health. *Health Disparities: Challenge and Opportunity.* NIH Publication No. 99-4544;July 1999.

9. Delaker J. U.S. Census Bureau, Current Population Reports, Series. *Poverty in the United States: 1998.* Washington DC: U.S. Government Printing Office; 1999;60–207.

10. William DR. Race, socioeconomic status, and health. The added effects of racism and discrimination. *Ann N Y Acad Sci.* 1999;896:173–188.

11. Nichens HW. Health promotion and disease prevention among minorities. *Health Affairs.* 1990 summer;133–143.

12. Nichens HW. The role of race–ethnicity and social class in minority health status. *Health Services Res.* 1995;30(1 Pt 2):151–162.

13. Nickens HW. The role of race–ethnicity and social class in minority health status. In: Harrington C, Estes C, eds. *Health Policy and Nursing.* 2nd ed. Boston: Jones and Bartlett; 1997:31–40.

14. Poldenak AP. Black–white differences in mortality in 38 standard metropolitan areas. *Am J Public Health.* 1991;81:1480–1482.

15. Ren XS, Amick BC, Williams DR. Racial/ethnic disparities in health: The interplay between discrimination and socioeconomic status. *Ethn Dis.* 1999;9(2):151–165.

16. Amaro H, Jenkins W, Kunitz S, Levy J, Mixon M, Yu E. Panel I: Epidemiology of minority health. *Health Psychol.* 1995;14(7):592–600.

17. Flack GM, Amaro H, Jenkins W, Kunitz S, Levy J, Mixon M, Yu E. Epidemiology of minority health. *Health Psychol.* 1995;14(7):592–600.

18. Kawachi I. Social capital and community effects on population and individual health. *Ann N Y Acad Sci.* 1999;896:120–130.

19. Fiscella K, Franks P, Gold MR, Clancy CM. Inequality in quality: Addressing socioeconomic, racial, and ethnic disparities in health care. *JAMA.* 2000;283(19):2579–2584.

20. Chin JL. Culturally competent health care. *Public Health Reports.* 2000;115:25–33.

21. Bushy A. Resiliency and social support. In: Sebastian JG, Bushy A. *Special Populations in the Community: Advances in Reducing Health Disparities.* MD: Aspen Publishers, Inc.; 1999:189–195.

22. Keller CS, Stevens KR. Cultural considerations in promoting wellness. *J Cardiovascular Nurs.* 1997;11(3):15–25.

23. National Literacy and Health Program. *Directory of Plain Language Health Information.* Ottawa, Canada: Canadian Public Health Association; 1999.

24. Coe K, Keller C. Health protective behaviors of young African-American women: Should we be using a kinship model to teach health behaviors? *J Human Ecology.* 1996;5:61–70.

25. Kluckhohn FR, Strodtbeck FL. *Variation in Value Orientations.* Westport, CT: Glenwood Press; 1961.

26. Murdaugh CL, Russel RB, Sowell R. Using focus groups to develop a culturally sensitive videotape interaction for HIV positive women. *Journal of Advanced Nursing.* 2000;32,1507–1513.

27. Office of Minority Health Resources Center. Assessing culture competence in health case: Recommendations for national standards and an outcome-focused research agenda [cited Jan 7, 2000]. Available from: *www.omhc.gov/clas/index.htm.*

28. Giger J, Davidhizar R. Transcultural nursing: assessment and intervention. St. Louis: Mosby. 1995.

29. Giger J, Davidhizar R, Poole VL. Health promotion among ethnic minorities: The importance of cultural phenomena. *Rehab Nurs.* 1997;22(6):303–307.

Part III

Planning for Prevention and Health Promotion

6

Assessing Health, Health Beliefs, and Health Behaviors

- Nursing Frameworks for Health Assessments
- Assessment of the Individual Client
  - A. Physical Fitness Evaluation
  - B. Nutritional Assessment
  - C. Health-Risk Appraisal
  - D. Life-Stress Review
  - E. Spiritual Health Assessment
  - F. Social Support Systems Review
  - G. Health-Beliefs Review
  - H. Lifestyle Assessment
- Assessment of the Family
- Assessment of the Community
- Directions for Research in Health Assessment
- Directions for Practice in Health Assessment
- Summary

A thorough assessment of health, health beliefs, and health behaviors is the foundation for tailoring a health protection–promotion plan to a given client. Assessment provides the database for making clinical judgments concerning the client's health strengths, health problems, nursing diagnoses, and desired health or behavioral outcomes, as well as the interventions likely to be effective. This information determines the nature of the client–health professional encounter. The portfolio of assessment tools used depends on characteristics of the client, including developmental stage and cultural orientation. A number of tools presented in this chapter can be used with older children and adolescents as well as with adults of all ages. Some of the tools cited have been developed specifically for youth. The nurse should assess the cultural appropriateness of the various tools for target populations before using them. Additional assessment instruments for areas such as functional status, coping, information seeking, and self-care activities as well as related research are described by Frank-Stromborg[1] and Wilkin, Hallam, and Doggett.[2] Nursing clinics, community health centers, and primary care centers should maintain an up-to-date resource file of assessment tools so that the assessment portfolio for any given client can be customized. In this chapter, the primary focus is on assessment of the individual. However, approaches for assessing families and communities are also discussed.

Nursing Frameworks for Health Assessment

Health assessment as performed by the nurse is a collaborative process with the client, which promotes mutual input into decision making and planning to improve the client's health and well-being. The desired outcomes of health assessment are to (1) identify health assets, (2) identify health-related lifestyle strengths, (3) determine key health-related beliefs, (4) identify health beliefs and health behaviors that put the client at risk, and (5) determine how the client wants to change to improve the quality of life. The initial assessment provides a valuable baseline against which subsequent assessments can be compared.

Several frameworks for nursing assessment and diagnosis are available. At this point, it is important to differentiate between nursing assessment and nursing diagnosis as they are used in this book. *Nursing assessment* is a systematic collection of data about client health status, beliefs, and behaviors relevant to developing a health protection–promotion plan. *Nursing diagnosis* is a clear specification of areas that may be enhanced to maximize health status.

A number of "accepted" nursing diagnostic classification systems (taxonomies) have been developed by nursing groups to guide clinical decisions in nursing. These taxonomies focus primarily on the individual and aspects of illness. Positive health states or strengths of the individual, family, or community are not adequately addressed in these taxonomies, and they are being expanded to include diagnoses appropriate to aspects of wellness and family and community-focused needs. Nursing must continue to expand its taxonomies to further undergird wellness activities as the knowledge about health promotion and health protection continues to expand.

The North American Nursing Diagnosis Association (NANDA)[3] provides a nursing diagnosis taxonomy structured around the nine human response patterns of exchanging, communicating, relating, valuing, choosing, moving, perceiving, knowing, and feeling. The

NANDA defining characteristics of each diagnosis, as well as related factors and risk factors, provide guidance as to what the critical assessment areas are in relation to that diagnosis. Following health assessment, the NANDA classification provides one means for clearly labeling some of the issues and problems identified. A limited number of diagnoses that address family and wellness have been added to the North American Nursing Diagnosis Association's (NANDA) classification of over 160 nursing diagnoses.

Gordon[4] grouped the NANDA diagnoses under 11 functional health patterns to assist in classifying nursing diagnoses. Gordon's functional health patterns for classifying nursing diagnoses are health perception–health management, nutritional–metabolic, elimination, activity–exercise, sleep–rest, cognitive–perceptual, self-perception–self-concept, role–relationship, sexuality–reproductive, coping–stress tolerance, and value–belief. A major strength of Gordon's work is the provision of guidelines for the conduct of a nursing history and examination to assess clients' functional health patterns. As assessment proceeds, diagnostic hypotheses are generated to direct targeted or more detailed data collection. The reader should refer to the *Manual of Nursing Diagnoses: 1998–1999* for the recommended formats for assessment of functional health patterns in adults, infants, and young children, families, and communities.[4]

An attempt to develop diagnoses related to community nursing resulted in the Omaha Visiting Nurse Association System.[5] Omaha incorporates the needs of individuals and families in categories of environment, psychosocial, physiologic, and health behavior needs. The Omaha system categories are referenced by keywords such as *individual, family,* and *health promotion.* Although the Omaha system addresses health promotion in the individual and family, it does not apply to the health behavior needs of groups,[6 (pp. 124–130)] so the Omaha system is of limited use in assessing communities.[7]

Nursing Diagnosis for Wellness: Supporting Strengths[8] is the published guide most focused on assessment of client strengths related to health promotion. This guide incorporates some of the NANDA diagnostic categories but expands to include wellness diagnoses organized according to the functional health patterns proposed by Gordon. Examples of wellness nursing diagnoses (client strengths) include nutrition, adequate to meet or maintain body requirements (nutrition–metabolic); exercise level, appropriate to maintain wellness state (activity–exercise); and spiritual strength (value–belief). Case studies and sample care plans illustrate how diagnostic statements can provide direction for health protection–promotion care planning.

Assessment of the Individual Client

Assessment of the individual client in the context of health promotion expands beyond physical assessment to also include a comprehensive examination of other client health parameters, health beliefs, and health behaviors. The components of health assessment focusing on individual clients are (1) functional health patterns, (2) physical fitness evaluation, (3) nutritional assessment, (4) health-risk appraisal, (5) life-stress review, (6) spiritual health assessment, (7) social support systems review, (8) health-beliefs review, and (9) lifestyle assessment. A description of assessment areas that have special relevance for health promotion and protection follows.

Physical Fitness Evaluation

Physical activity is an important part of personal health status that is discussed in detail in Chapter 8. Because of the sedentary lifestyles that, for many individuals, begin early in childhood and continue into adulthood, evaluation of physical fitness is a critical part of any nursing assessment. It is applicable to clients of all ages, with restrictions on some areas of testing for individuals who are physically compromised. It is important to differentiate between *skill-related physical fitness* and *health-related physical fitness.* Skill-related fitness is defined by those qualities that contribute to successful athletic performance: agility, speed, power, and reaction time. Health-related fitness includes qualities found to contribute to one's general health, including cardiorespiratory endurance, muscular endurance, body composition, and flexibility, which are briefly discussed below.[9]

CARDIORESPIRATORY ENDURANCE

This aspect of fitness reflects the ability of the circulatory and respiratory systems to adjust to and recover from exercise efficiently. There are a number of approaches to assessing cardiorespiratory endurance. Two approaches are presented here. For children and adolescents between the ages of 10 and 16 years, a *1-mile run–walk test* can be used. This consists of having the individual walk or run 1 mile at a steady pace over the entire distance. One mile can be measured out on either an outdoor or indoor track. Youths should be encouraged to practice the run the day before and warm up just before the run. Health fitness standards for a 10-year-old boy is a range of 9 to 11½ minutes and for a 16-year-old boy, 7 to 8½ minutes. The range for girls of the same ages is 30 seconds to 1 minute more in each category.[10]

The *step test* is a field version of the laboratory stress test for adults. If the step test is conducted in a clinic setting, the electrocardiogram may be monitored. The availability of a physician for emergency backup is suggested if the client is over 40 years of age, is obese, or has a history of cardiovascular difficulties. The step test is not as physiologically stressful as the laboratory stress test, but caution should be exercised in testing individuals with high-risk profiles for cardiovascular disease. For the step test, a step 16 to 17 inches high is recommended. The step rate should be 24 steps per minute for men and 22 steps per minute for women. Each step consists of the following sequence: left foot up; right foot up; left foot down; right foot down. Apical or carotid pulse rates are measured after stepping for 3 minutes at the prescribed cadence. With the client comfortably seated in a chair following step testing, pulse rates are counted for 15 seconds from 5 to 20 seconds into recovery and multiplied by 4 to obtain recovery heart rate. In the 95th percentile, recovery rate will be 140 for women and 124 for men. In the 10th percentile ranking, recovery rate will be 184 for women and 178 for men.[11]

MUSCULAR ENDURANCE

As a test of muscular endurance, bent-knee sit-ups can be used (Figure 6–1). The number of *sit-ups per minute* is counted. Older adults or those with cardiovascular disorders must be observed carefully for fatigue during endurance testing. Sit-ups should be terminated if signs of distress occur in the client. Between 36 and 45 years old, men are rated as excellent if they can perform 42 or more sit-ups, women if they can perform 39 or more sit-ups. Men and women are below average if they can perform only 21 and 12, respectively. For over 46 years of age, men are rated excellent if they can perform 38 or more sit-ups, women if they can

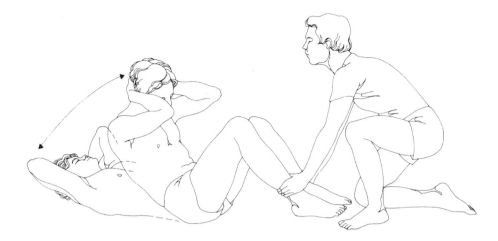

FIGURE 6-1 Bent-knee sit-ups

perform 24 or more sit-ups. Men and women are below average if they can perform only 18 and 11, respectively.[12]

The sit-up test may not be the test of choice because the hip flexer muscles are involved in addition to the abdominal muscles. Sit-ups must be performed accurately to prevent injury. The push-up muscular endurance test and the bench press test may also be used to evaluate muscle endurance. The nurse must determine which muscular endurance test to use based on the client's health history. Procedures for conducting a push-up muscular endurance test and the bench press are found in ACSM's *Guidelines for Exercise Testing and Prescription*.[9(p 49–85)]

BODY COMPOSITION

Hydrostatic weighing underwater is considered the "gold standard" of indirect body fat estimates. However, because of the complex and expensive equipment needed and the time and potential anxiety involved, it is seldom used in the clinical setting. Anthropometry is used most frequently to assess body composition by measuring skin folds. Approximately half of the body fat is subcutaneous so total body fat can be estimated by this method. A quality pair of skin-fold calipers is needed, and measures should be taken at the chest, midaxillary, triceps, subscapular, abdomen, suprailiac, and thigh sites (Figure 6–2). Duplicative measures should be taken at each of the sites and the average values summed. All the measurements should be taken on the right side of the body. For young adults, at the 50th percentile, the sum of skin folds is 21 for men or 9.4% body fat; the sum of skin folds for women is 30 or 22.8% body fat.[10] Marked deviation above or below these values should alert the health care provider to assess for either too much or too little nutrient intake for body requirements.

FLEXIBILITY

Flexibility is also an important component of physical fitness. It is the ability to move muscles and joints through their maximum range of motion. Flexibility may decrease with age

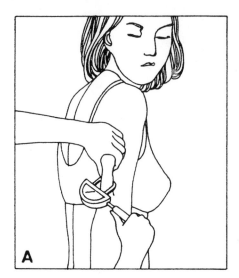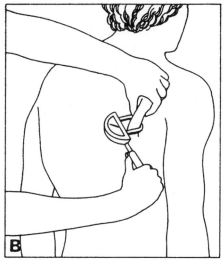

FIGURE 6-2 Skin-fold sites A. Triceps. B. Subscapula

or as a result of chronic illness. The lack of ability to flex or extend muscles or joints often reflects poor health habits, such as sedentary lifestyle, inappropriate posture, or faulty body mechanics. Loss of flexibility greatly decreases the client's ability to move about with ease and comfort.

Trunk flexion measures the client's ability to stretch the back and thigh muscles. The sit and reach test can be used to measure flexion. The client sits on a floor mat or on a flat examining table with legs fully extended and feet flat against a box (Figure 6–3). Arms and hands are extended forward as far as possible and held for a count of three. With a ruler, the distance that the client can reach beyond the proximal edge of the box can be measured in inches. If the client cannot reach the edge, the distance of the fingertips from the edge is measured and reported as a negative number. The desired range for men is +1 to +5 inches; for women, +2 to +6.[12]

The data collected during physical fitness evaluation can be used to assist the client in planning an appropriate exercise or physical activity program. Careful attention to assessment will optimize the fit of the exercise prescription to the physical capabilities of the client.

Nutritional Assessment

Effective planning for health promotion requires evaluation of the nutritional status of clients. Comprehensive nutritional assessment requires the use of four different types of assessment tools: anthropometric, biochemical, clinical, and dietary.[9] Anthropometric assessment includes height and weight measures, a circumference of various areas of the body, as well as skin-fold thicknesses to be compared with standard values. Height should be measured wearing 1-inch heels. Weight should be taken with lightweight clothing. The best method for determining healthy weight is the body mass index (BMI).[13] The BMI does not

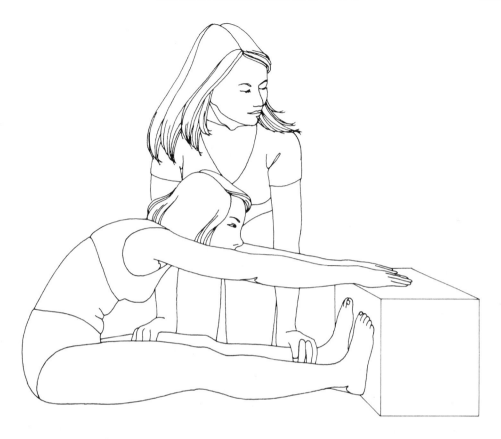

FIGURE 6-3 Trunk flexion

determine body fat distribution, but screens for overweight or obesity.[14] The BMI table is presented in Table 6–1 and the classification standards in Table 6–2. In addition to BMI, skin-fold measurements provide a simple criterion for obesity. Triceps skin-fold thickness indicative of obesity for children, adolescents, and men and women of differing age groups are presented in Table 6–3. Deviations from any of the norms on the measurements should be noted by the nurse and recorded as a part of the nutritional assessment. In addition to the BMI and anthropometric measures, the nurse can use the waist to hip ratio to assess the amount of fat distributed in the abdomen versus the fat distributed below the waist. The ratio is represented by the waist circumference over the hip circumference. The higher the value, the greater the risk for health problems.[13(p 381)]

Biochemical assessment can be conducted through blood or urine analyses to identify nutritional deficiencies. In addition to laboratory tests for cholesterol, triglycerides, glucose, and high-density lipoproteins, tests for protein (creatinine index, serum protein, serum albumin, total lymphocyte count, blood urea nitrogen, and uric acid), for serum or plasma vitamin levels (water-soluble, fat-soluble), and for minerals (calcium, sodium, potassium, iron, phosphorus, and magnesium) may be used to assess nutritional status.[15]

TABLE 6-1 Body Mass Index (BMI) Table

BMI	19	20	21	22	23	24	25	26	27	28	29	30	31	32	33	34	35
Height								Weight (in pounds)									
4'10"(58")	91	96	100	105	110	115	119	124	129	134	138	143	148	153	158	162	167
4'11"(59")	94	99	104	109	114	119	124	128	133	138	143	148	153	158	163	168	173
5' (60")	97	102	107	112	118	123	128	133	138	143	148	153	158	163	168	174	179
5'1" (61")	100	106	111	116	122	127	132	137	143	148	153	158	164	169	174	180	185
5'2" (62")	104	109	115	120	126	131	136	142	147	153	158	164	169	175	180	186	191
5'3" (63")	107	113	118	124	130	135	141	146	152	158	163	169	175	180	186	191	197
5'4" (64")	110	116	122	128	134	140	145	151	157	163	169	174	180	186	192	197	204
5'5" (65")	114	120	126	132	138	144	150	156	162	168	174	180	186	192	198	204	210
5'6" (66")	118	124	130	136	142	148	155	161	167	173	179	186	192	198	204	210	216
5'7" (67")	121	127	134	140	146	153	159	166	172	178	185	191	198	204	211	217	223
5'8" (68")	125	131	138	144	151	158	164	171	177	184	190	197	203	210	216	223	230
5'9" (69")	128	135	142	149	155	162	169	176	182	189	196	203	209	216	223	230	236
5'10"(70")	132	139	146	153	160	167	174	181	188	195	202	209	216	222	229	236	243
5'11"(71")	136	143	150	157	165	172	179	186	193	200	208	215	222	229	236	243	250
6' (72")	140	147	154	162	169	177	184	191	199	206	213	221	228	235	242	250	258
6'1" (73")	144	151	159	166	174	182	189	197	204	212	219	227	235	242	250	257	265
6'2" (74")	148	155	163	171	179	186	194	202	210	218	225	233	241	249	256	264	272
6'3" (75")	152	160	168	176	184	192	200	208	216	224	232	240	248	256	264	272	279

Evidence Report of Clinical Guidelines on the Identification, Evaluation, and Treatment of Overweight and Obesity in Adults, 1998. NIH/National Heart, Lung, and Blood Institute (NHLBI).

TABLE 6-2 Body Mass Index (BMI) Table

Classification	Men	Women
Normal	24–27	23–26
Moderately Obese	28–31	27–32
Severely Obese	>31	>32

Data from Department of Health and Human Services, *The Surgeon General's Report on Nutrition and Health.* DHHS (PHS) Publication 88-50210. Washington DC: U.S. Government Printing Office, 1998.

TABLE 6-3 Triceps Skin-Fold Thickness Indicating Obesity (mm)

Age (yr)	Males	Females
5	≥12	≥15
10	≥13	≥17
15	≥15	≥20
20	≥16	≥28
25	≥20	≥29
30 and above	≥23	≥30

Clinical examination can detect physical signs in the skin, muscular and skeletal systems, eyes, and tongue that suggest malnutrition. For an overview of physical signs suggestive of malnutrition, refer to *Nutrition in Health Maintenance and Health Promotion for Primary Care Providers* by Y. M. Gutierrez.[14] (pp. 242-244)

Clients' current dietary patterns should be assessed. Clients should be instructed to keep a record of everything eaten for three days during the week prior to their clinic appointment or home visit. The record can be kept on a food intake record that allows the listing of the types of foods and amounts consumed during regular meals and snacks.[16] When such a record is kept accurately, daily food choices can be compared with the *Food Guide Pyramid* from the U.S. Department of Agriculture's Human Nutrition Information Service (presented in Chapter 9) or analyzed using published daily food guides or the many computerized dietary analysis packages available. The nurse should be prepared to explain the *Food Guide Pyramid* to the patient as a basis for dietary planning. Once the usual dietary patterns of the client have been identified, the nurse can provide needed nutritional assistance to the client (see Chapter 9). Further, the nurse should work with nutritionists to prepare materials that inform the client about the latest thinking in use of nutritional supplements, including vitamins and minerals (calcium, iron, etc.) as well as protein or complex carbohydrates.

Poor eating patterns, obesity, and malnutrition occur in *all* socioeconomic classes. In addition, dietary risk factors for chronic disease are widespread in the American population. Therefore, assessment of nutritional status and dietary habits is a critical part of comprehensive health assessment for all clients including individuals, families, and specific target groups such as high school students, pregnant women, and the elderly. The reader is referred to the PACE Project for a patient-centered nutrition guide.[17]

Health-Risk Appraisal

The purpose of health-risk appraisal (HRA) is to provide an estimate of health threats to which clients may be particularly vulnerable because of genetic makeup, family history, and lifestyle.[18] Personal risk profiles are determined for clients using information from their health history, laboratory diagnostics, physical fitness evaluation, nutritional assessment, and lifestyle assessment. Risk factors can generally be classified according to the categories in Figure 6–4.

The assumptions underlying risk appraisal follow: (1) Each person is faced with certain quantifiable health hazards as a member of a specific group, (2) the client's risk is comparable to the average risk or mortality experience for a group with similar characteristics, and (3) knowledge of risk and related anxiety or concern are the sources of motivation for health-behavior change. It is assumed that providing information concerning mortality risk (estimated probability of death from a particular disease within the next 10 years) prior to the development of signs and symptoms of disease stimulate individuals to change their lifestyles to avert illness.

It is an accepted fact that the risk of developing any disease generally increases the greater the number of risk factors present and the greater their intensity. Through health-risk appraisal, clients are given an indication of what might occur *on average* if they have the health experience of their current referent group (personal risk age) and what improvements they could make in their mortality profile (achievable or target risk age) if they adopted more positive behaviors of other groups (e.g., stopping smoking, using seat belts, decreasing alcohol use, exercising, decreasing saturated fat intake).

The accuracy of mortality predictions from this method have been questioned, because population data do not accurately reflect the risk profile for a specific individual. Smith and colleagues[19] reported that health-risk appraisal (HRA) overestimates the probability of mortality from coronary heart disease. Further, risk appraisal in and of itself is unlikely to result in reductions in risk. If clients are to alter behavior significantly, risk appraisal must be linked to behavior-change programs and other appropriate community health resources. It is unethical to apprise individuals of their risk level without providing supportive counseling and resources to facilitate behavior-change efforts. The lifestyle changes to be made should be arrived at collaboratively by the nurse and the client. Predictions of premature death or shortened life expectancy may cause anxiety and depression in older adults who believe that it is too late to change risk status. Thus, in the decision to use risk appraisal with clients, both the advantages and disadvantages of this assessment tool must be considered.[20]

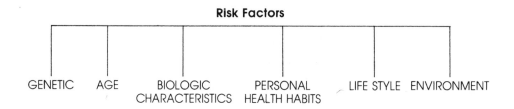

FIGURE 6-4 Categories of risk factors

Paper-and-pencil as well as computerized forms of HRAs are available from several commercial sources. Most appraisals also provide computerized analysis of individual risk based on national mortality data for selected health problems. These health problems usually include one or more of the 10 leading causes of death, with increasing attention being given to the social morbidities, such as death from violence and depression leading to suicide. Examples of risk-appraisal instruments include those focused on a single disease, such as the Cardiac Risk Factor Questionnaire developed by the Executive Health Group[21] and those focused on a number of health problems, such as the University of Minnesota Health Risk Appraisal developed by Raines and Ellis.[22(appB)]

Many companies use HRA as the "starter" for their health promotion and risk reduction program. Occupational health nurses often identify risk factors such as obesity, smoking, and high blood pressure, which are precursors of serious diseases and premature death. Through subsequent interventions, nurses aim to decrease employee illness, absenteeism, and disability and thus decrease health care costs for the company.[23] The Centers for Disease Control and Prevention conducted a review of the current HRA literature and previous reviews. On the basis of this review, evidence suggested that the HRA is effective when it is a component of a comprehensive work-site health promotion program. Future research is suggested to focus on awareness and commitment to change health behaviors rather than on behavioral outcomes.[24]

Life-Stress Review

Stress has been identified as a potential threat to mental health and physical well-being and has been associated with the occurrence of illness (heart disease, cancer, gastrointestinal disorders, etc.) in numerous studies. Psychoneuroimmunology as a field focuses on understanding the disruptive effects of stress on the neural and immune systems. Because of its apparent centrality to health, life stress should be evaluated as a part of comprehensive health assessment. The Derogates Stress Profile (DSP)[25] is used to assess personal and professional stresses in adults and adolescents. The Perceived Stress Scale[26] assesses moods and feelings about life stressors. The Hassles and Uplifts Scales measure day-to-day stressing or destressing experiences rather than major life events.[27] The State-Trait Anxiety Inventory[28] is a tool for assessing the extent of acute and chronic tension and anxiety that clients experience, whereas the Stress Warning Signals Inventory[21(p 182)] provides clients with information about how they respond to stressful events so that they can break the stress cycle and reduce negative physical and psychological outcomes. Stress Charting assists clients to pinpoint what aspects of their lives may be most stressful. Several of these instruments are described below.

STRESS SCALES

The DSP[25] is a comprehensive 77-item instrument designed to screen an adult's or adolescent's response to stress in the following dimensions: time pressure, driven behavior, attitude, relocation, work environment, family relationships, hostility, anxiety, depression, and health. Assessing a person's vulnerability to stress and strengths to cope provides an essential measure of mental and physical well-being. The Perceived Stress Scale[26] is a 10-item scale that is very easy to administer and score. It contains phases that describe how a person might feel about life stressors. The summed score is a measure of global stress.

Hassles and Uplifts Scales

Hassles are defined as the irritating, frustrating, distressing demands that to some degree characterize everyday life (traffic jams, losing things, arguments). Uplifts, the counterparts of hassles, are defined as the positive experiences or joys of life, such as getting a good night's rest, receiving a letter from a friend, or spending time with a pet. It has been proposed that assessment of daily hassles and uplifts may be a better approach to the prediction of health or illness outcomes than the usual assessment of life events. If negatively toned stressors such as hassles cause neuroendocrine changes that predispose to illness, positively toned experiences such as uplifts may buffer stress disorders. [27]

Kanner and Feldman explored the effects of hassles and uplifts, as well as perceived control of those events, among a group of 140 adolescents in relation to the experience of depression. Fewer hassles and more uplifts were related to less depression. Further, those adolescents who felt they had control over hassles and uplifts in their lives were less depressed than those who reported less control.[29] In a study of Navajo Indians, major life events and daily hassles were measured among adults presenting for either inpatient or outpatient care at a selected U.S. Indian Health Service facility. The number of outpatient visits and hospital admissions were monitored during the subsequent two years. Both major life events and daily hassles increased risk of hospital admission, whereas daily hassles were also predictive of increased use of outpatient services. These findings support the potential cross-cultural validity of the impact of daily hassles on health status and related health care use.[30] Hassles and uplifts scales have been developed for both children and adults.[27,29]

State-Trait Anxiety Inventory

Another instrument suggested for use as part of the life-stress review is the State-Trait Anxiety Inventory, which consists of 20 items pertaining to the amount of tension or anxiety the client feels at that moment (state), and 20 items concerning the way the client generally feels (trait). Sample questions from the inventory are presented in Figures 6–5 and 6–6. Clients respond by rating themselves on a 4-point scale for each item. A State-Trait Anxiety Inventory for Children, "How I Feel Questionnaire," has also been developed. Children respond by rating themselves on a 3-point scale.[31] Both instruments and administration manuals are available from Mind Garden, Palo Alto, California. The State-Trait Anxiety Inventories provide an efficient yet reliable means for assessing feelings of tension or stress experienced by child and adult clients.

Stress Warning Signals Inventory

In order to assist clients in understanding how they respond to stress, they must be made aware of the symptoms that provide personal feedback concerning an elevated stress level.[21] Once clients are aware of their own stress signals, they can use stress-management techniques presented in Chapter 10 more effectively. Symptoms of stress may be physical, behavioral, emotional, or cognitive as shown in Figure 6–7.

Stress Charting

The Menninger Foundation Biofeedback Center, in its stress management seminar, uses a stress-charting exercise that allows clients to list sources of stress. After listing as many stressors as possible, the client is instructed to write the number associated with each stressor in the section of the circle that describes the area of life in which the stressor occurs. If it is a stressor that is particularly troublesome, the client should place the number closer to the

Directions: Statements that people have used to describe themselves are given below. Read each statement and then blacken in the appropriate circle to the right of the statement to indicate how you *feel* right now, that is, *at this moment*. There are no right or wrong answers. Do not spend too much time on any one statement but give the answer which seems to describe your present feelings best.

① = **Not at All**; ② = **Somewhat**;
③ = **Moderately So**; ④ = **Very Much So**

I feel at ease	①	②	③	④
I feel upset	①	②	③	④
I feel nervous	①	②	③	④
I am relaxed	①	②	③	④
I am worried	①	②	③	④

FIGURE 6-5 Sample items from the self-evaluation questionnaire: State Anxiety Inventory (From Spielberger C, Gorsuch R, Lushene R, The State-Trait Anxiety Inventory, copyright © 1968, with special permission.)

Directions: A number of statements that people have used to describe themselves are given below. Read each statement and then blacken in the appropriate circle to the right of the statement to indicate how you generally feel. There are no right or wrong answers. Do not spend too much time on any one statement, but give the answer that seems to describe how you generally feel.

① = **Not at All**; ② = **Somewhat**;
③ = **Moderately So**; ④ = **Very Much So**

I wish I could be as happy as others seem to be	①	②	③	④
I am "calm, cool, and collected"	①	②	③	④
I feel that difficulties are piling up so that I cannot overcome them	①	②	③	④
I am inclined to take things hard	①	②	③	④
I am content	①	②	③	④

FIGURE 6-6 Sample items from the self-evaluation questionnaire: Trait Anxiety Inventory (From The State-Trait Anxiety Inventory, Spielberger C, Gorsuch R, Lushene R, copyright © 1968, with special permission.)

Stress Warning Signals

PHYSICAL SYMPTOMS

☐ Headaches
☐ Indigestion
☐ Stomachaches
☐ Sweaty palms
☐ Sleep difficulties
☐ Dizziness

☐ Back pain
☐ Tight neck, shoulders
☐ Racing heart
☐ Restlessness
☐ Tiredness
☐ Ringing in ears

BEHAVIORAL SYMPTOMS

☐ Excess smoking
☐ Bossiness
☐ Compulsive gum chewing
☐ Attitude critical of others

☐ Grinding of teeth at night
☐ Overuse of alcohol
☐ Compulsive eating
☐ Inability to get things done

EMOTIONAL SYMPTOMS

☐ Crying
☐ Nervousness, anxiety
☐ Boredom—no meaning to things
☐ Edginess—ready to explode
☐ Feeling powerless to change things

☐ Overwhelming sense of pressure
☐ Anger
☐ Loneliness
☐ Unhappiness for no reason
☐ Easily upset

COGNITIVE SYMPTOMS

☐ Trouble thinking clearly
☐ Forgetfulness
☐ Lack of creativity
☐ Memory loss

☐ Inability to make decisions
☐ Thoughts of running away
☐ Constant worry
☐ Loss of sense of humor

Do any seem familiar to you?

Check the ones you experience when under stress. These are your stress warning signs.

Are there any additional stress warning signals that you experience that are not listed? If so, add them here.

_____

_____

_____

_____

FIGURE 6-7 Stress warning signals (From Benson H, Stuart EM. *The Wellness Book.* New York: Birch Lane Press, 1992, with permission.)

center of the circle. The center of the circle represents the client. The stress-charting exercise appears in Figure 6–8. After completion of this portion of the life-stress review, the client should be aware of (1) the stresses that he or she is experiencing in daily living, (2) the areas of life in which multiple stressors are occurring, and (3) the personal closeness or distance of each stressor from the self.

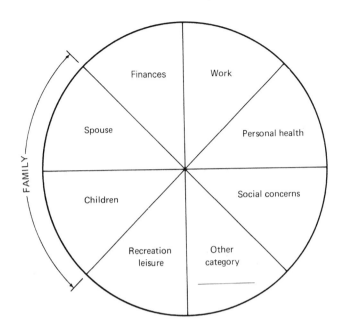

List of stressors:

1. _____
2. _____
3. _____
4. _____
5. _____
6. _____
7. _____
8. _____
9. _____
10. _____
11. _____
12. _____
13. _____
14. _____
15. _____
16. _____

FIGURE 6-8 Stress charting (Adapted with permission from Walters D, Biofeedback Center, The Menninger Foundation, Topeka, KS.)

In the 1990s, instruments were developed that focus on measuring coping strengths and mastery of stress in children and adults. Ryan-Wenger developed the Schoolager's Coping Strategies Inventory to measure the type, frequency, and effectiveness of children's stress-coping strategies. Children between 8 and 12 years of age were asked in group discussions to identify the kinds of things that they do when they are experiencing stress. The resulting instrument and its psychometric evaluation are described by the developer.[32] Younger[33] reports on the development and testing of an instrument to measure mastery of stress in adults. Mastery is defined as a human response to difficult or stressful circumstances in which a person gains competence and control over the experience of stress. This 89-item instrument yields both a stress score and mastery score and is appropriate for administration to adults 19 years of age or older.

Life-stress assessment, as well as assessment of mastery of stress and coping strategies, provides information valuable in planning effective stress-management interventions with the client. Increased self-awareness resulting from this component of health assessment facilitates the use of stress-management and relaxation techniques described in Chapter 10.

Spiritual Health Assessment

Spiritual health is the ability to develop one's spiritual nature to its fullest potential, including the ability to discover and articulate one's basic purpose in life, to learn how to experience love, joy, peace, and fulfillment, and how to help ourselves and others achieve their fullest potential. In a holistic approach to health assessment, it is critical to appraise the spiritual health of clients, because spiritual beliefs to which individuals subscribe affect their interpretations of life events and health. McBride, Brooks, and Pilkington[34] measured the relationship between a patient's spirituality and health experiences using the Index of Core Spiritual Experiences in 462 patients. Results showed a significant correlation between health and spirituality supporting the importance of assessing spirituality. The Spiritual Involvement and Beliefs Scale (SIBS)[35] is another instrument designed to be used across religious traditions to assess actions as well as beliefs. A 26-item modified Likert instrument, it is easy to administer and score.

Areas of spirituality to be assessed include relationship with a higher being, relationship with self, and relationships with others.[36]

I. Relationship with a higher being
   A. The importance of God or a higher being in the client's life
   B. Use of prayer and spiritually oriented readings as a means of dealing with life situations
   C. Belief in life after death or continuing spiritual existence
   D. Participation in individual or group worship activities
II. Relationship with self
   A. Existence of personal life goals that give meaning to life
   B. Spiritual beliefs that engender hope and zest for living
   C. Awareness of life priorities
   D. Commitment to spiritual growth

III. Relationships with others
   A. Extent of concern about the spiritual well-being of others
   B. Openness to sharing thoughts, feelings, and spiritual beliefs with others
   C. Respect for other individuals as spiritual beings

Questions related to spiritual assessment are usually asked toward the end of the interview when the client and nurse are more at ease with each other. Clients should be informed that assessing their spiritual well-being is integral to evaluating their overall health.

Social Support Systems Review

A number of instruments for reviewing social support systems are presented in Chapter 11 and so are not presented here. Social support configuration can be analyzed using the support systems review as in Figure 11–3 or depicted using support diagramming as in Figure 11–4. McDermott[37] describes 28 social support instruments representative of the broad spectrum of instruments used in social support research. Many of these instruments can also be used effectively in clinical settings, as well as in research.

Health-Beliefs Review

Health-belief measures can be classified as health specific or behavior specific. The health beliefs selected for assessment with any given client will depend on the areas of health and health behavior of most concern to the client. Although many health-belief measures of potential clinical use exist, only a few examples are identified here. The constructs in Table 6–4[(38–44)] have been shown through research to be related to actual performance of health-protecting or health-promoting behaviors in various populations. The behavior-specific measures almost always are more powerful than the health-specific measures in explaining and predicting the occurrence of health behaviors.

Clients' scores on a personally tailored portfolio of health-belief measures can provide an indication of readiness and motivation to engage in particular health behaviors. The health beliefs to be assessed should be determined through preliminary discussions between the nurse and client.

Lifestyle Assessment

Increasing evidence indicates that there is a great deal that individuals can do to maintain and enhance their well-being and prevent the early onset of disabling health problems by engaging in a health-promoting lifestyle. A thoughtful review of health habits with subsequent follow-up counseling and education can greatly increase the motivation and competence of clients to care for themselves in a responsible manner.

HEALTH-PROMOTING LIFESTYLE PROFILE II

In the context of health, lifestyle is defined as discretionary activities with significant impact on health status that are a regular part of one's daily pattern of living. Health-promoting behavior is an expression of the human actualizing tendency that is directed toward optimal well-being, personal fulfillment, and productive living. The 52-item Health-Promoting Lifestyle Profile II (HPLP-II), a revision of the original instrument, consists of six subscales,

TABLE 6-4 Health-Belief Measures and Examples of Instruments

Measure	Instrument
Health-Specific Beliefs	
Health locus of control	The multidimensional health locus of control scale (MHLC)[a]
	Assesses beliefs in internal, chance, and powerful others locus of control of health
Health care competence	Perceived health competence rating scale[b]
	Assesses perceived capability to care for one's own health
Definition of health	Laffrey health conception scale[c]
	Assesses one's conception of health in four domains: clinical, role performance, adaptive, and eudaimonistic
Intrinsic motivation	Health self-determinism index[d] for health behavior
	Health self-determinism index for children[e]
	Assesses active, independent decision making regarding health behavior and the self-satisfaction that the behavior engenders
Behavior-Specific Beliefs	
Exercise self-efficacy	Exercise self-efficacy scale[e]
	Assesses confidence in ability to continue exercise on a regular basis
Exercise benefits and barriers	Exercise benefits–barriers scale[f]
	Expected outcomes and barriers to exercise[g]
	Assesses perceptions of the "pros" or positive outcomes of exercise as well as the barriers, hurdles, or constraints to exercise
Social support for exercise	Exercise social support scale[h]

[a]Wallston et al.[38]
[b]Smith et al.[39]
[c]Laffrey[40]
[d]Cox[41]
[e]Cox[42]
[f]Sechrist et al.[43]
[g]Steinhardt et al.[44]
[h]A Garcia, MA Brode, personal communication.

which are intended to measure major components of a healthy lifestyle: health responsibility, physical activity, nutrition, interpersonal relations, spiritual growth, and stress management. Means can be derived for each subscale separately or a mean obtained on the total instrument as a measure of overall health-promoting lifestyle. Although this instrument is frequently used in research, it can provide important information about a client's lifestyle when used in primary health care. The instrument, scoring instructions, and psychometric information can be obtained from Dr. Susan Noble Walker, College of Nursing, University of Nebraska Medical Center. Sample items for each of the subscales appear in Table 6–5.

The profile of means on the HPLP-II can provide information useful in developing an individualized health promotion plan that identifies lifestyle strengths and resources as well

TABLE 6-5 Health-Promoting Lifestyle Profile II Subscales and Sample Items

Subscale	Sample Item
Health responsibility	Read or watch TV programs about improving my health.
	Question health professionals in order to understand their instructions.
Physical activity	Exercise vigorously for 20 or more minutes at least 3 times a week (brisk walking, bicycling, aerobic dancing, using a stair climber).
	Get exercise during usual day activities (such as walking during lunch, using stairs instead of elevators, parking car farther away from destination and walking).
Nutrition	Choose a diet low in fat, saturated fat, and cholesterol.
	Eat 2 to 4 servings of fruit each day.
Interpersonal relations	Spend time with close friends.
	Settle conflicts with others through discussion and compromise.
Spiritual growth	Feel connected with some force greater than myself.
	Am aware of what is important to me in life.
Stress management	Take some time for relaxation each day.
	Pace myself to prevent fatigue

as areas for further growth. There is a need for development of additional lifestyle assessment tools that are appropriate for children, adolescents, and families. An adolescent version is being designed to identify health-enhancing behaviors, positive steps that enhance health, and well-being.[45] Psychometric testing is in progress.

STAGE-OF-CHANGE ASSESSMENT

In relation to any given behavior change, clients may be at one of several stages. Based on various studies of behavioral changes from smoking cessation to exercise adoption, recurring stages seem to emerge. Prochaska and colleagues propose in the transtheoretical model that the stage of behavior change will determine the behavioral plan for intervention that is likely to be most effective. Stages of change for positive health behaviors can be assessed with the True-False questions presented in Table 6–6.[46]

Following completion of Lifestyle Assessment, the interest of the client in making various changes can be assessed as well as the stage of the client in relation to each behavior.

TABLE 6-6 Questions for Assessing Stages of Behavior Change

1. I currently do not (specify exact behavior, e.g., exercise 30 minutes three times a week, eat 2 to 4 servings of fruit daily) and do not intend to start in the next 6 months. (Precontemplation)
2. I currently do not (specify behavior), but I am thinking about starting to do so in the next 6 months. (Contemplation)
3. I have tried several times to (specify behavior) but am seriously thinking of trying again in the next month. (Planning)
4. I have (specify behavior) regularly for less than 6 months. (Action)
5. I have (specify behavior) regularly for more than 6 months. (Maintenance)

Prochaska and colleagues propose that "staging" a client in relation to various health behaviors will allow for more precise tailoring of interventions.

 ## Assessment of the Family

Assessment of the family, as well as assessment of the individual, is critical to successfully planning for health-behavior change. The family is the primary social structure for health promotion within society. It is within the context of the family that health behaviors are learned and the rudiments of health-enhancing or health-damaging lifestyles emerge. The family acts as a powerful mediating factor in determining how its members cope with a wide range of health concerns and challenges.[47] Thus, the family is a logical unit of assessment and intervention for health promotion, because it has the primary responsibility for (1) developing self-care and dependent-care competencies of the family, (2) fostering resilience of family members, (3) providing social and physical resources to the family group, and (4) promoting healthy individuation while maintaining family cohesion. Although women generally carry the major responsibility for health decision making and health education for the family, the task of fostering health and healthy behaviors should be "mainstreamed" as an integral part of family functioning.

In assessment of the family, the varying family forms that exist today, such as one-parent families and blended families, must be taken into consideration. The milieu for the promotion of health is likely to differ significantly across families, depending on their composition, structure, socioeconomic status, living environment, and cultural context. Healthy family traits can be expressed in many different ways. There is no one correct way to spend quality time together, promote physically active families, or express affection. Family strengths can have many different modes of expression. When conducting a family health assessment, the nurse must be attuned to this wide range of variation among families as well as variations produced by transitions in family life.[48] Several approaches to assessment that can be used in all types of families are described briefly here.

Using a systems approach, Whall proposed health assessment guidelines for families. She suggested that the following categories be assessed: (1) individual subsystems (developmental, biologic, psychologic, and social characteristics), (2) interactional patterns (relationships, communication patterns, roles, and attachment patterns), (3) unique characteristics of the whole (group psyche, capacity for change, belief systems, group dynamics, developmental needs, typologic actions, and economics), and (4) environmental interface synchrony. The full-length assessment tool appears in Whall's original work.[49]

Friedman has described a structural–functional approach to family assessment.[47] Within this framework, the family is viewed as a system with the following features: value structure, role structure, power structure, communication patterns, affective function, socialization function, health care function, and family coping function. This approach to assessment is based on systems theory and provides insight concerning the internal processes of the family as well as the relationship of the family to the environment and larger social system. Family decision-making patterns in relation to health are identified in assessing power structure and health care function.

Wright and Leahey[50] provide a thorough description of the Calgary Family Assessment Model (CFAM), which they have adapted specifically for nurses to use when assessing families. Their model for assessment consists of the following major categories: family structural assessment, family developmental assessment, and family functional assessment.

In structural assessment, the family is analyzed in terms of both its internal and external structures. Aspects of the internal structure include family composition, rank order, subsystem, and boundary. Components of the external structure are culture, religion, social class status and mobility, environment, and extended family.

Through family developmental assessment, the nurse appraises the current stage of the family in relation to family developmental history.[50] Wright and Leahey's assessment of family development focuses primarily on the traditional family developmental cycle, but they also discuss assessment of alterations in the family developmental life cycle brought about by separation, divorce, single parenthood, and remarriage by divorced persons.

Family functional assessment is dichotomized as instrumental functioning and expressive functioning. *Instrumental functioning* refers to the routine activities of everyday living, whereas *expressive functioning* is elaborated as emotional communication, verbal communication, nonverbal communication, circular communication, problem solving, roles, control, beliefs, and alliances and coalitions.[50] The reader is referred to Wright and Leahey's book for a detailed discussion of the family assessment model that they propose.

Mischke-Berkey and colleagues[51] propose a family health assessment scheme that focuses on assessment of tensions and stress created by situations in normal family life and on family health issues. The Neuman Health-Care Systems Model provides the blueprint for this assessment tool. Flexible and normal lines of defense as well as lines of resistance are important concepts in this assessment framework.

The Darlington Family Interview Schedule and Darlington Family Rating Scale have been described in detail by Wilkinson.[47] The interview explores the family's view of health issues or problems; children's health, development, emotional behavior, relationships, and conduct; parents' physical and psychologic health, marital harmony (if two-parent family), social support, and parenting skills; parent–child relationships in terms of care and control; and family functioning in terms of closeness, power hierarchies, emotional atmosphere and rules, developmental stage, and strengths. A rating scale is used to summarize the data as a basis for developing a strategy for care. The rating scale provides a succinct presentation of child, parent, and family information.

An excellent compilation of approximately 20 measures of family functioning that is potentially useful in practice has been prepared by Sawin and colleagues.[52] Examples of instruments described in this compilation are the Feetham Family Functioning Survey, the Family Adaptability and Cohesion Scale, and the Family Hardiness Index. These instruments can be used in health assessment of families as a basis for developing a health protection–promotion plan. Information provided on each instrument includes description with sample items, psychometric properties, cross-cultural uses, gender sensitivity, applicability to variant family structures, list of selected studies using the instrument, critique, and source for accessing the tool. The reader is referred to this excellent resource for further information on family assessment tools developed by nurses and other professionals.

A major gap in family assessment tools is the lack of an instrument that measures family dimensions of health-related lifestyle. Nurse scientists need to direct their attention to the development of valid and reliable tools to assess families' aggregate health behaviors. Areas suggested for assessment in such an instrument appear in Table 6–7.

In summary, family assessment complements individual assessment; thus, the two should be considered as interrelated processes. To provide further guidance to nurses in working with families, a format for developing a family health protection–promotion plan is presented in Chapter 7.

Assessment of the Community

A third essential component of health assessment is community analysis or appraisal. Community analysis is the process of assessing and defining needs, opportunities, and resources involved in initiating community health action programs. It is critical to recognize that analysis is done *with* the community, not *on* the community. Local citizens and organizations must be involved in the assessment process in order to have "ownership" of the program and to build widespread commitment to community action.[53] It is important to recall at this point that *Healthy People 2010* objectives are essentially community oriented. The underlying premise of the 2010 initiative is that the health of individuals and their community is bound together. All sectors of the community must be activated to achieve the broad national goals set for the year 2010: increase quality and years of healthy life and eliminate health disparities. Objectives focused on injury and violence prevention, educational and community-based programs, occupational safety and health, environmental health, and maternal, infant, and child health all require community assessment and intervention.[54]

A community is a social system that encompasses the collective human energies of individuals, families, and nonfamilial groups. It is the context in which aggregates and individuals either "bloom" or lie dormant. The community is a system with complex relationships among interdependent subsystems. Clark specifies the critical attributes of a community as group orientation in which the group's goals take priority over those of individual members; common bonds between members such as lifestyle, ethnicity, or culture; and significant social interaction among individuals that make up the community.[6] Communities have both health strengths and resources as well as health issues or problems. Communities must be competent in meeting their responsibilities to provide for the highest level of well-being of their members. Characteristics of the community must be assessed to determine what the community health assets and challenges are.

Goeppinger[55] has identified five approaches to collecting data about communities: informant interviewing (directed conversation with community members); participant observation (sharing in community life activities); mobile survey (observation while driving about); secondary analyses (use of preexisting data); and community surveys (organized data collection efforts). Because community citizens constitute a critical primary data source, informant interviewing should always be used as one approach to data collection. An assessment methodology that combines at least three to four of these data collection methods is more likely to provide a holistic picture of the community than an assessment that relies on only one or two approaches.

One approach to community assessment is to collect information about the following community subsystems and their interrelationships: (1) values and culture, (2) politics, (3) education, (4) recreation, (5) transportation, (6) religion, (7) communications and media, (8) welfare, (9) economics, (10) utilities, (11) business and labor, (12) social life, (13) safety and protection, and (14) health. In assessing the health subsystem, population growth patterns, functional activity status, nutritional status, dominant lifestyle patterns, coping ability, community stressors, goal setting and achievement capabilities, and risk factors need to be assessed in addition to traditional indices of morbidity, mortality, and accessibility of health care resources.

The nature of the assessment should be determined by the time available and the way in which the data will be used. Spradley and Alexander[56] describe a continuum of assessment important for the nurse to consider to economize on time and effort. In a comprehensive assessment, all relevant information about the community is synthesized from existing documents and primary data collection. This approach is costly and time-consuming so it should not be undertaken unless such a comprehensive study is absolutely essential before high-priority program goals can be addressed. A familiarization assessment is much more efficient and provides a broad rather than in-depth overview of the community at large. The windshield survey is an example. The nurse drives through the community and identifies multiple dimensions, including housing quality, recreation facilities, and the people residing in the area.[57] Problem-oriented assessment begins with a single problem and assesses the community in terms of that problem, for instance, neighborhood violence. Aspects of the community relevant to that health issue are assessed to determine their contributory, ameliorative, or preventive effects. Subsystem assessment is focused on a particular sector of the community and permits an in-depth assessment of that sector. For example, the subsystem might be education to determine the impact of educational programs on the health and productivity of the community.[56]

Data collection methods are numerous and varied. Existing records should be mined for as much data as possible before primary data collection is instituted. Key informants knowledgeable about the community provide another important data source. When primary data collection is necessary, focus group interviewing often is the method of choice because of the rich interactive data that can be obtained using this method. Survey data can also be important as information from a large segment of the population on key assessment questions is provided.

Screening is another method of collecting data about the community. Screenings are conducted to detect a particular, unrecognized health problem in individuals who are members of a group at risk for a certain disease or health problem. The data from screenings are an important component of the community assessment. The purpose of large screenings is to uncover health problems in populations in an efficient and economically feasible manner. There are three considerations the nurse must be concerned about when participating in or planning a screening. Screenings should be conducted only if the following factors are present: (1) The specific population has a high prevalence of the disease or health problem, (2) there is a successful treatment for the problem, (3) treatment is available if the condition is identified, and (4) the screening instruments are valid and reliable.[20] As with other components of the community assessment, the cost of conducting screenings must be considered in the decision. For example, conducting a screening to detect osteoporosis requires special equipment and the cost is high due to the number of machines needed to manage large screenings in a time-efficient manner. The reader is referred to the *Clinician's Handbook of Preventive Services*[58] developed by the Office of Disease Prevention and Health Promotion.

Community assessment provides the data regarding a community's health status from which community diagnoses are derived. Thus, community assessment is a primary building block for planning, implementing, and evaluating community health promotion and prevention programs. The components of a community assessment have been identified by Clark and have been organized and further expanded by this author in Table 6–7. Examples of assessment instruments[59,60] are available in most community health textbooks.

Assessment of communities is a complicated and time-consuming task. It requires collaboration on the part of many individuals in the community besides health professionals. However, such assessment is critical to the identification of community strengths and resources as well as to the diagnosis of community problems or deficits. Successful implementation of community health promotion and prevention programs depends in large part on accurate assessment of community characteristics.

Table 6–7	Components of Family Assessment

Nutrition

1. Meals prepared in the home are generally consistent with the food guide pyramid.
2. Healthy snacks are consumed in the home.
3. Knowledge about healthy eating habits is shared among family members.
4. Mutual assistance occurs among family members for maintenance of recommended weights and avoidance of overweight and underweight.
5. Family members praise each other for healthy eating.
6. Family members encourage each other to drink 6 to 8 glasses of water per day.
7. Family members base purchase decisions on nutritional labels on food.

Physical Activity

1. Many family outings consist of vigorous or moderate physical activity.
2. Exercise equipment is available within the home.
3. Use of home exercise equipment is part of "family time."
4. Family members expect each other to be physically active.
5. A family membership is held in recreational facilities or programs.
6. Time together is seldom spent watching television or playing video games.
7. Family prefers to spend as much time out of doors as possible.

Stress Control and Management

1. Family manages time well to minimize stressful demands on members.
2. Family often relaxes, shares stories, and laughs together.
3. Emotional expression is encouraged within the family.
4. Family members share stressful experiences with each other.
5. Family members offer each other assistance with difficult tasks.
6. Family members seldom criticize each other.
7. Periods of relaxation and sleep are considered important by the family.

Health Responsibility

1. A schedule for preventive care visits is maintained by the family.
2. Family often discusses news and articles about health topics.
3. Family members are encouraged to seek health care early if a problem develops.
4. Personal responsibility for health is encouraged by the family.
5. Family feels a sense of responsibility for the health of the family and each member.
6. Health professionals are consulted about health promotion as well as care in illness.
7. Appropriate protective behaviors are openly discussed and encouraged (abstinence, use of condoms, hearing protection, eye protection, sunscreen, helmets).

Family Resilience and Resources

1. Worship or spiritual experiences are a regular part of family activities.
2. Family members share a sense of "togetherness" despite difficult life events.
3. Family has a common sense of purpose in life.
4. Family members encourage each other to "keep going" when life is difficult.
5. Growth in positive directions is mutually encouraged within the family.

TABLE 6-7 continued

6. Health is nurtured as a positive family resource.
7. Personal strengths and capabilities are nurtured.

Family Support

1. Family has a number of friends or relatives that they see frequently.
2. Family is involved in community activities and groups.
3. Family members frequently praise each other.
4. In times of distress, the family can call on a number of other families or individuals for help.
5. Disagreements are settled through discussion rather than verbal abuse or physical violence.
6. Family members model healthy habits for each other.
7. Professional support services are sought when needed.

TABLE 6-8 Components of Community Assessment

Human Biology

1. Composition of population by age, gender, and race
2. Population patterns of longevity
3. Genetic inheritance patterns by gender and race
4. Disease incidence and prevalence compared to prior years, and to state and national statistics
5. Health status indicators (immunization levels, nutritional status, mobility)

Environment

1. Physical environment (urban/rural/suburban, housing, water supply, parks and recreation, climate, topography, size, population density, aesthetics, natural or manmade resources, goods and services, health risks)
2. Psychologic environment (productivity level, cohesion, mental health status, communication networks, intergroup harmony, future orientation, prevalence of stressors)
3. Social environment (income and education levels, employment, family composition, religious affiliations, cultural affiliations, language(s) spoken, social services, organization profile, leadership and decision-making structures)

Community Lifestyles

1. Consumption patterns (eg. nutrition, alcohol)
2. Occupational groups
3. Leisure pursuits
4. Comunity health attitudes and beliefs
5. Patterns of health-related behaviors in aggregates
6. History of participation in community health action

Health System

1. Health care services available (health promotion, prevention, primary care, secondary care, tertiary care, mental health)
2. Accessibility of promotive and preventive care (low income, homeless, varying racial and ethnic groups)
3. Financing plans for health care

(Adapted from Clark MJ,[14,app] with permission.)
Clark MJ. *Nursing in the Community.* Stamford, Conn: Appleton & Lange; 1996.

Directions for Research in Health Assessment

Research that develops and tests new measurement and assessment tools for the health, health beliefs, and health behaviors of individuals and aggregates from diverse racial, cultural, and socioeconomic backgrounds is of high priority. The tools used in both clinical practice and research must be reliable and valid. Assessment tools should be based on theoretical or conceptual frameworks that provide the infrastructure for development of individual items and scales.

Directions for Practice in Health Assessment

Nurses must continue to develop and use diagnostic systems to document areas for improvement of the health status of the community. Nurses who use nursing classification systems and collect data with valid and reliable assessment instruments contribute to evidenced-based practice. Assessment data about health status, beliefs, and behaviors provide the basis for clinical judgments and influences appropriate individual, family, and community interventions. Nurses must use their knowledge and influence to ensure that a portfolio of assessment instruments is available and used in the work setting. The nurse must know how to administer assessment instruments and explain the value of conducting systematic assessments to the client. The busy work environment may discourage the use of some assessment instruments because they require time to administer and to follow up. One way the nurse can manage the time issue is to seek innovative ways to communicate with clients through videotapes played and loaned to clients and brochures that explain assessment procedures. As the knowledge about assessment grows, practicing nurses must keep up-to-date and current about new assessment tools and strategies that can be quickly performed and yet yield accurate data. Nurses can influence the quality of the health promotion plan of the individual, family, and community through a commitment to thorough assessment of health, health beliefs, and health behaviors.[59]

SUMMARY

Health assessment is carried out at the individual, family, and community levels. Because assessment is time intensive for the nurse and the client, tools for use must be carefully selected according to the client's characteristics and presenting health issues. The nurse and client should determine what assessments are needed and combine them into a portfolio for that particular client.

Information technology will increasingly make computerization of assessment tools possible. Thus, clients may be able to complete self-assessments at home as time allows, with transmission of the information via computer in advance of health care visits.

QUICK REFERENCE GUIDE FOR WEB SITES RELATED TO TOPICS IN CHAPTER 6

Special Tools

1. Tufts University Nutrition Navigator steers you to the best diet and nutrition sites. (*www.navigator.tufts.edu*) Government Sponsored Sites

2. Healthfinder (*www.healthfinder.gov*) Gateway to consumer health and human services information.

3. Centers for Disease Control (*www.cdc.gov*)

4. National Center for Health Statistics (*www.cdc.gov/nchswww*)

5. National Cancer Institute (*cancernet.nci.nih.gov*)

6. National Institutes of Health (*www.nih.gov*)

7. PubMed (*www.ncbi.nlm.nih.gov/PubMed*) Corporate Sites

8. Healthtouch (*www.healthtouch.com*) Information about prescription and over-the-counter medications.

REFERENCES

1. Stromborg FM. *Instruments for Clinical Nursing Research*. Boston, MA: Jones & Bartlett; 1997:111–151.

2. Wilkin D, Hallam L, Doggett M. *Measures of Need and Outcome for Primary Health Care*. Oxford: Oxford University Press; 1993.

3. North American Nursing Diagnosis Association. *Nursing Diagnosis: Definitions & Classifications 1999–2000*. Philadelphia: 3rd Edition Publisher: NANDA (North American Nursing Diagnosis Association 1999.

4. Gordon M. *Manual of Nursing Diagnosis: 1998–1999*. St. Louis: Mosby Year Book; 1999.

5. Martin KS, Norris J. The Omaha System: A model for describing practice. *Holist Nurs Pract*. 1996 Oct;11(1): 75–83.

6. Clark MJ. *Nursing in the Community*. Stamfort, CT: Appleton & Lange; 1999:124–130.

7. Moorhead SA, McCloskey JC, Bulecheck GM. Nursing interventions classifications. A comparison with the Omaha System and the Home Healthcare Classification. *J Nurs Adm*. 1993; Oct;23(10):23–29.

8. Houldin AD, Saltstein SW, Ganley KM. *Nursing Diagnosis for Wellness: Supporting Strengths*. Philadelphia: J.B. Lippincott Co.; 1987.

9. American College of Sports Medicine. *Guidelines for Exercise Testing and Prescription*. 6th ed. Baltimore, MD: Lippincott, Williams & Wilkins; 2000.

10. Cooper KH. *Fit Kids! The Complete Shape-Up Program from Birth through High School*. Nashville, TN: Broadman & Holman Publishers; 1999.

11. Katch FI, McArdle WD. *Nutrition, Weight Control and Exercise*. 4th ed. Philadelphia: Lea & Febiger; 1992.

12. Golding LA, Myers CR, Sinning WE. *The Y's Way to Physical Fitness*. 3rd ed. Champaign, IL: Human Kinetics; 1989.

13. American College of Sports Medicine. *ACSM's Resource Manual for Guidelines for Exercise Testing and Prescription*. 3rd ed. Baltimore, MD: Williams & Wilkins: A Waverly Company, 1998.

14. Gutierrez YM. *Nutrition in Health Maintenance and Health Promotion for Primary Care Providers*. San Francisco: University of California, San Francisco School of Nursing; 1994.

15. Jeejeebhoy KN. Nutritional assessment. *Nutrition*. July–Aug; 16(7–8):585–590.

16. Evans SN. Nutritional assessment. A practical approach. *Nurs Clin North Am*. 1997;2000 Dec;32(4):637–650.

17. Patient-Centered Assessment and Counseling for Exercise & Nutrition (PACE) 1999 by San Diego State University Foundation and San Diego Center for Health Interventions.

18. Hyner GC, Peterson KW, Travis JW, Dewey JE, Foerster JJ, Framer EM, eds. S*PM Handbook of Health Assessment Tools*. Pittsburg, PA: The Society of Prospective Medicine & The Institute for Health and Productivity Management. 1999.

19. Smith KW, McKinlay SM, Thorington BA. The validity of health risk appraisal instruments for assessing coronary heart disease risk. *Am J Public Health*. 1987;77:971–974.

20. Anderson ET, McFarlane, JM. *Community as Partner: Theory and Practice in Nursing*. 2nd ed. Philadelphia: J. B. Lippincott Co.; 1996.

21. Benson H, Stuart EM. *The Wellness Book*. New York: Birch Lane Press; 1992:379.

22. Clark MJ. *Nursing in the Community*. Stamford, CT: Appleton & Lange; 1996.

23. Sherman Z. Health risk appraisal at the worksite. *Am Assoc Occupational Health Nurs J*. 1990;38(1):18–24.

24. The impact of worksite-based health risk appraisal on health-related outcomes: A review of the literature. *Am J Health Prom*. 1996 July–Aug;10(6):499–508.

25. Derogatis LR, Fleming MP. *Evaluating Stress. The Derogatis Stree Provile (DSP): A Theory Driven Approach to Stress Measurement*. Lanham, MD: Scarecrow Press; 1997:113.

26. Cohen S, Kessler RC, Gordon LU. *Measuring Stress*. New York: Oxford University Press; New York:1995.

27. Selye BL. Stress, coping, and health. In: Rice V; ed. *Handbook of Stress, Coping, and Health*. Thousand Oaks: Sage Publications; 2000.

28. Spielberger CD, Gorsuch RL, Lushene R, et al. *Manual for State-Trait Anxiety Inventory*. Palo Alto, CA: Consulting Psychologists Press, Inc.: 1983.

29. Kanner AD, Feldman SS. Control over uplifts and hassles and its relationship to adaptational outcomes. *J Behav Med*. 1991;14:187–201.

30. Zyzanski SJ, Wright AL. Life events and daily hassles and uplifts as predictors of hospitalization and outpatient visitation. *Soc Sci Med*. 1992;34:763–768.

31. Spielberger CD, Edwards CD, Lushene RE, et al. *State-Trait Anxiety Inventory for Children—Preliminary Manual*. Palo Alto, CA: Mind Garden; 1973.

32. Ryan-Wenger NM, Sharrer VW, Wynd CA. In: Rice V, ed. *Handbook of Stress, Coping, and Health*. Thousand Oaks: Sage Publications; 1999.

33. Younger JB. Development and testing of The Mastery of Stress Instrument. *Nurs Res*. 1993:42:68–73.

34. McBride JL, Arthur G, Brooks R, Pilkington L. The relationship between a patient's spirituality and health experiences. *Fam Med*. 1998 Feb;30 (2):122–126.

35. Hatch RL, Burg MA, Naberhaus DS, Hellmich LK. The Spiritual Involvement and Beliefs Scale. Development and testing of a new instrument. *J Fam Pract*. 1998 Jun;46(6):476–486.

36. Greenstreet WM. Teaching spirituality in nursing: A literature review. *Nurse Educ Today*. 1999 Nov;19(8):649–658.

37. Perrin KM, McDermott RJ. Instruments to measure social support and related constructs in pregnant adolescents; a review. *Adolescence*. 1997 Fall;32(127):533–557.

38. Wallston KA, Wallston BS, Devellis R. Development of the multidimensional health locus of control (MHLC) scales. *Health Educ Monogr.* 1978;6:161–170.

39. Smith MS, Wallston KA, Smith CA. The development and validation of the Perceived Health Competence Scale. *Health Educ Res.* 1995;10(1):51–64.

40. Laffrey SC. Development of a health conception scale. *Res Nurs Health.* 1986;9:107–113.

41. Cox C. The Health Self-Determinism Index. *Nurs Res.* 1985;34:177–183.

42. Cox C. The Health Self-Determinism Index for Children. *Res Nurs Health.* 1990;31:237–246.

43. Sechrist KR, Walker SN, Pender NJ. Development and psychometric evaluation of the Exercise Benefits/Barrier Scale. *Res Nurs Health.* 1987;10:357–365.

44. Steinhardt MA, Dishman RK. Reliability and validity of expected outcomes and barriers for habitual physical activity. *J Occup Med.* 1989;31:536–546.

45. Pender NJ. The Adolescent Lifestyle Profile (ALP): Assessing health-related behaviors. (1997) Unpublished manuscript.

46. Prochaska JO, Velicer WF, Rossi JS et al. Stages of change and decisional balance for 12 problem behaviors. *Health Psychol.* 1994;13(1):39–46.

47. Friedman MN. *Family Nursing: Research Theory and Practice.* 4th ed. New York: Appleton-Century-Crofts; 1998.

48. Gershwin MW, Nilsen JM. Healthy families: Forms and processes. In: Gilliss CL, Highly BL, Roberts BM, et al., eds. *Toward a Science of Family Nursing.* Menlo Park, CA: Addison-Wesley Publishing Co., Inc.; 1989:77–91.

49. Whall AL. Nursing theory and assessment of families. *J Psychiatr Nurs.* 1981;19:30–39.

50. Wright LM, Leahey M. *Nurses and Families: A Guide to Family Assessment and Intervention.* Philadelphia: F. A. Davis Co.; 2000.

51. Mischke-Berkey K, Warner P, Hanson S. Family health assessment and intervention. In: Bomar PJ, ed. *Nurses and Family Health Promotion: Concepts, Assessments, and Interventions.* Baltimore, MD: Williams & Wilkins; 1996.

52. Sawin KJ, Harrington MP, Wood P. *Measures of Family Functioning for Research and Practice.* New York: Springer; 1995.

53. Haglund B, Weisbrod RR, Bracht N. Assessing the community: Its services, needs, leadership, and readiness. In: Bracht N, ed. *Health Promotion at the Community Level.* Newbury Park, CA: Sage Publications; 1999.

54. *Healthy People 2010.* Washington DC: U.S. Public Health and Human Services publications PHS 91-50212.

55. Goeppinger J. Community as client: Using the nursing process to promote health. In: Stahope M, Lancaster J, eds. *Community Health Nursing: Process and Practice for Promoting Health.* St. Louis: Mosby; 1996.

56. Spradley BW, Alexander JA. *Community Health Nursing: Concepts and Practice.* Philadelphia: J.B. Lippincott Co., 1996.

57. Helvie C. *Advanced Practice Nursing in the Community.* Thousand Oaks: Sage Publications; 1998.

58. *Guide to Clinical Preventive Services: Report of the U.S. Preventive Services Task Force.* 2nd ed. Baltimore, MD: 1996. AMA Council on Scientific Affairs.

59. Hitchcock JE, Schubert DE, Thomas SA. *Community Health Nursing: Caring in Action.* Albany, NY: Delmar Publishers; 1999.

60. Aspen Reference Group. *Community Health: Education and Promotion.* Gaithersburg, MD: Aspen Publishers, Inc.; 1997.

$\underline{7}$

Developing a Health Protection and Promotion Plan

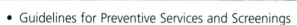

- Guidelines for Preventive Services and Screenings
- The Health-Planning Process
  - A. Review and Summarize Data from Assessment
  - B. Reinforce Strengths and Competencies of the Client
  - C. Identify Health Goals and Related Behavior-Change Options
  - D. Identify Behavioral or Health Outcomes
  - E. Develop a Behavior-Change Plan
  - F. Reiterate Benefits of Change
  - G. Address Environmental and Interpersonal Facilitators and Barriers to Change
  - H. Determine a Time Frame for Implementation
  - I. Commit to Behavior-Change Goals
- Revisions of the Health Protection–Promotion Plan
- Community-Level Health Protection–Promotion Plan
- Directions for Research in Behavior Change
- Directions for Practice in Health Planning
- Summary

Clients should be active participants in interpreting the assessment data and in health care planning. Client collaboration with the nurse in planning for care promotes positive perceptions of worth and affirms the ability of individuals, families, or communities to self-regulate and function on their own behalf in improving health and creating conditions supportive of healthy lifestyles. The role of the nurse is to *assist* clients with health planning rather than to *control* the process. During assessment, the nurse and client develop a mutual understanding of (1) the health and risk status of the client; (2) current health-behavior patterns of the client; (3) attitudes and beliefs that affect health and health-related behaviors of the client; (4) expectations of important referent groups; (5) behavioral options potentially available to the client; (6) the interaction of social-ethnic-cultural background with health practices; (7) potential or actual barriers to health-protecting and -promoting self-care; and (8) existing support systems for health-promoting behaviors. Developing a systematic plan for behavior change provides an opportunity for the client to express stabilizing and actualizing tendencies in purposeful ways directed toward increasing wellness and enhancing life satisfaction.

Health planning is a dynamic process in which flexibility to meet the changing needs of clients is critical. The plan systematically lends direction but does not dictate goals that must be attained or behaviors that must be learned. The health protection–promotion plan should be reasonable in terms of both demands on the client and the time frame allocated for accomplishment of desired health or health-related goals. Knowledge, skills, and strengths of the client should be utilized in the planning process. Capitalizing on positive health practices currently a part of personal or family lifestyle creates a sense of competence or efficacy as well as the behavioral control essential to successful behavior change. The nurse and the client should together assess the stage of change (precontemplation, contemplation, preparation, action, and maintenance) for behaviors the client wishes to modify. The client can then discuss with the nurse strategies for change that are likely to be most effective. The plan should be revised as needed to make behavior change a positive growth experience for clients. The ultimate goal of health planning and implementation is to make health protection and health promotion a way of life that individuals, families, and communities can manage and enjoy.

Innovative developments in information technology increasingly allow personalization of assessment and intervention protocols to the unique characteristics and needs of individual clients. Nurses should be actively involved in the design of health assessment and health-planning software that is interactive and client friendly.

Guidelines for Preventive Services and Screenings

With increasing emphasis on the prevention of disease, varying sets of guidelines for the delivery of preventive services to individuals and families throughout the life span have been developed. These guidelines focus on clinical care directed toward protection from specific diseases such as AIDS or behavioral morbidity such as substance abuse. The 1995 *Guide to Clinical Preventive Services,* 2nd edition, recommended screenings as an important component of health protection. The value and benefits of age-specific periodic screenings based on gender and individual risk factors are available from the Office of Disease Prevention and Health Promotion Web site odphp.osophs.dhhs.gov/ bubs.guidecps. The U.S. Preventive Services Task Force identified counseling clients about their personal health habits as one of the most important components of the health visit.[1] Nurses in all settings where primary care is delivered should become familiar with the following sets of guidelines to make sure that their clients benefit from "state-of-the-science" preventive services: *Guide to Clinical Preventive Services*[1], *Clinician's Handbook of Preventive Services: Put Prevention into Practice,*[2] *AMA Guidelines for Adolescent Preventive Services: Recommendations and Rationale,*[3] and *Bright Futures: Guidelines for Health Supervision of Infants, Children, and Adolescents.*[4] These publications provide recommendations and rationale for a wide array of preventive maneuvers.

The Health-Planning Process

The process for developing a health protection–promotion plan is outlined below, with each step in the process discussed separately. These nine steps actively involve both the client and the nurse in the health-planning process:

1. Review and summarize data from assessment.
2. Reinforce strengths and competencies of the client.
3. Identify health goals and related behavioral change options.
4. Identify behavioral or health outcomes that will indicate that the plan has been successful from the client's perspective.
5. Develop a behavior change plan based on the client's preferences, on the stages of change, and on "state-of-the science" knowledge about effective interventions.
6. Reiterate benefits of change and identify incentives for change from the client's perspective.
7. Address environmental and interpersonal facilitators and barriers to behavior change.
8. Determine a time frame for implementation.
9. Commit to behavior-change goals and to structure the support needed to accomplish them.

Review and Summarize Data from Assessment

During assessment, a wealth of information is shared between nurse and client. The reduction of this information to manageable proportions is accomplished by summarizing qualitative data and calculating scores and subscores on the various instruments employed in assessment of a specific client. From assessment activities, the nurse and client should have information available in the following domains as a basis for planning and action:

1. Physical health status
2. Status in relation to functional health patterns

3. Physical fitness
4. Nutritional status
5. Major health risks
6. Sources of life stress
7. Spirituality
8. Social support
9. Key health beliefs
10. Health-related lifestyle
11. Family health beliefs and practices
12. Environmental and community supports or constraints for health behaviors

The nurse during one or more clinic appointments or home visits can guide clients through the data summary process. Both nurse and client should retain a copy of the assessment summary for continuing reference during the health-planning process.

Reinforce Strengths and Competencies of the Client

Each individual or family seen by the nurse already has in place a system of health care practices compatible with its cultural orientation. Thus, the nurse and client should achieve consensus on areas in which the client is already taking informed and responsible health action as well as on areas for further development of self-care competencies. Clients bring unique strengths to the health-planning task. These assets should be identified, acknowledged, and reinforced by the nurse. Because clients will carry out health behaviors in ways that fit their cultural beliefs, preferences, and current levels of knowledge and skill, existing cultural practices supportive of health should be integrated into the overall health plan. The client's sense of cultural or ethnic pride should be reinforced during the health-planning process.

Through teaching, guidance, and support, the nurse nurtures and enhances existing competencies to meet health needs. Self-care requirements and resources of individuals will vary according to age, gender, developmental stage, and health status. The self-care needs of families may vary by family composition, developmental tasks being confronted, and role demands. Although clients will differ in their self-care and self-management competencies, it is important that the nurse emphasize to all clients their own importance as "primary self-care agent." Promoting client responsibility for health does not negate the importance of the nurse working to change the larger social infrastructure to make health-promoting options more available to communities. Personal change and social change are both essential for effective health protection and promotion.

A sample health protection–promotion plan for an individual client is presented in Figure 7–1 and one for a family in Figure 7–2. In both planning tools, sections in which client strengths can be identified are provided.

Designed for: ___James Moore___

Home Address: ___714 George___

Home Telephone Number: ___222–3333___

Occupation (if employed): ___building services supervisor___

Work Telephone Number: ___445-6666___

Cultural Identification: ___African American___

Birth Date: ___3/14/55___ Date of Initial Plan: ___1/15/2001___

Client strengths:	Satisfactory peer relationships, spiritual strength, adequate sleep pattern
Major risk factors:	Elevated cholesterol, mild obesity, sedentary lifestyle, moderate life change, multiple daily hassles, few reported uplifts
Nursing diagnoses: (derived from assessment of functional health patterns)	Diversional activity deficit; altered nutrition: more than body requirements; caregiver role strain (elderly mother)
Medical diagnoses: (if any)	Mild hypertension
Age-specific screening recommendations: (derived from Guide to Clinical Prev. Services)	Blood pressure, cholesterol, fecal occult blood, malignant skin lesions, depression
Desired behavioral and health outcomes:	Become a regular exerciser (3x/week), lower my blood pressure, weigh 165 lb

continued on next page

FIGURE 7-1 Example of an Individual Health Protection–Promotion Plan

Personal Health Goals (1 = highest priority)	Selected Behaviors to Accomplish Goals	Stage of Change	Strategies/ Interventions for Change
1. Achieve desired body weight	Begin a progressive walking program	Planning	Counter-conditioning Reinforcement management Patient contracting
	Decrease caloric intake while maintaining good nutrition	Action (eating 2 fruits and 2 vegetables daily; using low-fat dairy products for last 2 months)	Stimulus control Cognitive restructuring
2. Decrease risk for hypertension-related disorders	Change from high- to low-sodium snacks	Contemplation	Consciousness raising Learning facilitation
3. Learn to manage stress effectively	Attend relaxation classes and use home relaxation tapes	Contemplation	Consciousness raising Self-re-evaluation Simple relaxation therapy
4. Increase leisure-time activities	Join a local bowling league	Contemplation	Support system enhancement

FIGURE 7-1 Example of an Individual Health Protection–Promotion Plan (*continued*)

Designed for (family name): ___The Marshalls___

Home Address: ___1718 Green St.___

Home Telephone Number: ___777-4444___

Occupations of Employed
Members of Household: ___Mother—Dental assistant___

Work Telephone Number: ___883-7777___

Family Form: ___One-parent family___

Cultural Identification: ___Asian American___

Family Members:	Position in Family	Birth Date	Occupation/ Student/Retired
	Joan (Mother)	9/35	Dental assistant
	Dana (Daughter)	4/87	Student
	Tiffany (Daughter)	7/91	Student
	Eric (Son)	1/94	Student

Date of Initial Plan: ___1-15-2001___

Family strengths:	Open communication patterns, intrafamily cooperation, healthy snacks consumed at home
Major risk factors:	Mother recently divorced, oldest daughter has driver's license, high life change for family, minimal family physical activity
Nursing diagnoses:	Family coping: potential for growth
Medical diagnoses for family members:	None
Desired behavioral and health outcomes:	Active family outings, avoidance of early sexual activity and binge drinking among adolescent family members, injury prevention for children, adjustment to new family form

continued on next page

FIGURE 7-2 Example of a Family Health Protection–Promotion Plan

Family Health Goals (1 = highest priority)	Selected Behaviors to Accomplish Goals	Stage of Change	Strategies/ Interventions for Change
1. Healthy adjustment to single-parent family status	Realign family responsibilities	Action (divorced 3 mo)	Social liberation Family process maintenance Caregiver support
	Increase spiritual resources (increase church attendance)	Contemplation	Spiritual support Helping relationships
	Discuss life purpose and goals among family members	Planning	Self-re-evaluation Self-esteem enhancement Anticipatory guidance
2. Develop more active family lifestyles	Plan active family outings (biking, recreation center)	Planning	Exercise promotion Environmental re-evaluation Modeling
3. Foster healthy sexuality among preadolescent and adolescents	Provide age-appropriate information	Action	Anticipatory guidance Parent education: adolescent stage
	Enhance self-esteem through praise, expression of affection, and assistance with skill development	Maintenance	Self-esteem enhancement Helping relationships

FIGURE 7-2 Example of a Family Health Protection–Promotion Plan
(*continued*)

| 4. Encourage adolescents to avoid alcohol use | Hold family meetings to discuss binge drinking, drinking and driving, use of nonalcoholic alternatives | Contemplation | Parent education: adolescent stage Self-responsibility facilitation Substance use prevention |

FIGURE 7-2 Example of a Family Health Protection–Promotion Plan (*continued*)

Identify Health Goals and Related Behavior-Change Options

The next step in the planning process is to identify personal or family health goals, prioritize them, and review related behavior-change options. Systematically reviewing the range of changes that are possible to achieve important health goals can assist clients in making informed choices concerning the behavioral changes on which they will focus in the initial health protection–promotion plan. Providing relevant information but letting the client determine priorities for change constitutes educative–supportive care by the nurse. Clients should not be made to feel guilty or inadequate in regard to current health practices. During health counseling sessions, the nurse should create enthusiasm and excitement about growth in positive directions and about enjoyment of new health-related experiences.

Many clients will initially place high priority on areas of health protection in which the threat of illness is tangible and easily understood. Decreasing risk for specific chronic health problems fits the medical orientation to which most Americans have been socialized. A high level of client interest in risk reduction indicates to the nurse that health protection is likely the most meaningful area for emphasis in early health planning. Mastery of specific health protection measures will often motivate clients to consider making additional lifestyle changes directed toward health promotion in order to experience a higher level of health and well-being.

Clients often give important emotional cues concerning the behaviors they wish to change. Examples of such cues include:

"I hate myself when I gorge on fattening foods!"

"I get mad at myself for being so uptight!"

"I feel very sad when I think of how little time our family spends together."

The more open an individual or family is in discussing health concerns with the nurse, the higher the probability of developing a meaningful health protection–promotion plan. Often areas that the client is reluctant to discuss; such as marital relationships, human sexuality, spirituality, and family cohesiveness; are the most crucial areas for behavior change in order to enhance well-being. A "safe" climate should be created in which the client can discuss health issues of highest personal concern with assurance that communication will remain confidential.

Identify Behavioral or Health Outcomes

It is critical that the nurse and client together determine the desired health outcomes from implementation of the health protection–promotion plan. Clear identification of outcomes both energizes and guides the client in health behaviors. The client's perceptions concerning the outcomes desired should determine the criteria that will be used to evaluate whether the plan and its implementation have been successful. Have I reached my goal or made significant progress toward it is a critical question that must be asked periodically by the client to evaluate the viability of the health protection–promotion plan.

Research literature that supports the link between particular interventions and desired outcomes should influence the nursing process and the plan that is developed. For example, the factors or strategies that have been shown to affect the likelihood of maintaining a healthy diet should be integrated into the plan for persons wishing to address nutritional issues. The nurse should be cautious about the outcomes selected. For example, a behavioral goal of eating only at meals may be easier to attain than a goal of losing a certain number of pounds. Weight will most likely be lost if the plan is followed, but tangible behaviors are more under the control of the client and thus easier to reinforce and manage. Long-term outcomes can be set but achieved through a progressive set of short-term outcomes that move the client toward the desired endpoints.

Develop a Behavior-Change Plan

A constructive program of change is based on the client taking "ownership" of those behavior changes selected for implementation within everyday life. The client should be assisted in examining major value–behavior inconsistencies that exist. Alternative actions that are both healthful and enjoyable to the client need to be substituted for the behaviors that are inconsistent with personal values. It is unfortunate that what individuals and families have learned to prefer or value within the American lifestyle frequently can be detrimental to health. Values clarification can be a useful tool in the development of a behavior-change plan.[5–7]

At this point, clients should select from all the behavioral options available those behaviors that are appealing and that they are willing to try. This brings clients full circle from assessing current health status and lifestyle, through considering health goals and behavioral options, to actually identifying those behavior changes they are willing to adopt in order to accomplish desired goals and achieve health outcomes. The client's priorities for behavior change will reflect personal values, activity preferences, estimates of cognitive and psychomotor skills, affective responses to the various behavioral options, expectations for success in learning and carrying out the various behaviors, and ease with which the selected behaviors can be integrated into lifestyle. The stage of change of the client in relation to each of the selected behaviors should be assessed.

Appropriate strategies and interventions to facilitate behavior change can be identified from the nursing intervention classification systems,[8–11] from transtheoretical model literature,[12] or from literature in nursing and the behavioral sciences on behavior change. The nurse should develop expertise with implementing behavior-change interventions, including the activities that constitute the intervention and the appropriate sequencing of those activities. As the expert health care provider with skill in behavior-change facilitation, the nurse can assist the client in gaining the self-change skills needed for the adoption and maintenance of positive health behaviors.

Reiterate Benefits of Change

Although clients are aware of the changes they want to make and the benefits of change, these benefits need to be frequently reiterated by both the nurse and the client. The client should keep a list of benefits from the changes being made in a highly visible place so that they can be reviewed frequently. This may be on the refrigerator, the bathroom mirror, the dashboard of the car, or the computer at the workplace. Keeping health benefits "in front" of the client is a reminder that the behaviors in the health promotion plan are personally worthwhile and directed toward important life goals.

The benefits of change may include both health-related and non-health-related outcomes anticipated by the client. Although nurses tend to think in terms of health benefits, sensitivity to non-health-related benefits of change such as increased popularity or more time with friends is important as these may be central to the client's motivation to engage in health protection–promotion planning and implementation.

Address Environmental and Interpersonal Facilitators and Barriers to Change

Environmental features and interpersonal relationships that support positive change should be used to bolster the client's efforts to modify lifestyle. Facilitators can be used to counter barriers to change and encourage the client when problems occur in the behavior-change process. Both instrumental and emotional support from their social network are important in encouraging clients to persist with change efforts when the going gets difficult or competing demands or preferences vie for attention.

All individuals and families experience barriers to changing behavior. Although some obstacles cannot be anticipated, others can be planned for and their potential negative impact considerably weakened. If the client is aware of possible barriers and has formulated plans for dealing with them if they arise, successful behavior change is more likely to occur.

Barriers to effective health behavior can arise from clients' internal conflicts, from significant others, or from the environment. Internal barriers to change may be lack of motivation, fatigue, boredom, giving up, lack of appropriate skills, or disbelief that behavior can be successfully changed. Family members can impose considerable barriers if they encourage continuation of health-damaging behaviors or if they actively discourage attempts at behavior change. Environmental barriers that may inhibit positive change include lack of space or appropriate setting in which to carry out the selected activity; dangers within the immediate environment, such as heavy traffic or high crime rate; or inclement weather. The nurse can assist the client in dealing with these environmental barriers or in locating another setting appropriate for health activities.

Determine a Time Frame for Implementation

Progress toward healthier lifestyles needs to be made over a period of time in order to allow new behaviors to be learned well, integrated into one's lifestyle, and stabilized. Attempting to change or initiate a number of new behaviors all at once may result in confusion, discouragement, and the client's abandonment of the health protection–promotion plan. Whether the client is attempting to reduce risk for chronic diseases or to enhance health status, gradual rather than abrupt change is desirable. Just as health education for self-care must proceed at the pace of the learner rather than at that of the nurse, changes in behavior must be sequenced in reasonable steps appropriate for the client.

Developing a time plan for implementation allows appropriate knowledge and skills to be mastered before a new behavior is implemented. For example, it is difficult to warm up before brisk walking or jogging if the client has no idea of what appropriate warm-up exercises are. The time frame for developing a given behavior may be several weeks or several months. If the client is rewarded for accomplishing short-term goals, this provides encouragement for continuing pursuit of long-term goals and desired outcomes. A meaningful plan requires that deadlines be set for accomplishing specific goals. Adherence to deadlines should be encouraged, with changes made only when the time frame must be shortened or lengthened to make it more conducive to permanent behavior change.

Commit to Behavior-Change Goals

Through identification of new behaviors that the client is willing to try, a verbal commitment is made to change. However, the client may be more motivated to follow through with selected actions if the personal commitment is formalized. A commitment to change can be formalized in a number of ways. They are (1) nurse–client contract agreements like those that appear in Figures 7–3 and 7–4, (2) self-contracts such as those shown in Figures 7–5 and 7–6, (3) public announcements to family members and friends of intentions to engage in new behaviors, (4) integration of new health behaviors into daily or weekly calendar, and (5) purchase of necessary supplies (e.g., low-fat foods, relaxation audiotapes) and equipment (e.g., exercise bike, walking shoes).

Behavioral contracts contain specific information about (1) the change to be made, (2) the way the change is to be accomplished, (3) the individual or family members who are to engage in the change, (4) the time frame for behavior change, and (5) the consequences of meeting or not meeting the terms of the agreement. A *nurse–client contract* provides direction for the helping relationship through identification of mutual objectives and responsibilities of each party to the contract. Contracts allow clients to participate actively in their own care by choosing goals that can be realistically accomplished. Generally, the client is responsible for carrying out certain behaviors, whereas the nurse is responsible for providing information, training, counseling, or specific reinforcement rewards. The nurse, as the health care professional involved in the contract, bears the additional responsibility of providing helpful input and continuing feedback to the client concerning the adequacy of performance of activities identified in the contract. It is also critical that the nurse be consistent and conscientious in managing the reinforcement–reward contingencies of the contract.

Nurse–Client Contract and Agreement

Statement of Health Goal: _Decreased feelings of stress and tension_

I _Jim Johnson_ promise to _use progressive relaxation_
(client)

techniques (four-muscle groups) upon arriving home from work each day
(Client Responsibility)

for a period of _one week_ , whereupon,

Kathy Turner will provide _a copy of_
(nurse)

Herbert Benson's book, Relaxation Response
(Nurse Responsibility)

on _Saturday, March 7th_ to me.
(date)

If I do not fulfill the terms of this contract in total, I understand that the designated reward will be withheld.

Signed: _____
(client)

_____
(date)

_____
(nurse)

_____
(date)

FIGURE 7-3 Sample nurse–client contract for an individual client

---

Nurse–Client Contract and Agreement

Statement of Health Goal: _____ *Improve eating habits* _____

We _____ *The Nichols* _____ promise to __*eat two servings of*__
              (family)

_____ *vegetables and two servings of fruit daily* _____
         (family responsibility)

for a period of _____ *one week* _____ whereupon,

_____ *Lana Buxton* _____ will provide _____ *guest passes* _____
         (nurse)

_____ *Riverbanks Zoo* _____
         (nurse responsibility)

on _____ *Friday, April 10th* _____ to us.
         (date)

If we do not fulfill the terms of this contract in total, We understand that the designated reward will be withheld.

    Signed: _____
                  (family representative)

             _____
                        (date)

             _____
                       (nurse)

             _____
                        (date)

FIGURE 7-4 Sample nurse–client contract for a family

```
                           Self-Contract

Personal Health Goal: _____ Change Dietary Habits _____

I _____ Doris Downs _____ promise myself that I will _follow_

_____ the sample menus for a 1,200 calorie diet for breakfast, lunch, and

_____ dinner _____ for a period of _____ four days _____ ,

whereupon I will _____ buy myself a new pair of earrings _____

on _____ Wednesday, June 8th _____ .



         Signed _____


         Date   _____
```

FIGURE 7-5 Sample individual self-contract

```
                           Self-Contract

Family Health Goal: _____ Get more exercise _____

We _____ The Stones _____ promise each other that we will ___ go ___

_____ swimming at the "Y" once a week _____ for a period of __ three weeks __

whereupon we will _____ buy the newest version of Trivial Pursuit _____

on _____ Friday, February 10th _____ .


         Signed: _____

                 _____

                 _____



         Date    _____
```

FIGURE 7-6 Sample family self-contract

Failure in fulfilling this commitment will destroy the trust and confidence placed in the nurse by the client.

In a nurse–client contract with a family, the agreement may be made to brisk walk, jog, or bicycle together two to three times each week or to modify their nutritional practices, such as increasing vegetables in their diet to three to four servings per day. Family members, because of their continuing contact and emotional bonding, can serve as important sources of encouragement, reinforcement, and reward for one another.

The extent to which the contract has worked must be evaluated. Did the client accomplish the goal fully, partially, or not at all? If failure occurred, what were the reasons? How could the contract be reorganized so that the probability of successful completion is high? Does the contract need to be renegotiated? Should the contract be terminated? Careful analysis of the contracting process and evaluation of subsequent outcomes will permit the nurse and client to design contracts that successfully move clients toward desired health goals.

In a *self-contract* the client is responsible both for the behavioral commitment and for reinforcement of identified behaviors. Self-contracting is an effective approach for enhancing the client's control over behavior, thus creating a sense of independence, competence, and autonomy. The client does not become overly dependent on the nurse for reinforcement but instead serves as the source of rewards for positive health behaviors. Rewards may be extrinsic such as tangible objects (magazine, cosmetics) or experiences (warm bath, telephone call to a friend), or intrinsic (self-praise, feelings of pride). Rewards selected should be highly desirable to the client in order to have reinforcement value. A reward–reinforcement plan can be developed as illustrated in Figure 7–7.

Success in fulfilling the agreements in the contract enhances the client's self-esteem and problem-solving abilities. The client gains increased confidence in meeting future health needs. In reality, it is the client who must learn to manage a self-reward system that is supportive of new positive health practices.

Publicly announcing intentions to engage in a new behavior to family members and close friends is still another way of solidifying commitment to a particular course of action. The expectations of significant others that the client will follow through with the designated behavior can trigger personal encouragement and emotional and instrumental support on the part of significant others that enhance motivation for behavior.

Integrating new behaviors into one's calendar is an important way of building them into daily routines. For example, exercise time can be scheduled during the lunch hour and the appointment for exercise kept just like an appointment with one's boss or coworker. Lack of time is a frequent excuse for being unable to follow through with newly adopted behaviors. When time is actually scheduled to accomplish health behaviors, the probability of their occurrence is significantly enhanced.

Purchasing necessary supplies and equipment is still another way of making a commitment to behavior change. When equipment is purchased and a monetary investment is made, clients are much more likely to follow through with the desired behavior. For example, people who have exercise equipment and exercise videos in their home are more likely to be active than persons who do not.

Behavior: Learn to Use Progressive Relaxation as One Approach to Handling Stress	
Component of Behavior	**Reward or Reinforcement**
Attend first class session at 9 A.M. Saturday at the County Health Department	Watch the football game in the afternoon on TV
Use relaxation audiotape at home for 20 minutes of practice	
Sunday	Call John and visit for a while
Monday	Spend an hour at the driving range
Tuesday	Buy a new paperback novel
Wednesday	Praise myself for having practiced relaxation each day thus far
Thursday	Invite Harry and Jim over to play pool
Friday	Take my family to a movie
Attend second class session at 9 A.M. Saturday at the County Health Department	Take an orange juice break afterward with Bret, a class member
Practice relaxation techniques for 20 minutes providing my own cues rather than using the tape	
Sunday	Go for a short drive and enjoy the scenery
Monday	Spend 30 minutes reading my new novel
Tuesday	Buy myself a new bottle of aftershave lotion
Wednesday	Praise myself for persistence and successful practice
Thursday	Allow myself to linger in a warm shower longer than usual
Friday	Go biking with the family
Keep my weekly record of relaxation practice	The nurse will provide a copy of *Relaxation Response* by Herbert Benson

FIGURE 7-7 Reward-reinforcement plan

Revisions of the Health Protection–Promotion Plan

A schedule for periodic review of the health protection–promotion plan should be established. Revisions should be carried out during counseling sessions, with both the client and the nurse contributing to the process. Impetus for changes in the plan may result from mastery of target behaviors, changes in client's values and priorities, or awareness of new options available to the client. Outdated plans fail to provide impetus or direction for change and thus become uninteresting and meaningless to the client. Periodic revision and updating of the health plan provides a systematic approach for movement of the client toward higher levels of health behavior and health.

Community-Level Health Protection–Promotion Plan

For progress toward some health goals, community-level plans and interventions may be the most effective way to engage members in improving their health. Important health concerns such as youth and family violence, initiation of tobacco use, unintended pregnancy in adolescents, and unintentional injuries may require broad-based planning and intervention. School-based curricular[13,14] and community programs[15,16] may be the most effective way to address these health problems. The nurse must be aware of community-based initiatives and encourage client participation. The nurse may also serve as a consultant to communities implementing programs and be an advocate for developing community-based health plans and interventions.[17,18]

Directions for Research in Behavior Change

Many nursing research questions relative to planning for health protection and health promotion can be identified. Nurses are in a pivotal position to address these questions and create new knowledge about the behavior-change process. Questions to be addressed include

1. How can face-to-face and computerized feedback from health assessment be combined to optimize level of motivation for health protection and promotion planning?
2. To what extent do nurses reinforce clients' positive cultural health practices during health counseling?
3. During what stages of change for a given health behavior is intrinsic motivation likely to be more effective than extrinsic motivation?
4. What factors affect the tempo of behavior change at different life stages?
5. To what extent does successful behavior change increase beliefs concerning self-esteem, self-efficacy, and behavioral control?

6. To what extent does a community intervention improve the health of its members?

7. What community-based interventions are effective in improving the health of special populations?

Directions for Practice in Health Planning

Developing a plan to counsel clients about their health behaviors is a major responsibility of nurses in practice. The nurse must possess the skills necessary to be able to implement all of the steps outlined in order to guide clients to participate in developing a realistic, positive plan. Nurses with a working knowledge of current guidelines will insure that accurate, up-to-date information is incorporated into the plan. Understanding all information obtained from the assessment may mean that other disciplines are consulted to help interpret information or recommend appropriate goals. An interdisciplinary approach in which multiple experts are available enables the client and nurse to set appropriate goals and strategies to meet these goals. Support is critical during the change process, so the nurse also needs to learn to identify family and other significant support for the client, and to develop creative strategies to incorporate their support into the plan. The plan must be adapted to life-span issues, gender differences, as well as socioeconomic status. Knowledge of cultural issues that may play a role is key to the design of a culturally sensitive, age- and gender-appropriate plan. Last, whenever possible, technology should be incorporated when developing the plan. Interactive software that provides feedback on meeting goals and achieving outcomes and provides an opportunity for ongoing review of the plan may motivate clients, as they see the immediate results of their input. Developing a health protection–promotion plan is straightforward, but complex, and the nurse will need to continually update skills to assist clients in this important process.

SUMMARY

The health protection–promotion plans presented in this chapter provide individuals and families with a systematic approach to improving health practices and lifestyle. All clients should be provided with a health portfolio that contains a summary of their health assessment, their health protection–promotion plan, and other relevant health records. It is imperative that clients take home all the information and planning documents needed to follow through successfully with their desired behavior changes. Focusing on outcomes desired by the client will energize and direct implementation of the plan. Adjusting the plan as needed to insure client success is vital to effective health-protective and -promoting care. Community-level plans that address broad-based health concerns are being developed. Increasing evidence supports the efficacy and effectiveness of developing health protection-–promotion plans at the community level.

REFERENCES

1. U.S. Preventive Services Task Force. *Guide to Clinical Preventive Services.* 2nd ed. Baltimore, MD: Williams & Wilkins; 1995.'

2. U.S. Public Health Service. *Clinician's Handbook of Preventive Services: Put Prevention into Practice.* Waldorf, MD: American Nurses Publishing; 1994.

3. American Medical Association. *AMA Guidelines for Adolescent Preventive Services: Recommendations and Rationale.* Baltimore, MD: Williams & Wilkins; 1994.

4. Green M, ed. *Bright Futures: Guidelines for Health Supervision of Infants, Children, and Adolescents.* Arlington, VA: National Center for Education in Maternal and Child Health, 1994.

5. Chitty K. *Professional Nursing: Concepts and Challenges.* Chattanooga, TN: University of Tennessee at Chattanooga, 1997; 178–180.

6. Townsend MC. *Psychiatric Mental Health Nursing : Concepts of Care.* 3rd ed. Oklahoma City: 1996; 81–83.

7. Potter PA, Perry AG. *Fundamentals of Nursing: Concepts, Process and Practice.* St. Louis: Mosby; 1997:312–315.

8. McCloskey JC, Bulecheck GM, eds. *Nursing Interventions Classification (NIC): Iowa Intervention Project.* St Louis: Mosby Year Book; 2000.

9. Bowles KH, Naylor MS. *Nursing Intervention Classification Systems.* Philadelphia: *Image J Nurs Sch.* 1996 winter; 28(4):303–308.

10. Moorhead SA, McCloskey JC, Bulecheck GM. Nursing Interventions Classification. A Comparison with the Omaha System and the Home Healthcare Classification. *J Nurs Adm.* 1993 Oct;23(10):23–29.

11. Henry SB, Holzemer WL, Randell C, Hsieh SF, Miller TJ. Comparison of Nursing Interventions Classification and Current Procedural Terminology Codes for Catagorizing Nursing Activities. *Image J Nurs Sch.* 1997 second quarter; 29(2):133–138.

12. Nigg CR, Burbank PM, Padula C, Dufresne R, Rossie JS, Velicer WF, Laforge RG, Prochaska JO. Stages of change across ten health risk behaviors for older adults. *Gerontologist.* 1999 Aug;39(4):473–482.

13. Institute of Medicine. *Schools and Health: Our Nation's Investment.* Washington, DC: National Academy Press; 1997.

14. U.S. Department of Health and Human Services. *Healthy People 2010.* (Conference Edition, Educational and Community–Based Programs). Washington, DC: U.S. Government Printing Office; 2000.

15. Rivara FP, Thompson DC, Thompson RS, et al. The Seattle Children's Bicycle Helmet Campaign: Changes in helmet use and head injury admissions. *Pediatrics.* 1994; 93:567–569.

16. Davidson LL, Durkin MS, Kuhn L, et al. The impact of the Safe Kids/Healthy Neighborhoods Injury Prevention Program in Harlem, 1988 through 1991. *Am J Public Health.* 1994;84:580–586.

17. Murdaugh CL, Vanderboom C. Individual and community models for promotion wellness. *J Cardiovasc Nurs.* 1997 Apr;11(3):1–14.

18. Tessaro I. The natural helping role of nurses in promoting healthy behaviors in communities. *Adv Pract Nurs Q.* 1997 Spring;2(4):73–78.

Part IV

Interventions for Prevention and Health Promotion

8

Physical Activity and Health

- Health Benefits of Physical Activity
- Genetic and Environmental Effects on Activity Level
- Life-Span Patterns of Physical Activity
- Determinants of Physical Activity in Children and Adolescents
- Determinants of Physical Activity in Adults
- The Process of Physical Activity Behavior Change
- Interventions in Primary Care to Promote Physical Activity
- Tailoring Physical Activity Interventions
- Intensity of Physical Activity
- Risks of Physical Activity
- Interventions in the Community to Promote Physical Activity
- Directions in Physical Activity Research
- Directions for Practice to Promote Physical Activity
- Summary

Regular physical activity is essential for healthy, energetic, and productive living. Modern life with its automobiles, televisions, computers, video games, and low levels of physical activity in school and work environments necessitates the commitment of significant leisure time to physical activity in order to gain resultant health benefits. Furthermore, the competitive aspects of sports stressed in many school athletic programs results in few children and adolescents making a lifelong commitment to physical activity. *Physical activity* is defined as any bodily movement produced by skeletal muscles that results in expenditure of energy (expressed as kilocalories) and includes a broad range of occupational, leisure-time, and routine daily activities. These activities can require either light, moderate, or vigorous effort.[1] *Leisure physical activity* is physical activity undertaken during discretionary time. *Lifestyle physical activity* is characterized as integration of numerous short bouts of moderate activity into daily living. *Exercise* is leisure-time physical activity conducted with the intention of developing physical fitness.[2] *Physical fitness* is a measure of a person's ability to perform physical activities that require endurance, strength, or flexibility and is determined by a combination of level of physical activity and genetically inherited physical characteristics.[2] The term *physical activity* will be used in this chapter to encompass a broad range of activities that if performed regularly can improve health. Because of the centrality of physical activity to health, this chapter focuses on the benefits of physical activity, guidelines for activity, the determinants of physical activity for children and adults, primary care and community interventions to promote physical activity, and the importance of health providers routinely incorporating physical activity counseling into the care of clients of all ages.

Maintenance of regular physical activity is largely dependent on sources of personal and social motivation within a person's day-to-day environment. Family and peers play a powerful role in encouraging active lifestyles. Many individuals begin physical activity on their own; some are able to continue this important health behavior. Others rely on the school or work environments to create programs that help them achieve their physical activity goals. Many others cycle through periods of activity and inactivity, never establishing regular physical activity patterns. Within the last decade, there has been an alarming increase in the prevalence of obesity among both adults and adolescents. Among adults, obesity increased from 25% of the population in the late 1970s to 33% in the early 1990s.[3] The cost of obesity to U.S. business in 1994 was estimated at $12.7 billion (health expenditures, sick leave, life insurance , and disability insurance).[4] The 1996 National Longitudinal Study of Adolescent Health found 24% of white adolescents, 31% of black and Hispanic adolescents, and 42% of Native American adolescents to be overweight ($\geq$ 85th percentile). These are larger proportions than have been found in prior waves of the study.[5] Obesity and being overweight result, in part, from inactivity.

Healthy People 2010, the 10-year health plan for the American people, identifies the important goals of improving health, fitness, and quality of life of Americans through daily physical activity. The report notes the disparity in level of physical activity among population groups. The percent of the population reporting no leisure time activity is higher among women than men, among African Americans and Hispanics than whites, among older than younger adults, and among the less affluent than the more affluent. Participation in all types of physical activity declines strikingly during the adolescent years. In *Healthy People 2010,* a total of 15 physical activity objectives are identified to be achieved by the end of the decade. Selected objectives include[6]:

- Increase from 15% (baseline) to 30% the proportion of adults who engage regularly, preferably daily, in moderate activity for at least 30 minutes per day.
- Increase from 20% (baseline) to 30% the proportion of adolescents who engage in moderate physical activity for at least 30 minutes on 5 or more days per week.
- Increase from 64% (baseline) to 85% the proportion of adolescents who engage in vigorous physical activity that promotes cardiorespiratory fitness 3 or more days per week for 20 or more minutes per occasion.
- Increase from 32% (baseline) to 50% the proportion of adolescents who spend at least half of school physical education class time being physically active.
- Increase from 60% (baseline) to 75% the proportion of children and adolescents who view television two or fewer hours per day.
- Increase the proportion of work sites offering employer-sponsored physical activity and fitness programs.

Achieving these goals would increase the level of health and well-being of persons of all ages and increase the prevalence of healthy lifestyles in the population.

Health Benefits of Physical Activity

Regular physical activity contributes to physiologic stability and high-level functioning and assists individuals in actualizing their physical performance potential. Regular activity also decreases the risk for obesity, heart disease, diabetes, hypertension and stroke, and is associated with a decreased risk for colon cancer. Being physically active enhances psychological well-being, reduces the risk of depression, improves mood as well as self-concept and self-esteem. Over 40 well-designed research studies provide evidence of the causal link between inactivity and cardiovascular disease. Indeed, millions of Americans are at risk for a wide range of chronic diseases and mental health problems that might well be prevented by active lifestyles. Among children and adolescents, weight-bearing exercise is needed for normal skeletal development and attainment of peak bone mass. Regular physical activity can increase strength and agility and prevent falls among older adults and increase their independence in activities of daily living. It can improve the functional capacity of individuals with disabilities.[6] Despite the need for research to increase knowledge concerning the actual mechanisms connecting physical activity and health, studies indicate a variety of beneficial effects from regular patterns of activity that cannot be ignored.

To achieve health benefits, regular physical activity of moderate to vigorous intensity is essential. Moderate-intensity activity refers to a level of effort that burns 3.5 to 7 kilocalories per minute (kcal/min) or 3 to 6 metabolic equivalents (METS). Activities at this level include walking briskly, bicycling on level terrain, swimming, or dancing. Vigorous-intensity activity is at a level of effort that burns more than 7 kcal/min or greater than 6 METS. Such activities include jogging, swimming continuous laps, or bicycling uphill. The minimum amount of activity required for health benefits burns approximately 150 kcal of energy per day or approximately 1,000 kcal per week. The time needed each day to achieve this goal depends on the intensity level of the activity and the number of days of activity each week.[2]

It is difficult to sort out the health benefits solely from physical activity, because being active may trigger other health behaviors such as changes in dietary and smoking habits and adoption of more effective methods of coping with stress. Proposed positive effects of regular physical activity are summarized in Table 8–1. For a detailed discussion, see Bouchard and colleagues.[7]

TABLE 8-1 Positive Effects of Physical Exercise

Cardiopulmonary and Blood Chemistry Effects

Reduce systolic and diastolic blood pressure
Increase blood oxygen content
Decrease total cholesterol
Increase high-density lipoproteins
Reduce serum triglycerides
Increase peripheral blood circulation and return
Reduce resting heart rate by increasing stroke volume
Increase blood supply to heart and myocardial efficiency
Increase heart rate recovery after exercise

Immunologic–Oncologic Effects

Reduce incidence of selected types of cancer
Improve prognosis posttreatment for cancer
Increase circulating leukocytes

Endocrine and Metabolic Effects

Improve glucose tolerance
Decrease reactivity to psychosocial stressors
Decrease body fat
Increase endogenous opioid peptides, particularly beta-endorphins
Enhance oxidation of fatty acids
Increase metabolism rate

Musculoskeletal Effects

Increase lean muscle mass
Maintain bone mass
Prevent or ameliorate chronic back and joint pain
Increase muscle strength and endurance

Psychosocial Effects

Improve self-concept
Improve body image
Decrease anxiety and depression
Improve mental alertness
Enhance general mood and psychologic well-being

Genetic and Environmental Effects on Activity Level

The interaction between genetic and environmental influences on level of physical activity is receiving increased attention from researchers. Familial resemblance in physical activity was examined among 100 children 4 to 7 years of age, 99 mothers, and 92 fathers. Caltrac accelerometers were used to measure movement on 9 days for 10 hours per day. Active fathers or mothers compared to inactive fathers or mothers were more likely to have active children with an odds ratio of 3.5 and 2.0, respectively. When both parents were active, the children were 5.8 times more likely to be active than with two sedentary parents.[8] These results suggest that some combination of genetic factors transmitted to children from parents as well as role models within the environment result in a genotype–environment interaction, predisposing children to be active or inactive. In analyzing the habitual physical activity of 1,610 members of 375 families in the Quebec Family Study, investigators estimated that 29% of the variance was explained by genetic factors and 71% by environmental factors. These results indicate some inherited differences in predisposition to be spontaneously active.

The fitness response to varying levels of physical activity also may be genotype dependent. In studying pairs of monozygotic twins, there was two to twelve times more variation between genotypes than within genotypes in responses to exercise training. This suggests that unidentified genetic characteristics may account for these differences. Obesity and regional fat distribution, factors that may contribute to activity or inactivity, have definite heritability components. The estimated variance due to genotype is 5% for body mass index and 25% for percent body fat and truncal abdominal fat.[9] Rapid advances in the field of genetics will offer new and vital information for nurses concerning the effects of the genotype–environment interaction both on predisposition to physical activity and on health-related fitness responses from physical activity. Scientific breakthroughs in understanding genetic individuality will become increasingly important in assessing differences in risk for diseases associated with inactivity.

Life-Span Patterns of Physical Activity

Interest in life-span patterns of physical activity has been fueled by the realization that a number of risk factors for cardiovascular disease including obesity, high blood pressure, and elevated cholesterol are often evident early in childhood. Further, of the four major risk factors for coronary heart disease, elevated cholesterol, smoking, hypertension, and inactivity, the latter—lack of regular physical activity—is the most prevalent in the population. A survey conducted by the Centers for Disease Control and Prevention (CDC) indicated that only 40% of the population are active enough to gain physical and mental health benefits.[10]

Habits of physical activity begun early in life are likely to persist over time. It is much easier to focus on developing positive physical activity patterns initially than on changing unhealthy behaviors once they are stabilized as habits. Although vigorous activity is likely to result in the most health benefits, the accumulation of 30 minutes or more of moderate physical activity on most days of the week may be more acceptable to currently sedentary individuals. Lifestyle activity provides flexibility for increasing energy expenditure through altering patterns of daily activities such as walking to work or school, taking the stairs, and being active during lunchtime or after school or work. Activities other than participation in organized sports are attractive to a broader range of the population.[11]

Understanding the determinants of physical activity in various age groups is essential to effective intervention and counseling by health care providers to promote active lifestyles. Physical activity declines by 50% during the adolescent years, with females becoming increasingly more sedentary than males.[12] More research is needed that examines developmental transitions in physical activity attitudes and beliefs from childhood through adulthood to explain variability in physical activity behavior for individuals across the life span.

Determinants of Physical Activity in Children and Adolescents

A commonly held misperception is that children and adolescents are perpetually active and physically fit. Nothing could be further from the truth. Various studies indicate that greater than one-third of youths have adopted sedentary lifestyles by 10 years of age. The long-term goal of physical activity research among youths is to identify factors influencing level of activity as a basis for designing culturally appropriate interventions to increase activity and improve related short- and long-term health outcomes. Of particular interest are the ways in which developmental and social transitions, which occur with great rapidity during late childhood and early adolescence, affect participatory patterns. Pubertal changes (onset of menarche, changing patterns of body fat distribution) and social transitions (moving from elementary school to junior high school and on to senior high school) undoubtedly exert important influences on sports participation and patterns of physical activity. To date, most studies have been cross-sectional, identifying only correlates or potential influences on physical activity. Longitudinal studies are needed to identify changing activity patterns and probable influences on physical activity across childhood and adolescence. Prediction of physical activity behavior is difficult as influences may fluctuate in their predictive importance for different gender, race, or socioeconomic groups and at different developmental time points. Thus it is important to specify clearly the group(s) being studied and their stage of development.

Physical activity patterns and related influences vary by gender across many studies. Among 732 fourth and fifth graders, significant declines in physical activity occurred over 20 months. Gender-specific factors appeared to influence this decline. For boys, changes in attitude toward physical education, perceived competence or self-efficacy, parental transport to activities, and level of activity of the parent were related to the decline. For girls, changes in activity preferences and parental transport to activities were related to the decline.[13] Sallis and colleagues in studying 198 sixth graders found that for boys, physical activity self-efficacy, social norms regarding physical activity, and involvement in community sports organizations predicted level of physical activity. For girls, only physical activity self-efficacy predicted activity level.[14]

In a longitudinal study, 111 families with fifth and sixth grade children were followed for three years to determine influences on physical activity over time. In the first phase of the study, enjoyment of exercise was the only variable related to activity for girls. Three years later, exercise knowledge, mother's physical activity, and friend–family modeling and support were related to activity among girls. Initially for boys, enjoyment and friend–family modeling and support were related to level of activity. Three years later, physical activity self-efficacy, exercise knowledge, and interest in sports media correlated with physical activity. Trends in the data appeared to indicate that social support became more important for girls over time whereas personal interest and self-efficacy became more important for boys.[15] Determinants of physical activity differed for boys and girls and changed over the period of development that was studied. Continuing assessment of factors influencing physical activity as the children transitioned to middle school and high school would provide valuable information about gender-specific developmental changes in the determinants of physical activity.

Biddle and Armstong[16] identified interesting gender differences in psychologic correlates of physical activity. Among 11- to 12-year-old boys, activity was positively correlated with intrinsic motivation; that is, engaging in an activity for its own sake or for the sense of mastery and control. An opposite trend was found for the girls of the same age with approval by their teacher, or external motivation, being more important than the intrinsic challenge of the task. Garcia and colleagues, in applying the Health Promotion Model to physical activity behavior in a racially diverse population, found definite gender differences between physical activity beliefs and behaviors of fifth, sixth, and eighth graders. Compared to boys, girls reported less representation of self as athletic and lower levels of past and current physical activity. The benefits to barriers differential (benefits-of-physical activity score minus barriers-to-physical activity score), access to recreational facilities and programs, and gender were significant predictors of physical activity measured several weeks later. Grade, health status, physical activity self-efficacy, social support, and social norms appeared to exert indirect effects on physical activity by modifying the balance between perceived benefits and barriers to being active. Race influenced physical activity through differential access to recreational facilities.[17]

Family influences during childhood have a positive effect on the physical activity patterns that children develop. For example, more active parents have been shown to have more active children of both genders.[18] Role modeling of active lifestyles, social support for being active, and normative expectations that children will be active are likely to have positive effects on the physical activity patterns that children develop. McKenzie and colleagues[19] examined the activity patterns of 351 Anglo and Mexican American preschoolers at home and during recess. Ethnic differences were noted. Mexican American children were less active than Anglo children at home and during recess. This may be related to environmental factors, as Mexican American children spent more time in the presence of adults both at recess and at home and had access to fewer active toys. Thus, the effects of early physical activity experiences of children with parents and siblings on lifetime physical activity patterns need to be further explored and cannot be dismissed lightly.

A study of 2,285 children in fourth to sixth grades in a multiethnic, low-income urban neighborhood revealed that 20% of the girls and 25% of the boys were inactive. Children of Asian origin were less active than children in other ethnic groups. Socioeconomic status particularly influenced participation in organized sports outside of school where cost of participation and transportation may pose major problems to parents. Correlates of low levels of activity included no participation in organized sports at or outside of school, lower physical activity self-efficacy, and lack of parental support for engaging in physical activity. Physical activity programs should promote high levels of perceived competence (self-efficacy) among youths and involve parents in family-oriented activities. Further, interventions should be developed to encourage parents to be positive role models of physically active lifestyles.[20] In another study of 1,871 multiethnic high school students, boys reported a level of physical activity 41% higher than girls. The most common activities for boys were weight lifting, baseball, basketball, jogging, and bicycling. The most common activities for girls were dancing, walking, calisthenics, and baseball. African Americans reported twice as much dancing as did other groups and Asian Americans reported more tennis than did other groups. Boys reported more modeling and support from friends to be active than did girls. Girls reported more barriers to being active and disliked physical education more than did boys. In terms of ethnic differences, Asian American and Latinos reported the lowest level of neighborhood safety for physical activity, and African American and Latinos reported the fewest convenient facilities for physical activity. African Americans reported the highest level of television viewing per week.[21] Caution should be exercised in interpreting the findings of many multiethnic studies because ethnicity–race is often confounded with social class so differences may be due to class rather than cultural background. Studies of physical activity determinants among youth that clearly separate these social and economic influences are needed. A multiethnic, developmental approach to the promotion of physical activity takes into consideration the level of maturity of youth, their decision-making ability, and culture-specific sources of motivation.

According to a recent comprehensive review of 108 studies of correlates of physical activity,[22] factors that increase the likelihood of children (4 to 12 years) being active include *history of being active, preference for physical activity over sedentary pursuits, goals or intentions to be active, lack of barriers to physical activity, access to recreational facilities and programs,* and *time spent outdoors.* Among adolescents (13 to 18 years), *history of being active, achievement orientation, intention to be active, perceived physical competence, opportunities to be active such as involvement in community sports, sensation seeking,* and *not being sedentary after school and on weekends* is associated with a more active lifestyle. *Active parental support such as transport or payment of activity fees, encouragement from significant others,* and *level of activity of siblings* were important social influences on adolescents. More studies are needed of the determinants of activity in diverse groups of children and adolescents to better understand how to tailor effective programs. Nurses should address important correlates of physical activity in their counseling with children and adolescents as these influences when addressed have the potential for increasing the development of an active lifestyle.

Schools play a major role in promoting involvement of children in recreational activities that they can enjoy for a lifetime. By involving children on a daily basis in physical activity, teaching the personal value of regular activity, and encouraging continuing involvement in moderate or vigorous activities both at school and at home, schools contribute to the goal of an "active" generation. School-based programs should be supplemented by family-based activities, community-based recreational programs, and physical activity counseling by nurses and physicians in primary care. Family-based programs encourage parents to be active with their children in relationship-building experiences. For example, weekend family bike outings and parent–child aerobic or recreational activities create opportunities for parents to be role models for active lifestyles. Community-based programs such as community runs, community all-sports days, and neighborhood walking groups can establish norms of physical activity participation for youths. Childhood and adolescence are ideal periods in the life span to cultivate regular physical activity that can reap positive health benefits throughout life.

Determinants of Physical Activity in Adults

Most of the theories and models used in adult physical activity studies to date have their origins in social psychology: social cognitive theory, theory of reasoned action, theory of planned behavior, Health Belief Model, protection-motivation theory, and the Health Promotion Model. In a classic article, Godin and Shephard[23] reviewed the use of attitude –behavior models in promotion of physical activity. They identified *past behavior, self-efficacy, barriers to physical activity, outcome expectancies (positive and negative),* and *intentions* as useful in predicting level of physical activity among adults. However, they concluded their review by pointing out that attitude–behavior models seldom explain more than 35% of the variance in physical activity behavior. Models that sometimes explain more variance, do so inconsistently. They suggest that this may be due to the fact that the models used to study physical activity have focused on predisposing factors or those factors that result in the initiation of physical activity. Other factors that need to be studied include facilitating factors, such as accessibility and availability of facilities, and reinforcing factors, such as rewards and incentives that accompany or follow moderate or vigorous physical activity and contribute to its persistence. With advances in the field of genetics, the interaction of genetic makeup, psychologic factors, and environmental factors in the determination of level of physical activity in adults requires further investigation.

In a study of 2,020 adults, the determinants of exercise behavior were studied using the Health Promotion Model (HPM) as the framework. The sample consisted of subgroups of working adults, community-dwelling older adults, cardiac rehabilitation patients, and ambulatory cancer patients. Perceiving many benefits from exercise, few barriers to exercise, and good perceived health status predicted greater involvement in exercise behavior. In the two populations (working adults, older adults) in which exercise efficacy was tested, higher perceived efficacy predicted greater involvement in exercise behavior. Among working adults, level of prior exercise program participation was highly predictive of continuing participation. Among older adults, preference for a moderate to high level of physical exertion and being high in self-motivation also contributed to the explanation of exercise frequency. The variance in exercise predicted across the four subgroups ranged from 23% to 59%.[24]

Whereas in the past, most studies of physical activity focused on males, there is increasing interest in the determinants of physical activity among women. Interest in the health benefits of moderate physical activity, that is, accumulation of at least 30 minutes most days of the week, has particular importance for women who are more likely to adopt moderate compared to vigorous physical activity. It is estimated that only 40% of women participate in regular physical activity.[25] Women's roles such as multiple family obligations and work pressures decrease their time for physical activity. Zaravar and Nies found that as women experienced increased daily hassles related to household activity, family, friends, and personal life, there was a decrease in physical activity.[26] Unmarried women generally profile as more active than do married women with children at home. However, little is known about how physical activity is affected by role changes in women's lives such as parenthood, employment, children leaving home, or retirement.[27]

Lack of social support to be physically active from spouse or close friends can reinforce sedentary lifestyles. Low physical activity self-efficacy is characteristic of many females throughout the life span and may undermine efforts to increase level of activity. In some neighborhoods, safety issues and lack of facilities tailored to women's needs further impede adoption of active lifestyles. Home-based programs compared to structured health club programs are more accessible and affordable particularly for women with limited economic resources. Home-based programs should be fun and allow inclusion of other family members in physical activities. The occupational dimension of physical activity is important for women. Wylbur and colleagues found that women with higher occupational energy expenditure had higher HDL cholesterol and lower total cholesterol than did women with lower occupational energy expenditure. Because over 65% of women work outside the home, work sites provide a critical environment for promoting increased physical activity during work hours.[28]

A consistent finding is that after adoption, adults have difficulty maintaining regular exercise patterns, which results in a usual rate of dropout from organized programs of about 50% in the first three to six months. Further, those who might benefit most, such as overweight persons, are most susceptible to dropping out due to a low level of tolerance for physical activity. Influences on physical activity for middle-age adults include *past program participation, self-efficacy, benefits, barriers, spouse support, peer support, perceived available time,* and *access to facilities.*

Older adults merit special consideration in discussions of determinants of physical activity. Feeling better physically and improving fitness (endurance, muscle strength, balance) are frequent reasons given for participating in physical activity. Barriers to physical activity, an important consideration for the elderly, need further exploration because although work and family demands may lessen with age, convenience of facilities, cost, opportunities for physical activity with others, fear of resultant illness or injury, disability, and sensory impairment become more salient with age. Concern about existing medical conditions can be a further deterrent to an active lifestyle. Conn[29,30] found perceived barriers and self-efficacy expectations as well as age to be important predictors of participation in physical activity among older adults.

Shephard[31] suggests that focusing on personal beliefs rather than subjective norms (expectations of others) may be more effective in motivating older adults to be active. Further, providing transportation, facilitating companionship for physical activity, building on prior activity habits, and tapping existing skills that have developed over a lifetime can facilitate regular physical activity.

Older adults consist of the young old (65 to 74 years), middle old (75 to 84 years), and very old (over 85 years). Ability to be physically active as well as relevant determinants undoubtedly vary over this age spectrum. Almost all studies of determinants of physical activity in older adults have focused on the young old. In order to optimize physical activity potential for those 75 years of age or older, further studies of exercise capabilities and determinants are needed that investigate physical activity in the middle old and very old.

The Process of Physical Activity Behavior Change

The use of process models to specify the mechanisms underlying the adoption and maintenance of physical activity behavior is advocated by a number of investigators.[32,33] The transtheoretical model or stages of change model has been applied by Marcus and colleagues to physical activity behavior. This model proposes that individuals engaging in a new behavior move through a series of changes: precontemplation (not intending to make changes), contemplation (considering changes), planning or preparation (making minor changes), action (actively engaged in major behavior change), and maintenance (sustaining the behavior over time). The processes and strategies used to promote change are linked specifically to the stage of change of the client.[34] In testing the model on 1,172 participants in a work site health promotion project, Marcus and colleagues concluded that the constructs of the theory can be applied to physical activity. Experiential processes suggested as useful interventions in the precontemplation and contemplation stages include consciousness raising and self-reevaluation. Behavioral processes proposed as useful interventions in the preparation, adoption, and maintenance stages include helping relationships, counterconditioning, reinforcement management, and stimulus control. The study revealed that women were more likely than men to be in the contemplation or action stages and less likely to be in the maintenance stage. Working women with young children in the home were more likely to be in the lower stages of exercise adoption than were women without young children.[35] In a study of 286 women aged 50 to 64, precontemplators were significantly older, had lower exercise knowledge, perceived lower psychologic benefits from exercise, had lower family support for exercise, and did not perceive exercise as important compared to the action group. Both the precontemplation and the contemplation groups perceived more barriers to exercise than did the action group. Persons in maintenance also scored the highest on the pro scale (benefits of exercise) and lowest on the con scale (costs of exercising) as predicted by the theory.[36] Findings supported predictions based on the transtheoretical model.

Cardinal has proposed an extension of the transtheoretical model of physical activity behavior to include a sixth stage identified as the transformed stage. He defines the transformed stage as having participated regularly in physical activity for five or more years and being 100% confident in personal ability to remain physically active for life. In a study of 551 members of a physical education and recreation professionals organization, those in the transformed stage had a higher reported level of physical activity and a more positive attitude toward role modeling an active lifestyle than did those in the maintenance group.[37] Understanding the stages of physical activity behavior will provide important information for appropriately tailoring interventions to groups at differing points in the change process.

Interventions in Primary Care to Promote Physical Activity

Nurses and physicians in primary care have multiple opportunities to engage in physical activity counseling. The American Nurses' Association's *Clinician's Handbook of Preventive*

Services: Put Prevention into Practice[38(pp97–99)] recommends that every primary care visit be seen as an opportunity to promote an active lifestyle. In a recent national survey, 58% of the adult nurse practitioners surveyed indicated that they routinely advised clients to engage in moderate-intensity physical activity for a total of 30 minutes on most days of the week. This is the latest recommendation for sedentary adults from the American College of Sports Medicine and the Centers for Disease Control and Prevention.[39] Nursing diagnoses from the North American Nursing Diagnosis Association (NANDA) in the category of Activity-Exercise Pattern include diversional activity deficit and high risk for activity intolerance. The reader is referred to the NANDA taxonomy for further diagnostic information about definitions, defining characteristics, and etiologic or related factors.[40] Nursing interventions to address these diagnoses include behavior modification and exercise promotion.[41] Nursing outcomes or goals of client care achieved through these nursing interventions include improvements in circulatory status, endurance, muscle function, leisure participation, and physical fitness.[42]

Counseling in primary care should assist children and adolescents to select activities they enjoy and not focus solely on competitive sports. Children should be encouraged to engage in activities that can be carried into adulthood and can be easily incorporated into their daily life year-round. Appropriate safety equipment should be used in order to avoid injuries and youth should be counseled to avoid use of any anabolic steroids.

Adult clients in primary care should be asked about their physical activity habits at work, at home, and during leisure to determine if these activities are of sufficient frequency, intensity, and duration to confer health benefits. Adults should be assisted in planning a program of physical activity that is medically safe, enjoyable, convenient, realistic, and structured to achieve self-selected goals. Routine monitoring, follow-up, and booster sessions are essential to assist clients in maintaining their exercise programs. Home exercise programs may work for some adults, whereas for others structured programs may need to be offered at work sites or convenient community locations. Group activities may be particularly appealing to adults who prefer the social support and comradeship of group programs.

Few studies have been conducted of physical activity counseling interventions in primary care. Existing studies have focused primarily on delivery of the intervention by physicians rather than by nurse practitioners or collaborative nurse–physician teams. Calfas and colleagues[43] evaluated the Physician-Based Assessment and Counseling for Exercise (PACE) program developed to promote adoption of physical activity among sedentary adults.[44] The intervention protocol is based on social cognitive theory and the transtheoretical model. PACE incorporates proven behavioral change techniques, tailors physical activity counseling to the individual client, and incorporates both moderate and vigorous activity guidelines. The intervention is designed to alter factors known to influence physical activity such as self-efficacy, social support, perceived benefits, and perceived barriers. The protocol includes physical activity assessment forms, and stage-specific counseling protocols. For example, the "Getting Out of Your Chair" protocol is geared to working with clients in the precontemplation and contemplation stages, the "Planning the First Step" protocol to those in the preparation or planning stage, and the "Keeping the Pace" protocol to those in the adoption or maintenance stages. The physical activity assessment is completed by the client in the waiting room and scored by office personnel. The client is then given the appropriate counseling protocol for stage of exercise, and the assessment and protocol are placed on the client's chart for use by the primary care provider during the visit.

The provider counsels the client and arranges for appropriate follow-up by phone, mail, or office visit.

The effectiveness of the protocol for the contemplation stage was tested with 98 intervention and 114 control primary care clients who were sedentary at the beginning of the study. Intervention clients received the office-based intervention and a 10-minute booster phone call to answer questions and discuss progress. The control group received the regular office visit. A significant number of clients moved from the contemplation to action stage in the intervention compared with the control group. Intervention subjects increased 40 minutes per week in self-reported walking compared to a 10-minute-per-week increase in the control group. These results were supported by accelerometer readings. The study demonstrated that brief activity counseling in primary care followed by a booster phone call—both matched to the client's stage of physical activity—produced meaningful increases in activity among sedentary adults. By identifying the client's stage of physical activity prior to the visit, the primary care provider can efficiently tailor counseling to the client's specific needs.[43] Calfas and colleagues examined the possible mechanisms fostering physical activity change as a result of the intervention. They found that the intervention increased reported use of cognitive and behavioral processes to facilitate adoption of physical activity, but they did not find any increase in physical activity self-efficacy or social support for being active. The brevity of the intervention may have precluded these psychological and social effects. Studies are needed of other physical activity interventions structured to impact more directly an array of factors known to affect levels of physical activity.[45]

Adult and adolescent versions of the PACE+ Program that includes protocols for both physical activity and nutrition counseling are currently undergoing evaluation. These protocols have both provider-based and computer-based tailored components as well as individualized follow-up protocols.

The Activity Counseling Trial (ACT) is another major study of a primary care–based physical activity counseling intervention sponsored by the National Heart, Lung, and Blood Institute. This is a 5-year multicenter, randomized controlled trial with 874 adults in primary care between the ages of 35 and 75 years assigned to one of three educational interventions: standard care control, staff-assisted intervention, or staff–counseling intervention. Standard care consists of advice to exercise by a physician or health educator. The staff-assisted intervention includes advice but adds in-clinic counseling by a health educator and interactive mail follow-up. The staff–counseling intervention further adds telephone counseling and classes to the intervention components in the other two groups. Multiple outcomes over 24 months will be examined. Results will be published when the study is completed.[46,47]

Barriers to physical activity counseling sometimes cited by health professionals include lack of time, lack of reimbursement, absence of theoretically sound protocols to guide counseling with diverse groups, lack of perceived effectiveness as a counselor, and lack of proper training to fulfill this role. If nurses are to provide quality counseling to clients regarding their physical activity, they must work to overcome these barriers. Providers who model active lifestyles themselves are likely to be much more effective counselors than their sedentary counterparts. According to social learning theory, observation of others is a powerful mode for transmitting attitudes, beliefs, patterns of thought, and behaviors. Clients are quick to recognize the extent to which their provider has actually experienced the challenges and the "ups and downs" of adopting and maintaining a regular program of physical activity. The physical appearance of health care providers also provides powerful cues to clients as to whether they actually "practice what they preach."[48]

Tailoring Physical Activity Interventions

Interventions that tailor physical activity counseling and behavioral interventions to individuals based on motivational readiness and other psychological influences proven to affect physical activity are now being developed and tested. Information technology will revolutionize physical activity interventions in the next decade providing interactive, personalized, and Web-based formats for counseling. A review of 28 studies of media-based interventions indicated that mass-media campaigns had little impact on physical activity behavior. Interventions using printed self-help media and telephone contacts were effective in the short term in changing level of activity. Interventions with more intensive contacts and tailored to the target audience were most effective.[49] A review of tailored print communications found them to be superior to nontailored interventions in 75% of the studies reviewed.[50]

In a randomized, controlled study of 194 sedentary adults recruited from the community, Marcus and colleagues tested the efficacy of an individually tailored intervention matched to stage of readiness to change. This intervention consisted of individually tailored reports generated by a computer expert system and stage-matched self-help manuals. The initial assessment and interventions were mailed to participants. The control group was mailed a standard self-help intervention. At six months the group receiving the tailored intervention outperformed the control group on minutes of physical activity per week, reaching 30 or more minutes of moderate activity on most days of the week, and on reaching the action stage of physical activity. Surprisingly, there were no group differences in the psychological constructs associated with physical activity in other studies, for example, self-efficacy, decisional balance, processes of change.[51] In another controlled trial of 763 sedentary patients, brief advice and a pamphlet tailored to stage of change were given to the intervention group. The control group received brief advice and a standard pamphlet. There were no group differences in physical activity or movement across the stages of change.[52]

The effective content and processes in tailored interventions, the conditions under which they positively impact behavior, and the extent to which these interventions are effective with differing population groups are areas needing further exploration. The cost effectiveness of various tailoring methods for physical activity counseling also needs to be determined to optimize efficient use of time by health care providers.

Intensity of Physical Activity

Vigorous physical activity has been widely advocated with at least 20 minutes spent, three times per week at 60% or more of maximum heart rate. Recently, moderate physical activity (less than 60% maximum heart rate) has been proposed as having some of the same health-protective benefits as vigorous activity. The national recommendation for *moderate physical activity* is accumulating 30 minutes daily on most days of the week through a combination of activities. Because some people dislike strenuous physical activity, moderate activities may have fewer barriers to participation and therefore may be incorporated more easily into an individual's daily routine. Blair and colleagues[53] suggest that lifestyle exercise in which a person engages in numerous short bouts of physical activity throughout the day (stair climbing, walking to and from a distant parking place) resembles the physical activity measured in epidemiologic studies that have found cumulative energy expenditure to be inversely related to cardiac risk. Some combination of lifestyle physical activity and moderate or vigorous leisure-time physical activity is probably closer to the ideal for most individuals. Sedentary and active approaches to daily living are presented in Table 8–2.

Special considerations in optimizing tolerance of physical activity are warming up and cooling down properly. *Warming up* is important to increase blood flow to the heart and skeletal muscles, enhance oxygenation of tissues, and increase flexibility of muscles before physical activity. The warming-up period allows the heart rate and body temperature to increase gradually and the joints to become more flexible prior to physical activity. A gradual increase in heart rate reduces chances of arrhythmias. Warming up can include activities such as walking briskly, arm circles, jumping jacks, leg exercises, or wall push-ups. The warming-up period need take no longer than 7 to 10 minutes and should be followed immediately by moderate or vigorous physical activity. Following physical activity, a *cooldown* period is essential. Taking time to cool down for a period of 5 to 10 minutes following physical activity is important because activity raises heart rate, blood pressure, body temperature, and lactic acid within the muscles. Cooling down allows the heart rate to decrease gradually, preventing pooling of blood in muscles and resultant lightheadedness. It helps eliminate lactic acid within muscles and maintains blood flow to and from the muscle. During the cooling-down period, it is important to keep the lower extremities moving in activities such as slow walking, jogging, or cycling. At the end of the cooling-down period, the client's heart rate should be below 100.

TABLE 8-2 Sedentary and Active Approaches to Daily Living

Sedentary	Active
Take the elevator or escalator	Climb the stairs
Call on the telephone	Walk down the hall or walk next door
Drive to lunch	Walk to lunch
Sit in a chair throughout a meeting	Get up quietly and walk about the room
Park right next to your destination	Park some distance away from your destination
Remain sedentary at your desk	Take several minutes to do arm and leg exercises
Use the remote control for the TV	Get up and walk to the TV when you want to change the channel
Visit with your colleagues in the "break room"	Take a walking break and visit

Risks of Physical Activity

An overly aggressive approach to physical activity can exaggerate existing clinical conditions and put patients, particularly older adults, at risk for untoward effects. If an individual has an undiagnosed heart condition, strenuous physical activity could create arrhythmias. Persons with cardiovascular disease or other chronic conditions should be cautioned to avoid activity at levels that are physiologically untenable or result in untoward symptoms. Overstressing muscles and joints can result in muscle soreness and joint pain. Individuals over 50 years of age or with an existing chronic illness should be evaluated medically before starting regular physical activity. A program of gradually increasing physical activity is recommended, with much more emphasis for older adults on moderate rather than vigorous activity. Appropriate physical activity should optimize the benefits while minimizing the risks.

Interventions in the Community to Promote Physical Activity

Interventions to promote physical activity can occur in schools, work sites, community organizations, and families. These interventions generally reach a larger group than one-on-one primary care interventions. The many community physical activity intervention studies preclude an exhaustive review. Thus, in this section several examples of community interventions will be presented.

A school-based intervention, the Cardiovascular Health in Children Study, was conducted in 18 elementary schools in North Carolina. A sample of 2,109 third- and fourth-grade children was randomized by school to either a public health classroom-based intervention, a risk-based intervention for those with one or more cardiovascular risk factors, or a control group. All children in the classroom-based intervention received a physical activity intervention three times per week that included warm-up, 20 minutes of physical activity, and a cooldown period. In the risk-based intervention group, only at-risk children received the physical activity intervention. Posttest data were collected two weeks after the eight-week intervention. Both intervention groups improved their cardiovascular risk profiles. However, the classroom-based intervention was easier to implement and reached a wider group of children.[54]

The Child and Adolescent Trial for Cardiovascular Health (CATCH) compared 56 intervention schools given a multicomponent behavioral intervention over three grades with 40 control schools. Enhancement of physical education classes, home curricula, and family fun nights were part of the three-year physical activity program for the intervention group. The intensity of physical activity in physical education classes increased significantly more in the intervention group than in the control group. Although total minutes of activity did not differ between youths in intervention and control schools, reported vigorous activity was significantly higher in students at the intervention schools. These increases were maintained at follow-up testing three years later. The results of this study suggest that changes in physical activity initiated in elementary school can persist into early adolescence.[55,56]

Project Active is another example of a community-based intervention. This study focused on 235 sedentary men and women between the ages of 35 and 60 years of age. Volunteers were randomly assigned to a structured exercise program or a lifestyle physical activity program. Social cognitive theory and the transtheoretical model provided the theoretical basis for study interventions. Participants randomized to the structured program group received a traditional exercise program at 50% to 85% of maximal aerobic power for 20 to 60 minutes for 3 to 5 days per week. Individual supervised sessions were offered to this group at a state-of-the-art fitness center 5 days a week for 6 months. Participants in the lifestyle group were advised to accumulate at least 30 minutes of moderate-intensity physical activity on most days of the week. This group met and learned cognitive and behavioral strategies matched to their stage of change or level or motivational readiness. After six months of intervention, both groups were significantly more fit than at baseline. Of the structured group, 85% were meeting physical activity criterion for their group. Of the lifestyle group, 78% were meeting the physical activity criterion for their group. For both groups, those who increased their use of cognitive and behavioral strategies, increased in self-efficacy, perceived more benefits than barriers, and were more likely to achieve the physical activity criterion. Both groups experienced reduction in cardiovascular risk. The importance of this study is the finding that a lifestyle approach compared to a structured approach to physical activity achieved comparable results. Sedentary adults can make significant progress in becoming more fit and lowering cardiovascular disease risk without attending a traditional exercise program.[57,58,59]

Community interventions are an effective approach to increasing physical activity in population groups. These interventions if widespread throughout communities could contribute significantly to attaining the physical activity goals of *Healthy People 2010* by the end of the decade.

Directions in Physical Activity Research

This chapter has provided a research-based discussion of the benefits of physical activity, factors influencing physical activity among youth and adults, and physical activity interventions in primary care and in the community. Research is still needed to better understand how to tailor exercise programs to the needs of different populations. Particular focus should be placed on developing and testing interventions that assist very young children to adopt physical activity as enjoyable and rewarding. How to sustain physical activity in adolescence also needs further study. Focusing on behavior development rather than behavior change is critical as behaviors once developed during youth are highly resistant to change.

Directions for Practice to Promote Physical Activity

Throughout this chapter, benefits of physical activity, determinants of physical activity, and approaches for increasing physical activity have been emphasized. This information can guide evidence-based nursing practice in counseling persons of all ages about the adoption of regular physical activity. Within any given age, gender, or cultural group, nurses should start by assessing the client's level of physical activity and the influences known to predict physical activity. For example, when working with children, the nurse should assess pattern of physical activity; preferred activities; perceptions of barriers to being active; perceptions of self-efficacy; intentions to be active; availability of active parents, siblings, peers; access to safe recreational facilities; and time spent outdoors. For older adults, current health status, existing medical conditions, disabilities, fear of injury, preference for activities requiring exertion, as well as perceived benefits and self-efficacy for being active need to be assessed. Physical activity counseling and behavioral intervention programs can then be developed for the individual that focus on the most relevant sources of motivation as well as their personal concerns.

Tailoring the behavioral intervention program to the individual is likely to enhance its effectiveness. Nurses should consider developing or using existing computer-based tailoring programs to optimize their physical activity counseling effectiveness and efficiency. It is also important to follow up assessment and counseling in the office with mail or phone follow-ups at periodic intervals. These contacts should focus on assessing the stage of physical activity of the client, providing advice regarding appropriate strategies to increase or maintain activity, and helping them deal with any barriers to being active that they have encountered. Generally, in-office or phone follow-up is considered more effective than mail follow-up.

The nurse should work with the health care team to set up office systems that will facilitate regular physical activity counseling for all clients. Physical activity components of health promotion and prevention systems should consist of screening systems for assessing patterns of physical activity, clear agency guidelines for physical activity counseling, chart reminders for counseling at client visits, relevant client education materials, and follow-up protocols to "booster" interventions. When health care agencies systematize counseling protocols, physical activity counseling is much more likely to be carried out as an integral part of care by all health professionals.

Nurses can access Web sites that provide additional information concerning recommendations and considerations related to physical activity for different populations. Three suggested sites are the American College of Sports Medicine (www.acsm.org), the President's Council on Physical Fitness and Sports (www.surgeongeneral.gov/ophs/pcpfs.htm), and the Centers for Disease Control and Prevention (www.cdc.gov/nccdphp/dnpa).

Suggestions for future research include:

1. Investigate the influences in infancy and early childhood that promote the development of physically active lifestyles.

2. Explore how important developmental milestones or life transitions (e.g., school transition, marriage, pregnancy) influence readiness and opportunities to be physically active.

3. Explore the mechanisms that explain transition across stages of physical activity from precontemplation to transformation.

4. Investigate the influence of multiple roles and daily hassles on the adoption and maintenance of physical activity among women.

5. Investigate the interaction of genetic makeup, environment, and behavior on the adoption and maintenance of physical activity.

6. Test the effectiveness of computer-assisted physical activity interventions tailored to motivational readiness, age, gender, race–ethnicity, and socioeconomic status.

7. Test the effectiveness of family, school, work site, and community interventions to increase physical activity.

8. Test the effectiveness of changing both policies (environmental, educational, and health policies) and community environments to increase physical activity in populations.

SUMMARY

Nurses, as key health professionals, need to assume responsibility for using current and emerging knowledge to assist clients to develop lifelong habits of physical activity. Physical activity must be an integral part of personal lifestyle if it is to have optimum effects on health. Maintaining physical fitness can be enjoyable and rewarding for persons of all ages and contribute significantly to extending longevity and improving the quality of life.

SELECTED WEB SITES RELEVANT TO PHYSICAL ACTIVITY

A Guide from the National Institute on Aging—*http://weboflife.arc.nasa.gov/exerciseandaging/toc.html*

American College of Sports Medicine—*http://www.acsm.org*

American Heart Association—*http://www.americanheart.org/catalog/Health_catpage9.html*

Centers for Disease Control and Prevention, Division of Nutrition and Physical Activity—*http://www.cdc.gov/nccdphp/dnpa*

Mayo Clinic Rochester Aerobic Exercise and Fitness Guidelines—*http://www.mayo.edu:80/cv/wwwpg_cv/cv-whc/mc1952/mc1952.htm*

Office of the Surgeon General—*http://www.surgeongeneral.gov/ophs/pcpfs.htm*

The Cooper Institute—*http://www.cooperinst.org/7.html*

REFERENCES

1. U.S. Department of Health and Human Services, Center for Disease Control and Prevention, National Center for Chronic Disease Prevention and Health Promotion. *Physical Activity and Health: A Report of the Surgeon General.* Atlanta: U.S. Department of Health and Human Services; 1996.

2. U.S. Department of Health and Human Services. Public Health Service, Centers for Disease Control and Prevention, National Center for Chronic Disease Prevention and Health Promotion, Division of Nutrition and Physical Activity. *Promoting Physical Activity: A Guide for Community Action.* Champaign, IL: Human Kinetics; 1999.

3. Kuczmarski RJ, Flegal KM, Campbell SM, et al. Increasing prevalence of overweight among U.S. adults. *JAMA.* 1994;272:205–211.

4. Thompson D, Edelberg J, Kinsey KL, Oster G. Estimated economic costs of obesity to U.S. business. *Am J Health Prom.* 1998;13(2):120–127.

5. Popkin BM, Udry JR, Adolescent obesity increases significantly in second and third generation U.S. immigrants: The National Longitudinal Study of Adolescent Health. *J Nutri.* 1998;128:701–706.

6. U.S. Department of Health and Human Services. *Healthy People 2010* (Conference Edition, in Two Volumes). Washington, DC: U.S. Government Printing Office; January 2000.

7. Bouchard C, Shephard RJ, Stephens T, eds. *Physical Activity, Fitness and Health: International Proceedings and Consensus Statement.* Champaign, IL: Human Kinetics; 1994.

8. Moore LL, Lombardi DA, White MJ, Campbell JL, Oliveria SA, Ellison RC. Influence of parents' physical activity levels on activity levels of young children. *J Pediatr.* 1991;118:215–219.

9. Bouchard C, Perusse L. Heredity, activity level, fitness and health. In: Bouchard C, Shephard RJ, Stephens T, eds. *Physical Activity, Fitness and Health: International Proceedings and Consensus Statement.* Champaign, IL: Human Kinetics; 1994:106–118.

10. Karch B. A case for physical activity in health promotion. *Health Promotion: Global Perspectives.* 2000;2(6):1.

11. Marcus BH, Forsyth LH. How are we doing with physical activity? *Am J Health Prom.* 1999;14(2):118–124.

12. Rowland TW. *Exercise and Children's Health.* Champaign, IL: Human Kinetics; 1990:1–7.

13. Trost SG, Pate RR, Ward DS, Saunders R, Riner W. Correlates of objectively measured physical activity in preadolescent youth. *Am J Prev Med.* 1999;17(2):120–126.

14. Sallis JF, Alcaraz JE, McKenzie TL, Hovell MF. Predictors of change in children's physical activity over 20 months: Variations by gender and adiposity. *Am J Prev Med.* 1999;16(3):222–229.

15. DiLorenzo TM, Stucky-Ropp RC, Vander Wal JS, Gotham HJ. Determinants of exercise among children. II. A longitudinal analysis. *Prev Med.* 1998; 27:470–477.

16. Biddle S, Armstrong N. Children's physical activity: An exploratory study of psychological correlates. *Soc Sci Med.* 1992;34(3):325–331.

17. Garcia AW, Norton MA, Frenn M, et al. Gender and developmental differences in exercise beliefs among youth and prediction of their exercise behavior. *J School Health.* 1995; 65(6):213–219.

18. Moore LL, Lombardi DA, White MJ, et al. Influence of parents' physical activity levels on activity levels of young children. *J Pediatr.* 1991;118:215–219.

19. McKenzie TL, Sallis JF, Nader PR, et al. Anglo- and Mexican-American preschoolers at home and recess: Activity patterns and environmental influences. *Dev Behav Pediatr.* 1992;13(3):173–180.

20. O'Loughlin J, Paradis G, Kishchuk N, Barnett T, Renaud L. Prevalence and correlates of physical activity behaviors among elementary schoolchildren in multiethnic, low income, inner-city neighborhoods in Montreal, Canada. *Annals of Epidemiology.* 1999; 9:397–407.

21. Sallis JF, Zakarian JM, Hovell MF, Hofstetter CR. Ethnic, socioeconomic, and sex differences in physical activity among adolescents. *Journal of Clinical Epidemiology.* 1996; 49(2):125–134.

22. Sallis JF, Prochaska JJ, Taylor WC. A review of correlates of physical activity of children and adolescents. *Medicine and Science in Sports and Exercise.* 2000;32(2):963–975.

23. Godin G, Shephard RJ. Use of attitude-behaviour models in exercise promotion. *Sports Med.* 1990;10(2):103–121.

24. Pender NJ, Walker SN, Sechrist KR, et al. *The Health Promotion Model: Refinement and Validation.* Final Report to the National Center for Nursing Research, National Institutes of Health (Grant no. NR 01121). DeKalb, IL: Northern Illinois University Press; 1990.

25. Caspersen CJ, Merritt RK. Physical activity trends among 26 states, 1986–1990. *Medicine and Science in Sports and Exercise.* 1995;27(5):713–720.

26. Zaravar PW, Nies MA. Daily hassles and exercise frequency in women. *Home Health Care Management and Practice* 1997; 10(1):54–58.

27. Pinto BM, Marcus BH, Clark MM. Promoting physical activity in women: The new challenges. *Am J Prev Med.* 1996;12:395–400.

28. Wilbur J, Naftger-Kang L, Miller AM, Chandler P, Montgomery A. Women's occupations, energy expenditure, and cardiovascular risk factors. *J Women's Health.* 1999;8(3):377–387.

29. Conn VS. Older women: Social cognitive theory correlates of health behavior. *Women and Health.* 1997; 26(3):71–85.

30. Conn VS. Older adults and exercise: Path analysis of self-efficacy related constructs. *Nurs Res.* 1998; 47(3):180–189.

31. Shephard RJ. Determinants of exercise in people aged 65 years and older. In: Dishman R, ed. *Advances in Exercise Adherence.* Champaign, IL: Human Kinetics; 1994:343–360.

32. Prochaska JO, Marcus BH. The transtheoretical model: Applications to exercise. In: Dishman R, ed. *Advances in Exercise Adherence.* Champaign, IL: Human Kinetics; 1994:161–180.

33. Bock BC, Marcus BH, Rossi JS, Redding CA. Motivational readiness for change: Diet, exercise, and smoking. *Am J Health Behavior.* 1998;22(4):248–258.

34. Marcus BH, Dubbert PM, Forsyth LH, McKenzie TL, Stone EJ, Dunn AL, Blair SN. Physical activity behavior change: Issues in adoption and maintenance. *Health Psychol.* 2000;19(1)(suppl):32–41.

35. Marcus BH, Rossi JS, Selby VC, et al. The stages and processes of exercise adoption and maintenance in a worksite sample. *Health Psychol.* 1992;11:386–395.

36. Marcus BH, Pinto BM, Simkin LR, et al. Application of theoretical models to exercise behavior among employed women. *Am J Health Prom.* 1994;9(1):49–55.

37. Cardinal BJ. Extended stage model of physical activity behavior. *Journal of Human Movement Studies.* 1999;37:37–54.

38. American Nurses' Association. *Clinician's Handbook of Preventive Services: Put Prevention into Practice.* Waldorf, MD: American Nurses Publishing; 1994.

39. Burns KJ, Camaione DN, Chatterton CT. Prescription of physical activity by adult nurse practitioners: A national survey. *Nurs Outlook.* 2000;48:28–33.

40. North American Nursing Diagnosis Association. *Nursing Diagnoses: Definitions and Classification: 1999–2000.* Philadelphia: NANDA; 1999.

41. McCloskey JC, Bulechek GM, eds. *Nursing Interventions Classification (NIC).* 3rd ed. St. Louis: Mosby; 2000.

42. Johnson M, Maas M, Moorhead S, eds. *Nursing Outcomes Classification (NOC).* 2nd ed. St. Louis: Mosby; 2000.

43. Calfas KJ, Long BJ, Sallis JF, Wooten WJ, Pratt M, Patrick K. A controlled trial of physician counseling to promote adoption of physical activity. *Prev Med.* 1996;25:225–233.

44. *PACE Manual: Patient-Centered Assessment and Counseling for Exercise and Nutrition.* San Diego, CA: San Diego State University Foundation; 1999.

45. Calfas KJ, Sallis JF, Oldenburg B, French M. Mediators of change in physical activity following an intervention in primary care: PACE. *Prev Med.* 1997;26:297–304.

46. King AC, Sallis JF, Dunn AL, Simons-Morton DG, Albright CA, et al. Overview of the Activity Counseling Trial (ACT) intervention for promoting physical activity in primary care settings. *Medicine and Science in Sports and Exercise.* 1998;30(7):1086–1096.

47. Blair SN, Applegate WB, Dunn AL, Ettinger WH, Haskell WL. et al. Activity Counseling Trail (ACT): Rationale, design, and methods. *Medicine and Science in Sports and Exercise.* 1998;30(7): 1097–1106.

48. Pender NJ, Sallis JF, Long BJ, et al. Health-care provider counseling to promote physical activity. In: Dishman RK, ed. *Advances in Exercise Adherence.* Champaign, IL: Human Kinetics; 1994:213–235.

49. Marcus BH, Owen N, Forsyth LH, Cavill NA, Fridinger F. Physical activity interventions using mass media, print media, and information technology. *Am J Prev Med.* 1998;15(4):362–378.

50. Skinner CS, Campbell MK, Rimer BK, Curry S, Prochaska JO. How effective is tailored print communication? *Annals of Behavioral Medicine.* 1999;21(4):290–298.

51. Marcus BH, Bock BC, Pinto BM, Forsyth LH, Roberts MB, et al. Effects of an individualized, motivationally tailored physical activity intervention. *Annals of Behavioral Medicine.* 1998;20(3):174–180.

52. Bull FC, Jamrozik K, Blanksby BA. Tailored advice on exercise—Does it make a difference? *Am J Prev Med.* 1999;16(3):230–239.

53. Blair SN, Kohl HW III, Gordon NF. Physical activity and health: A lifestyle approach. *Med Exerc Nutr Health.* 1992;1:54–57.

54. Harrell JS, McMurray RG, Gansky SA, Bangdiwala SI, Bradley CB. A public health vs. a risk-based intervention to improve cardiovascular health in elementary school children: The cardio-vascular health in children study. *Am J Public Health.* 1999;89(10):1529–1535.

55. Luepker RV, Perry CL, McKinlay SM, Nader PR, Parcel GS, et al. Outcomes of a field trial to improve children's dietary patterns and physical activity: The Child and Adolescent Trial for Cardiovascular Health (CATCH). *JAMA.* 1996;275:768–776.

56. Nader PR, Stone EJ, Lytle LA, Perry CL, Osganian SK, et al. Three-year maintenance of improved diet and physical activity: The CATCH cohort. *Archives of Pediatric and Adolescent Medicine.* 1999;153:695–704.

57. Dunn AL, Marcus BH, Kampert JB, Garcia ME, Kohl HW, et al. Reduction in cardiovascular disease risk factors: 6-month results from Project Active. *Prev Med.* 1997;26:883–892.

58. Kohl HW, Dunn AL, Marcus BH, Blair SN. A randomized trial of physical activity interventions: Design and baseline data from Project Active. *Medicine and Science in Sports and Exercise.* 1998;30(2):275–283.

59. Dunn AL, Garcia ME, Marcus BH, Kampert JB, Kohl HW III. Six-month physical activity and fitness changes in Project Active, a randomized trial. *Medicine and Science in Sports and Exercise.* 1998;30(7):1076–1083.

9

Nutrition and Health

Good nutrition is important to the nurturance of health. Accumulating evidence indicates that eating patterns play a major role in preventing disease and in creating the capacity for energetic and productive living. Although much is yet to be learned through nutrition research about mechanisms underlying the relationship between nutrition and health, community-based health education programs and national dietary and food production policies are focused on promoting optimum nutrition among persons of all ages. One of the goals of *Healthy People 2010*[1] (www.health.gov/healthypeople) is to promote health and reduce chronic disease with diet and weight management. A significant number of the nutrition objectives relate to reducing the proportion of children, adolescents, and adults who are overweight or obese. The objectives that address nutrition and overweight measure in some way the implementation of the Dietary Guidelines for Americans.[2] Other nutrition objectives relate to increasing the quality of food choices made by children and adolescents at school and increasing the proportion of work sites that offer nutrition or weight management classes or counseling.

Of the 27 nutrition objectives in the *Healthy People 2000* initiative, targets for only 5 were met. These included 2 related to the availability of reduced-fat foods and the prevalence of growth retardation. A majority of the remaining objectives showed progress, including those related to intake of fruits, vegetables, grain products, total fat, saturated fat, availability of nutrition labeling, breast-feeding, nutrition education in schools, and work site nutrition and weight management programs. The objective to reduce salt intake in the elderly was not met. Of particular concern was the result that objectives to increase intake of calcium and reduce the number of overweight and obese persons moved away from the targets.[1, 3] The number of children and adults who are overweight or obese increased substantially.[1]

Because nurses are the health professionals most often in extended contact with clients, they are a valuable resource to individuals, families, and communities in providing information and assistance in regard to healthy nutrition. The professional nurse must be able to deal not only with therapeutic aspects of nutrition but also with nutrition as a critical element in prevention and health promotion. Nutritionists and psychologists are valuable colleagues of the nurse in planning sound nutrition education programs for individuals, families, or entire populations.

 # The Role of Nutrition and Diet in Prevention

Poor eating habits are often established during childhood. More than 60% of young people eat too much fat, and less than 20% eat the recommended amount of fruits and vegetables each day.[2] A study of the prevalence and trends over 23 years among children and adolescents (6 to 17 years old) in the U.S. population showed that 11% of children and adolescents were overweight in 1994 and an additional 14% had a body mass index (BMI) between the 85th and 95th percentiles with overweight defined at the 95th percentile. The prevalence of overweight did not differ based on race–ethnicity, income, or education.[4] There is evidence that among boys, there is a prepubertal increase in subcutaneous fat that is lost during adolescence, whereas prepubertal fat in girls continues through puberty and into adulthood.[5] The National Cholesterol Education Program (1991) guidelines for children over 2 years of age were studied to determine whether dietary fat and cholesterol intake in young children compared with recommended levels and to determine the relationship of diet to obesity. The subjects were 468 children, second to fifth graders. The mean percentages of intake from total fat, saturated fat, monounsaturated, and polyunsaturated fat were higher than the recommended levels.[6] A study of 200 obese children (BMI 30 or more) revealed that 35% of the parents did not believe their child to be obese and 53% reported they could control what their child ate. Parents expressed concern about heart disease as a consequence of childhood obesity but did not perceive their own child to be at risk.[7] Studies also document obesity in preschool children. Data collected from 309 charts of children enrolled in a Head Start program found 99 (32%) were obese.[8]

Overweight and obesity affect 55% of the adults in the United States. Over the last two decades, the percentage of obese adults has increased from 14.5% to 22.5% of the population. Approximately 25% of adult women and 20% of adult men are obese (BMI 30 or greater, which equates to 30 pounds or more).[9] African American and Hispanic women are more likely to be obese compared to white women, and the proportion of African American women who are obese is 80% higher than the proportion of African American men who are obese. Because weight management is difficult for most people, the goal of 15% or less of adults having a BMI of 30 or more is challenging.[1]

The overconsumption of saturated fats, cholesterol, sugar, and salt has been linked to four of the leading causes of death: coronary heart disease, some types of cancer, stroke, and Type II diabetes. These diseases cost the U.S. economy over $200 billion in health care expenses and lost productivity.[1] Evidence documents a *strong* link between diet and atherosclerotic cardiovascular diseases and hypertension and is *highly suggestive* for certain forms of cancer, especially those of the esophagus, stomach, large intestine, breast, lung, and prostate. Certain dietary patterns also appeared to predispose individuals to obesity, the risk of non-insulin-dependent diabetes mellitus, chronic liver disease, and possibly osteoporosis. Although these chronic diseases are complex, involving genetic and environmental determinants, modifications in diet may play a significant role in reducing the risk of occurrence.[10,11]

For example, about 1.5 million Americans suffer myocardial infarctions, nearly 500,000 die each year, and many more have angina pectoris.[12] Coronary heart disease (CHD) costs the U.S. economy approximately $100 billion annually. A number of factors influence the development of cardiovascular disease. Factors that offer little possibility for control are genetic predisposition, gender, and advancing age. Factors over which individuals can have control include high blood cholesterol, cigarette smoking, high blood pressure, excessive body weight, and long-term physical inactivity. Addressing controllable risk factors can decrease deposits of cholesterol and other lipids, resultant cellular reactions, and the thickening of coronary artery walls and subsequent risk of myocardial infarction and sudden death.[5]

A considerable amount of observational evidence from case-control and cohort studies provides evidence that dietary factors may be associated with both the occurrence of cancer and protection against cancer.[13] Dietary constituents suspect in the occurrence of cancer include excessive intake of fat, kilocalories, nitrites, mutagens (contained in smoked, charbroiled, fried, or pickled meats), meats, and alcohol. Milk; fruits; vegetables; dietary fiber; vitamins A, C, and E; carotenoids; folate; and calcium have been suggested as protectants against cancer. Cox[14] compared the diets of 210 randomly selected low-income African American and white women on intake of potentially cancer-promoting and cancer-protecting food components. For considerable numbers of the women in both groups, fat intake was above the recommended 30%, fiber intake was less than half the recommended amounts, and consumption of vitamins A, C, E; folate; calcium; fruits; vegetables; and milk were inadequate. Intake of meats and possible sources of nitrites were not excessive. Although the sample studied was relatively small, results of the study indicate the need for aggressive intervention programs to assist low-income populations to make healthy modifications in their dietary intake as a basis for possible protection against cancer.

The *Dietary Guidelines for Americans, 1998*[15] form the basis for a federal nutrition policy. In general these guidelines answer the question concerning how Americans over two years of age should eat for good health. Too many Americans eat too many calories; too much fat, cholesterol, and sodium; too few complex carbohydrates; and not enough fiber, which contributes to the high rates of chronic disease in the United States. The dietary guidelines for the prevention of chronic diseases appear in Table 9–1. The *Food Guide Pyramid,*[16] consistent with these guidelines and published by the U.S. Department of Agriculture, appears in Figure 9–1. The pyramid has replaced the Basic Four Food Groups and is useful for simple dietary screening and as a foundation for general nutrition education. Of calories consumed daily, 30% or less should be from fat (less than 10% saturated fatty acids, 10% polyunsaturated fatty acids, and 10% monounsaturated fatty acids). No more than 300 mgm of dietary cholesterol should be consumed daily. Fat content of some commonly eaten foods appears in Table 9–2. Implementation of these recommendations would result in an approximate reduction of 10% or more in the average blood cholesterol level of the U.S. population and lead to an approximate reduction of 20% or more in coronary heart disease, significantly improving the health and quality of life of the population. As fat in the diet is lowered, carbohydrate intake, primarily complex carbohydrates, should be increased to 50% to 60% of the diet, and protein should not exceed 10% to 20% of calories. Additional recommendations relevant to prevention of cancer include limiting intake of salt-cured, smoked, or nitrate-preserved foods.[15]

TABLE 9-1 Nutrition and Your Health: Dietary Guidelines for Americans

1. Eat a variety of foods.
2. Maintain a healthy weight.
3. Choose a diet low in fat, saturated fat, and cholesterol:
   30% or less of calories from fat;
   less than 10% of calories from saturated fat.
4. Choose a diet with plenty of vegetables, fruits, and grain products:
   3 or more servings of vegetables daily;
   2 or more servings of fruit daily;
   6 or more servings of grain products daily.
5. Use sugars only in moderation.
6. Use salt and sodium only in moderation.
7. If you drink alcoholic beverages, do so in moderation:
   1 drink per day for women
   1 drink per day for men

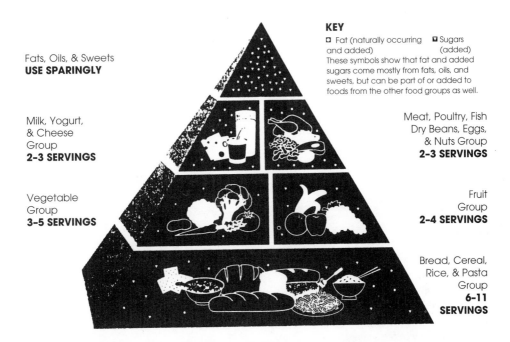

FIGURE 9-1 Food Guide Pyramid: A Guide to Daily Food Choices

(*Source:* U.S. Department of Agriculture–U.S. Department of Health and Human Services)

Most studies on diet and health focus on a single nutrient, food or food group. For example, studies have looked at Vitamin E intake and its relationship to heart disease. Researchers at Queen's College, New York City, studied dietary patterns using diet data from 42,000 women who participated in a two-year breast-cancer study. Those who ate more variety of foods from several of the recommended food categories were found to have a 30% lower death rate during six years of follow-up. It is possible that complex interaction among foods and nutrients in the overall diet produces some protective mechanism.[17]

Undernutrition is also a problem in many segments of the population, resulting in retardation in linear growth of preschool children. Chronic iron deficiency in childhood may have adverse effects on growth and development. The prevalence of iron deficiency is higher in African American children compared to white children and higher in children of families below the poverty level than in children of more affluent families. Inadequate calcium intake in youth may be related to failure to attain peak bone mass during the years of bone mineralization (up to age 20 years), possibly resulting in later predisposition to osteoporosis. Eating disorders resulting from undernutrition such as anorexia nervosa and bulimia are nutritional threats to the health of youth, particularly young women, which are not well understood. Anorexia nervosa affects one in 100 adolescents between 12 and 18 years old.[18] In the nursing home settings, the elderly may experience weight loss due to undernutrition because they are not adequately fed.[19] In a nonrandomized study of undernourished nursing home patients (defined by BMI, weight loss, and anthropometrics), those

TABLE 9-2 Fat Content of Some Foods

Foods	Fat Content (grams)	Total (kcal*)
Milks and Yogurt	per c	per c
skim milk (milk solids added	1	90
low-fat milk (1%)	3	100
low-fat milk (2%)	5	120
whole milk (3.3%)	8	150
low-fat yogurt, plain	4	145
low-fat yogurt, fruit-flavored	3	230
Table Fats	per tbsp	per tbsp
butter	12	100
margarine	12	100
whipped butter or margarine	8	65
mayonnaise	11	100
Creams	per tbsp	per tbsp
half-and-half	2	20
sour cream	3	30
nondairy whipped topping (frozen)	1	15
liquid nondairy coffee lightener	1	20
powdered nondairy coffee lightener	1 (per tsp)	10 (per tsp)
Desserts	per 1/2 c	per 1/2 c
ice cream (11% fat)	7	135
ice cream, soft serve	12	188
ice milk (4.3% fat)	3	93
sherbet	2 per portion	135 per portion
apple pie, 1/4 of 9″ pie	15	345
danish pastry, 4 1/4″ diam × 1″ deep	15	275
doughnut, glazed, 3 3/4″ × 1 1/4″ deep	11	205
Cheese	per 1 oz	per 1 oz
cheddar	9	115
American processed cheese	9	105
part-skim mozzarella	5	80
cottage cheese (4% fat)	5 (½ c)	118
cottage cheese (1% fat)	1 (½ c)	82
Meat, Fish, Poultry	per 3-oz serving	per 3-oz serving
ham, lean and fat	19	245
shrimp	1	100
rib roast, lean and fat	33	375
ground beef, 21% fat	17	235
ground beef, 10% fat	10	185
turkey, light meat	3	150

*Total kilocalories represent the kilocalories not only from fat but also from the protein and carbohydrate the food may contain.
Source: Nutritive Value of Foods, USDA Home and Garden Bulletin No. 72. Washington, DC: U.S. Department of Agriculture; 1981.

who gained at least 10 pounds due to increased nutritional supplements had fewer recurring infections and were less likely to die.[20] Further research is needed to explore mechanisms underlying nutritional problems as a basis for effective interventions.

Factors Influencing Eating Behavior

A wide variety of factors influence overt eating behavior. These factors can be classified as genetic–biologic, psychologic, sociocultural, and environmental. The multicausal nature of eating behavior makes it highly complex and resistant to change. Eating behaviors are an integral part of individual and family lifestyle. Effective modification requires consideration of the factors that determine eating behavior and the use of appropriate behavior change techniques.

Genetic–Biologic Factors

Some advances have been made in identifying the relationship between appetite and metabolic factors as they relate to fat and protein intake. Several new peptides have been identified that play a role in regulating energy expenditure, appetite, and metabolic factors.[21] Fuel metabolism generates signals that control food intake and evidence exists that the interaction of carbohydrate and fat fuel may play a role in overeating.[22] Also, the recent discovery of the "obese" (or "ob") gene offers the potential of understanding what stimulates and inhibits the processes of eating behaviors in humans. With this discovery, new drugs will be developed that will regulate appetite and calorie expenditure.[3] Genetics influence taste and account for some of the variation in the desire for certain foods by some people and not others[23] and appear to confer specific dispositions to the development of obesity.[24] Although one study found evidence that genetic factors influenced the frequency of food intake, no relationship was found to exist between genetic effects on weight gain and actual increase in weight.[25]

The biologic changes of aging have a marked effect on eating behavior. A progressive loss of taste buds on the anterior tongue occurs with age, resulting in decreased sensitivity to sweet and salty tastes. In contrast, taste buds sensitive to bitter and sour increase with age. This taste distortion may result in decreased enjoyment of food and decreased intake of nutrients. Decreased gastric secretions can result in limited absorption of iron, calcium, and vitamin B_{12}. Decreased gastric motility augments the need for foods high in fiber (fresh fruits, raw vegetables, whole-grain breads, and cereals) and increases the importance of water consumption to promote regularity in bowel evacuation. A decrease in basal metabolic rate with aging has also been associated with a decrease in caloric intake. Many elderly people also suffer from isolation and depression. Altered hypothalamic-pituitary-adrenal–axis regulatory mechanisms have been noted in depression, including excessive cortisol secretion and an elevation in corticotropin releasing factor, a potent inhibitor of food intake.[26]

In regard to other physiologic influences, energy requirements also appear to be highly salient biologic determinants of eating behavior. Individuals exhibit awareness and sensitivity to low energy levels. Fatigue, listlessness, and apathy can indicate a caloric intake that is inadequate to meet energy needs. More studies are needed to document how various biologic factors affect eating behavior.

Psychologic Factors

Increasing knowledge of proper nutrition by itself does not necessarily improve eating habits. Adolescents report that saturated fat and foods high in sugar should not be eaten in excess, but this knowledge has only a slight influence on the consumption of foods high in these constituents.[27] Motivation and other psychologic factors must be addressed among persons of all ages if healthy nutritional practices are to become a reality for a larger portion of the population. Psychologic factors can have positive or negative effects on eating behaviors. Perceiving many benefits from good dietary practices encourages individuals to select foods that are high in nutrients, low in fat and refined carbohydrates, high in fiber, and low in sodium and food additives. Health-conscious decisions about nutrition can be taught as early as preschool with systems such as "green" foods (foods high in nutrition), "red" foods (foods low in nutrition), and "yellow" foods (foods with limited but some nutritional value that are to be eaten sparingly). A positive self-concept also creates a psychologic climate that encourages persons of all ages to take care of themselves and control what they eat because they place a high value on their own health and well-being.

Emotions, such as depression, low self-esteem, and lack of personal control over one's life, particularly overeating behavior, can markedly impair nutritional practices. Negative emotions, such as anger, frustration, and insecurity, can lead to disturbances in eating behavior that lead to undernutrition (e.g., anorexia nervosa, bulimia) or overnutrition (obesity). These problems frequently are indicative of a personal search for comfort, security, and nurturance. Focusing on enhancing or modifying self-concept and reducing depression may well be necessary before nutritional behaviors can be changed. Provision of nutritional guidance without attention to coexisting psychologic states may exaggerate rather than ameliorate nutritional problems.

Habits constitute another important determinant of eating behavior. A habit is defined as a behavior that occurs often and is performed automatically or with little conscious awareness.[28] Habits are performed so frequently that many cues within the environment serve as signals for the behavior. They often result in a psychologic addiction to certain behaviors because they become a pervasive part of lifestyle. Such behaviors are known as consummatory because the response itself (eating) provides the reinforcement. People can also become psychologically addicted to the consequences of habitual behaviors such as the "energy spurt" experienced after the ingestion of highly refined sugars (doughnuts, sweet rolls, snack foods) or caffeine (sodas, coffee, chocolate). Habits can result in poor dietary practices because little or no conscious thought is given to eating behavior. Habits also depend on the availability of foods that can be readily consumed without preparation. Fast foods that are high in fats and refined carbohydrates and low in protein, minerals, and vitamins often meet this requirement. To change lifestyle behavior, most notably, modification of eating behavior, self-management skills are necessary. New attitudes and behavior must replace old habits.[29]

Sociocultural Factors

Social determinants of food choice include moral or health concerns (whether one chooses to eat genetically modified foods), optimistic bias (whether one believes others are at a greater risk for negative health outcomes), and ambivalent attitudes about healthy eating habits.[30] The dietary habits of young children are profoundly impacted by family food preparation and eating behaviors. Numerous organizations have recommended th⸝ cholesterol be restricted in the diets of children over two years of age (satur⸝ of calories, total fats to 30% of calories, and dietary cholesterol to less th⸝ African American children and children from low-income families have diets⸝ with recommendations.[31] Parental beliefs about good nutrition for children ꜟꜟꜟy ꜟꜟot match these recommendations and thus may actually contribute to an unhealthy diet. For example, in a study of 547 children between the ages of two and five, the major food source of saturated fat for the total group was whole milk, which contributed 16.1% for white children, 18.5% for African American children, and 26.9% for Hispanic children of saturated fat consumed. Many parents who drink reduced-fat or skim milk themselves will give their children over two years whole milk in the belief that it is better for them. When the diets of African American children were examined separately, their major sources of total dietary fat were franks, sausages, lunch meats, and bacon, with whole milk as a close second. This finding suggests cultural differences that may need to be considered in dietary counseling. Almost a third of total cholesterol consumed by children comes from eggs or egg products, with additional cholesterol added by whole milk, sweets, and beef. Children's diets could be considerably improved by changing the beliefs and practices of their care providers, including parents, other relatives, and day care or preschool personnel. Substituting 1% milk for all the whole milk consumed, skim milk cheese for whole milk cheese, and skim milk for all the low-fat milks consumed would markedly decrease total fat intake. Not all children will find the substitutes acceptable and not all will use them all the time. However, moderate changes in food consumption patterns would result in favorable changes in dietary intake for most children.[2]

Mass media are another aspect of an individual's sociocultural environment that exerts considerable influence over behavior, including health behaviors. Television and print media provide models of various behaviors that result in vicarious learning about the social desirability of behaviors and their positive and negative consequences. For example, in examining nutrition, dieting, and fitness messages in a magazine widely read by adolescent women from 1970 to 1990, Guillen and Barr[32] reported that both nutrition-related and fitness-related coverage emphasized weight loss and physical appearance. Less emphasis was placed on the role of good nutrition in improving health and well-being. The volume of content on nutrition and weight loss did not change over time but the hip:waist ratio of models decreased, becoming less curvaceous and more linear. This is a clear indication that the cultural norm expected of women, "thinness," is becoming **more** evident in media despite national concern about unhealthy nutrition practices among adolescent women that may lead to eating disorders. The peak onset of eating disorders occurs during adolescence. Ironically, in the same magazine, candy and snacks were the most frequently advertised food products. Rapid changes in body shape may make adolescents particularly vulnerable to these confusing messages. This is cause for concern, because early adolescence is a time of high nutritional demands due to high growth rates, energy demands, and calcium and iron requirements related to onset of puberty and menstruation.

Ethnic and cultural backgrounds serve as important influences on eating behavior. Ethnic foods are a source of pride and identity for many groups and may have deep emotional meaning for individuals because of their association with their country of origin or because of fond childhood memories of holidays on which particular foods were served. Food-consumption patterns of some ethnic groups provide good role models for other cultural groups within American society. For example, Choi and colleagues[33] found that when

‫ne nutrition and health status of elderly Chinese Americans in Boston were analyzed, these elderly subjects consumed a high-carbohydrate and low-fat diet, were physically active, and were seldom obese. Compared with elderly whites, they had lower mean blood pressures and blood levels of total and low-density lipoprotein (LDL) cholesterol. Interestingly, high-density lipoprotein (HDL) cholesterol was also lower. Even more interesting were the dietary attitudes and behaviors of Chinese American middle school students when compared to Chinese middle-school students living in China. Chinese students living in China consumed less meat, dairy products, fats, sweets and snacks, and fast foods and consumed more fruits, vegetables, and starches.[34] Story and Harris[35] assessed the meals and snack patterns, food practices and beliefs, and food preferences of 207 Southeast Asian refugee high school students to determine the extent to which they adhered to their traditional cultural diet rather than an American diet. Results of the study indicated that the youth maintained strong ties to their native foods and traditional meal patterns. Rice remained the staple food in their diet. Fruits, meats, and soft drinks, high-status foods in Southeast Asia, remained preferences. In terms of dairy products, white milk was positively viewed but cheese was disliked. Foods with little nutritional value such as candy bars, cakes, and potato chips were not consumed frequently. Overall, the Asian Americans had much healthier nutritional practices than did European Americans. Thus, the nurse should be alert to cultural groups that can serve as positive role models for healthy eating behaviors to other Americans. Sharing health-promoting cultural practices with the larger society is an important asset of the increasing cultural diversity in North America.

Recognition of and respect for individual food preferences is important for professional nurses in dealing with adults from a wide variety of cultural backgrounds. Suggestions for health promotion in diverse cultural communities that can be extrapolated to the promotion of good nutrition in various ethnic groups include:[36,37]

- Understand cultural beliefs about the interrelationships between food and health.
- Recognize how food consumption practices contribute to cultural identity.
- Assess the extent to which acculturation to dominant-group nutritional behaviors has taken place.
- Consult with nutritionists or nurses of similar ethnic backgrounds to clients.
- Form a group of lay consultants on nutritional practices from the target ethnic community.
- Recognize nutritional attributes of ethnic foods.
- Reinforce ethnic nutritional practices that are positive.
- Make recommendations, when necessary, for changing ingredients to lower saturated fats, cholesterol, and sodium or increase fiber while still retaining taste.
- Provide information on nutrient values of ethnic foods to clients.
- Work with ethnic restaurants to offer healthy choices that are acceptable to target populations.
- Promote increased consumption of nutritious ethnic foods among the general population.
- Incorporate healthy ethnic food choices into work site and school site cafeterias and vending machines.

The nurse should also be sensitive to the difficulties that ethnic groups may have in identifying the contents of foods packaged in the United States and in understanding nutrition labeling. Inability to obtain foods familiar to them and trying to eat foods that are unfamiliar can be a source of considerable frustration and distress. Lack of money, language barriers, day-to-day stresses of an unfamiliar environment, and confusing messages on mass media about nutritious foods often serve as barriers to good nutrition among members of varying ethnic groups.[38]

As part of their clients' sociocultural milieu, health professionals serve as important role models in terms of healthy eating patterns. Thus, nurses and other health professionals should not only advocate healthy diets for others but also put the dietary guidelines into practice as a part of their own lifestyles. Modeling recommended eating behaviors as well as struggling with the issues that surround maintenance of positive nutritional practices will indicate a sincerity and commitment to good health practices that speaks louder than words to the clients that they serve.

Environmental Factors

The American food environment is slowly changing to support healthier eating behavior on the part of all Americans. For example, new mandatory labels on all packaged foods contain more complete, useful, and accurate nutrition information than ever before. Improved labeling can assist individuals and families in making healthier food choices. Parents should include children and adolescents in grocery shopping and make them a part of the search for healthy, appealing foods. Learning by active decision making about food selections is one way to increase the nutrition awareness of youth. In 1994, nutrient content claims (e.g., reduced fat) and health claims (e.g., decreases cholesterol) on food-product labels became regulated to eliminate misleading statements. A section called Nutrition Facts on each packaged food product now provides per serving values of nutrient information. Daily value percentages of nutrients are derived from recommended daily allowances (RDAs) and are based on a 2,000 calorie diet.[39] Legislation and regulation to achieve truth in advertising and open disclosure of information on food constituents is an important step toward facilitating consumers' awareness and use of knowledge to make nutritious point-of-choice decisions about food purchases.

Many environmental barriers to healthful eating still remain. The complexities of modern life make it difficult for many individuals consistently to maintain access to foods rich in important nutrients. For example, Americans spend over 40% of their food budget on take-out, restaurant, and convenience foods. Foods prepared away from home are higher in fat, cholesterol, and sodium, and lower in calcium and fiber.[1] The major environmental factors influencing eating patterns appear to be accessibility, convenience, and cost. These factors can present barriers to positive nutritional practices during the action phase of health behavior. Seasonal variation in availability of foods such as raw vegetables and fresh fruits determines both accessibility and costs. Seasonal patterns in the types of fruits and vegetables used by clients need to be followed to maximize nutrient quality and minimize cost. Use of frozen fruits and vegetables in their natural juices rather than those canned during off-season is recommended to decrease the intake of sugar and salt. Home-frozen products are an important source of nutrients at reasonable cost.

Ease of preparation also plays an important role in food selection. Quick and effortless preparation techniques appeal to many families because of busy work schedules. In addition, attractiveness of prepared foods is an important consideration. Assisting the client in selecting nutritious foods that are quickly prepared and esthetically appealing increases the likelihood of sustaining positive eating behavior. Cost of food is also a critical consideration for many families, given the increasing numbers of families living at or below the poverty level. Sources of complex carbohydrates (fruits, vegetables, and grains) may exceed the cost of highly refined sugar products. Proteins also vary greatly in per-unit cost. Assisting families in identifying low-cost, high-nutrition options within their "choice" environments is an important responsibility of the nurse providing nutritional guidance to diverse populations.

In modern society, food additives are used to retard spoilage and prevent deterioration of quality, improve nutritional value, enhance consumer acceptability, and facilitate preparation. Types of additives include preservatives, coloring agents, flavorings, bleaching and maturing agents, and nutrition supplements. By law, labels of many products must list the manufacturer, packer, and distributor, and the amount of each ingredient. Even when ingredients are listed, information on the products is often by itself insufficient to guide knowledgeable food selection. Not only are potentially carcinogenic additives used in preparation of foods (e.g., nitrosamines in bacon and saccharin in low-caloric carbonated beverages), but unintentional food additives such as pesticides and other agricultural chemicals may appear in foods. A great deal of research must be done on the safety of large numbers of food additives. Unfortunately, some of the synergistic, cumulative, and long-term effects of many additives will be determined only after years of use and exposure within human populations.

Nutritional Needs of Special Populations

Infants and Children

The caloric and nutrient intake of children are critical for supporting growth and development. Infants whose diet is primarily mother's milk or infant formula consume 40% or more of their calories from fat, which is appropriate during infancy. When children reach two years of age, however, they should be encouraged to consume a diet lower in total fat, saturated fat, and cholesterol than the usual American diet (36% to 40%) as a basis for lowering risk for chronic diseases in later years.

Iron deficiency is also a problem for 21% of low-income children one to two years of age and for 10% of low-income children three to four years of age. Chronic iron deficiency may have adverse effects on both early and later growth and development. Anemia, an index of iron deficiency, can result in decreased physical ability, impaired body temperature regulation, lowered resistance to infection, and alterations in intellectual performance. A healthy start for infants means encouraging mothers to breast-feed or use iron-rich formulas for formula-fed infants. It is important that during pregnancy and lactation mothers maintain sufficient iron intake through iron-rich foods or supplements, as this increases the likelihood that their children will not be iron deficient during the early years of life.[39,40]

Research suggests that parents influence the dietary choices made by preschoolers. Parents have less influence on food choices made by school-age children.[1] Infants and children in child-care facilities should be provided with adequate nutrition. Cost consciousness on the part of caretakers should not interfere with the provision of good nutrition. It is

important that parents monitor the food provided to their children in care fac
are assured that healthy nutrition guidelines are followed.

Adolescents

Adolescence is a period of biologic and social change. Body size, composition, functions, and physical abilities are changing rapidly. Undernutrition slows height and weight growth and can delay puberty. Among adolescents, minimal dietary requirements are those that maintain an optimal rate of pubertal development and growth. Adolescents who are vigorously active also have increased energy needs. Thus, adolescents should consume diets providing more total nutrients than they consumed as young children. Moderation is a good rule as adolescents whose caloric intake is too high will gain weight, potentially leading to obesity. Those whose caloric intake is too low will experience loss of energy, weight loss, and, in the extreme, eating disorders that can lead to health problems and even premature death. Adolescents with chronic diseases such as diabetes have special nutrition needs, because absorption, metabolism, or excretion of particular nutrients may change both as a result of adolescent biologic changes and as a result of their disease.[41]

In terms of fat intake, adolescents should be given dietary counseling on how to reduce total fat to less than 30% of calories per day and cholesterol to less than 300 milligrams per day to lower risk factors for chronic disease. Because adolescents consume many fast foods at lunchtime or during the evening hours, selecting low-fat fast foods can be a real challenge. As an example of high-fat, fast-food meals, a meal of double burger with sauce, milkshake, and French fries contains 46% of total calories from fat. Because the goal should be less than 30% calories from fats, it is easy to see why consumption of such meals day after day can create conditions of high risk for cardiovascular disease as early as adolescence. There is accumulating evidence that this "risk" carries over into adulthood.[12]

Adolescent girls in the United States typically begin menstruating at 12 1/2 years of age. Menstrual losses increase the need for iron, as does physical activity. Thus, particular attention should be given to adequate intake of this mineral in the diet for women in general and, in particular, for female athletes. The mineral calcium helps to build strong bones. It is also thought that adequate intake of calcium throughout childhood to age 25 will reduce the risk of osteoporosis in later life. Thus, girls should receive counseling on selecting diets that ensure adequate calcium and iron intake.[12]

Adolescents have special nutritional needs that require the attention of adolescents themselves as well as that of their families and primary care health professionals. Nurses play a critical role in heightening awareness of the importance of good nutrition to overall adolescent health and performance. The challenge is to make nutritious food options appealing to adolescents who may eat primarily for taste rather than for nutritional or health reasons. Peer support for healthy eating practices is also critical, as the desire to be accepted by peers is extremely high during the adolescent years. Meal skipping contributes to poor nutrition and should be discouraged. Eating fast food but selecting lower-fat options creates opportunities for adolescents to be with their peers and yet limit fat intake. Pressure on fast-food establishments to offer healthier options is also essential to creating a supportive environment for healthy nutritional practices among adolescents. Schools have been increasingly used in the last few years by health professionals as a vehicle for early health promotion and prevention activities. As of 1992, 9 states mandated nutrition education as a separate activity and another 21 included it as a required topic in mandated subjects such as health. The remaining states did not require it.[42] Efforts on the part of major national health organizations should be directed toward ensuring that nutritional education is a part of all kindergarten through grade 12 education programs. Efforts should also be made to integrate nutrition concepts throughout the entire curriculum including into courses where it is not traditionally taught, such as math, chemistry, and history.[41]

Older Adults

Research on the nutritional needs of the elderly is expanding rapidly as the American population ages. Aging is thought to alter nutrient requirements for calories, protein, and other nutrients as a result of changes in lean body mass, physical activity, and intestinal absorption. Although many older Americans maintain healthy eating patterns, for some, changing nutritional needs may be accompanied by deterioration in diet quality and quantity, jeopardizing nutritional status, quality of life, and functional independence. Many elderly people skip meals and exclude whole categories of food from their diet because of reduced appetites, infrequent grocery shopping, lack of energy to cook, and difficulties in chewing and swallowing. For these individuals, supplementation may be required but should be initiated in consultation with health professionals. Too much self-medication can result in toxic levels of some vitamin and mineral supplements.

The interaction of foods and drugs must be considered. With polypharmacy common in older adults, some may take medications that interact with foods, decreasing nutrient absorption. Foods and drugs can interact, increasing the absorption of some foods and drugs and decreasing the absorption of others. The rate of absorption or the total level of absorption of drugs or nutrients may be affected. For example, crackers, dates, jelly, and other carbohydrates may slow down the rate of absorption of analgesics and limit their effectiveness in reducing pain. Milk, eggs, cereals, and dairy products can inhibit the absorption of iron. Antibiotics such as tetracycline are less readily absorbed when milk, dairy products, or iron supplements are taken. Prune juice, bran cereal, and high-fiber foods can increase intestinal emptying time to the point where some drugs cannot be adequately absorbed. There is a need for further exploration of food–drug interactions that commonly occur among the elderly.[43]

For individuals over 65 years of age, recommended eating patterns lower in saturated fatty acids, total fat, and cholesterol help maintain desired body weight and lower the risk of chronic heart disease (CHD); generally these are nutritionally adequate. High-fat diets contribute to the overall risk of CHD. Risk factors are as follows: being male or a postmenopausal female, having a family history of premature CHD, cigarette smoking, hypertension, high LDL cholesterol level, low HDL cholesterol concentration, diabetes mellitus, history of cerebrovascular or occlusive peripheral vascular disease, and severe obesity. All of these factors except cigarette smoking are influenced by diet in some way. Thus, there is international consensus among scientists that CHD is linked to nutritional patterns throughout life, with the damage manifest most frequently in middle-age and older adults. Daily activity along with an adequate diet can prevent premature mortality from heart disease and maintain vigor into old age.[39,44]

The diets of older Americans generally would be healthier if they contained more complex carbohydrates and fiber. Many elderly people have tooth or mouth problems that make eating fruits and vegetables difficult. Average daily fiber intake among the elderly is less than half the recommended 20 to 35 grams. Health benefits attributed to fiber include pr[?]tion, reduced risk of colon cancer, reduction of serum cholesterol, and i[?] response. Six servings of whole grains are the recommended minimum for th[?]

Energy requirements decline with reductions in body size, lean body m[?]olism rate, and decreased physical activity. Because physical activity maintains muscle mass, it is highly desirable to keep physically active in later years. Diets of the elderly may also be deficient in protein along with calories as the result of inability to chew meat or the cost of protein-rich foods. Infections, trauma, and other metabolic stresses may increase protein needs. Protein–calorie malnutrition can lower resistance to disease and delay recovery from illness.[39]

Older adults of limited economic means should be assisted in selecting low-cost foods that meet recommended nutritional requirements. They may need guidance on using label information to select foods and on how to prepare foods so that they are easier to chew and swallow. Nutrition is integral to quality of life for the elderly. Thus, it is a primary area for focus by nurses providing care to the elderly in primary care and long-term care settings.

Interventions to Change Eating Behaviors

The functional health pattern inclusive of eating behaviors is the Nutritional-Metabolic Pattern. Gordon[45] describes this area of functional assessment as patterns of food and fluid consumption relative to metabolic need. Nursing diagnoses relevant to health promotion include Altered nutrition: high risk for more than body requirements, Altered nutrition: more than body requirements, and Altered nutrition: less than body requirements. Diagnoses focus on the categories of obesity and undernutrition. An overview of definitions, defining characteristics, and etiologic or related factors can be found in Gordon's *Manual of Nursing Diagnosis: 1998–1999.*

Improving eating patterns involves changing knowledge, attitudes, and skills as well as the food consumption environment. The following strategies are recommended:

- Improving accessibility of nutrition information, nutrition education, nutrition counseling and related services, and healthful foods in a variety of settings and for all subpopulations
- Focusing on preventing chronic disease associated with diet and weight, beginning in youth
- Strengthening the link between nutrition and physical activity in health promotion
- Maintaining a strong national program for basic and applied nutrition research to provide a sound science base for dietary recommendations and effective interventions
- Maintaining a strong national nutrition monitoring program to provide accurate, reliable, timely, and comparable data to assess status and progress and to be responsive to unmet data needs and emerging issues
- Strengthening state and community data systems to be responsive to the data users at these levels
- Building and sustaining broad-based initiatives and commitment to these objectives by public and private sectors partners at the national, state, and local levels[1]

Altering nutrition education, the food acquisition environment, and food consumption patterns will all contribute to health. To alter nutrition education, there must be wide exposure of the general population at all ages to nutrition education through mass media, education at schools and work sites, do-it-yourself nutrition education packages, and nutrition counseling in primary health care services. New information technology must be used while at the same time making sure that nutrition education approaches are user friendly. Interactive computer nutrition programs, nutrition videos, and integration of healthy nutrition messages into packaging are all important in broad-based nutrition education. The dietary advice offered needs to evolve as scientific discoveries about the contribution of diet to health take place.[46,47,48]

The food acquisition environment still must undergo considerable change. It is affected by legislation and regulation regarding production of food and by availability of food options. Many populations at schools and work sites are captive and rely primarily on others to provide and prepare their food for a considerable part of the day. The availability of healthy options within the environment, such as from cafeterias and vending machines, greatly affect nutrition behaviors. Furthermore, healthy food choices must have appeal in terms of taste and texture. Widespread research in the food production industry is creating more food options that are both consistent with dietary recommendations and acceptable to the public.

Food consumption patterns are affected not only by knowledge and availability but also by the decision-making patterns of the individual or family. Kiosks at grocery stores and shopping malls to query about nutrients in specific foods as well as simple coding systems for fat, sodium, and fiber content all provide cues and easy assistance to consumers in making food selections.

Randomized Clinical Studies Outcomes

The development of randomized clinical trials to study long-term success of strategies for changing eating behavior is an increasingly important goal for scientists in the fields of nutrition and behavior. Although it is not always possible to generalize the findings of clinical trials to the general population due to the stringent criteria for inclusion of participants, the findings do make an important contribution to the knowledge about changing eating behaviors.[49,50]

In a review of dietary fat reduction research, Barnard found that studies that had the strictest fat intake reduction resulted in the greatest success. Some studies set less stringent fat restrictions to make the diet more acceptable to the study participants, and it appeared to minimize the degree of change needed and discouraged people from making the commitment to reduce their fat intake. Other study characteristics that predicted success were focus on participants who had cardiac problems, participants who initiated the program while in a hospital, family involvement, frequent monitoring, prepackaged meals, and meatless or vegetarian meals. Support groups were not found to contribute to reduction of fat intake. Barnard looked at a total of 18 studies that were one year or longer and found that the mean fat intake was 29 percent. This compared with a mean intake of 28 percent fat reported in 21 shorter studies showing that the length of the intervention did not make a difference in the reduction of the participants' fat intake. Brunner and colleagues[50] found similar outcomes in their review of several randomized, controlled intervention studies and

10 other studies. However, in all of the studies the greater the number of intervention contacts, the greater the positive change.

The Eating Patterns Study

The Eating Patterns Study[51] is a randomized controlled study of 2,111 patients in six primary care practices. The study participants were 90% white and had at least some college education. The primary care offices were randomized to have intervention or no intervention conditions. The low-intensity intervention included a self-help book, *Help Yourself,* introduced by a physician and a two-week follow-up letter. A food frequency questionnaire and a foods habit questionnaire were administered over the telephone at three-month and one-year intervals after the baseline data were collected. The control group offices received no intervention. Intake of fat was reduced in the intervention and control groups with the amount of reduction of fat significantly more in the intervention group controlling for age, gender, and baseline value. Participants in the intervention group had greater success than did others in the intervention group if they had the responsibility for food shopping and preparation, were motivated to change, and indicated they used the self-help book. The summary of research findings to date indicates that in large, intensive, community-based studies fat intake can be modified in participants who are well screened and motivated to change. In smaller studies with less intensive interventions, smaller changes are found to occur.[47]

Work Site Intervention Study

Sorenson and colleagues[52] studied the dietary fat, fiber, and fruit and vegetable intake in a two-year multi work site intervention. The intervention included joint planning and implementation of work site programs by workers and management, increased healthy foods available at the work site, and programs offered to support individual change. Questionnaires were used to collect data over time. The intervention resulted in an increased fruit and vegetable intake (0.23 servings per day) compared to the control sites (0.10 servings per day). Managers and professional staff increased their intake of fruits and vegetables more than did other workers, but they did not improve their fiber intake to the extent that others workers did. The number of community-based studies conducted to study fruit and vegetable intake is limited. The results of the few studies available show that small increases in fruit and vegetable consumption can be achieved.[47]

The Waianae Diet Program

The Waianae Diet Program[53] is an excellent example of a culturally sensitive program to change eating behaviors of the native Haiwaiian population, who have a disproportionately high rate of obesity. In 1993, the program received the Distinguished Community Health Promotion Program Award from the U.S. Secretary for Health and Human Services. The primary intervention is a three-week program of adhering to a strict, traditional Hawaiian diet with medical monitoring. Historical evidence suggests that prior to the adoption of western diets, Native Hawaiians had little cardiovascular disease or obesity.

The intervention includes a number of components. In the evenings, community participants come together to eat traditional foods such as taro (a starchy root similar to potato), poi (a mashed form of taro), sweet potatoes, yams, breadfruit, greens, fruit, seaweed, fish, and chicken. This diet approximates that of ancient Hawaiians, which was estimated to contain less than 10% fat, 12% to 15% protein, and 75% to 78% carbohydrates. Participants also attend educational sessions, which include cultural teachings, nutrition education, and motivational sessions. They are taught techniques for using the diet as a template for making food choices. A whole-person approach, with emphasis on spiritual aspects of living and group *ohana* (family-like) support, are additional features. Participants are particularly encouraged to act as role models for the modified eating behaviors they have learned. The program is viewed as a strategy for community empowerment, bringing community members together to address a problem they want to solve.

Early results suggest that the Waianae Diet Program[53] has been successful. Weight, cholesterol, low-density lipoproteins (LDL), triglycerides, glucose, and systolic and diastolic blood pressures have decreased significantly in participants. Long-term evaluation is necessary to determine if modified eating behaviors and their health benefits can be sustained. The unique aspects of the program offer particular insight into how changes in dietary behavior can be integrated into the cultural, spiritual, recreational, and social aspects of participants' life perspective. This whole-person approach, espoused by nursing, may decrease the problems with compliance to new dietary behaviors evident in so many prior studies.

The Partners in Prevention Nutrition Program

This intervention[46] used a stage-of-change approach based on the transtheoretical model developed by Prochaska and colleagues[54] to match tailored communications about dietary behavior to the needs of participants at different points in the change process. The 558 adult participants were recruited from four family practices in central North Carolina. The study sample was 73% female, 62.3% married, 19% minority (predominantly African American) with a mean education level of 13.6 years, average age of 40.8 years, and median income level of $30,000 to $39,000. A randomized trial was used with pretest and posttest measures to determine the impact of tailored versus nontailored nutrition education materials on consumption of fat, fruit, and vegetables. Current dietary intake, stage of change in regard to dietary behavior, self-efficacy for dietary change, beliefs concerning perceived susceptibility to diet-related diseases, perceived benefits of dietary change to avoid health problems, and other psychosocial and physical variables were assessed at baseline. Participants were categorized at baseline as being in one of the following stages: precontemplation (not seriously thinking about change), contemplation (seriously thinking about change within the next 6 months), preparation (planning to change within the next 30 days), or action or maintenance (currently trying to change). Participants were randomly assigned to one of three groups: tailored nutrition messages, nontailored nutrition messages, or a control group that received no nutrition messages. Messages were mailed to participants three weeks after collection of baseline data. The tailored intervention consisted of a one-time, mailed nutrition information packet customized to participant's stage of change, dietary intake, and psychosocial information. For example, contemplators received information designed to decrease barriers to change and increase self-efficacy. Those individuals already trying to change received tailored recipes and messages aimed at preventing relapse. The nontailored messages provided standard risk information about the relation of diet to disease and gave dietary recommendations based on the 1990 *Dietary Guidelines for Americans*.[15] The control group completed pretest and posttest surveys but received no nutrition information. Members of the tailored message group, when surveyed approximately six months later, had significantly decreased total fat by 23% compared to 9% in the nontailored group and 3% in the control group. The tailored group reported decreased saturated fat by 26%, compared to 11% in the nontailored group and 3% in the control group. The tailored message did not affect reported intake of fruits and vegetables. Also, more individuals in the tailored message group, compared to the other groups, remembered receiving and reading the nutrition information packet. Thus, the stage-of-change approach to dietary modification looks promising. Further research is needed to determine whether interventions based on the transtheoretical model can be used to promote maintenance of dietary changes.[46]

Maintaining Recommended Weight

Obesity is generally defined as a BMI of greater than or equal to 30kg/m.[9] Whereas the physical basis for excessive weight gain is relatively simple and straightforward (i.e., the ingestion of more calories than needed for energy expenditure), the actual causes of being overweight are complex. They include

1. Heredity
2. Cognitive factors (e.g., unrealistic personal standards and expectations)
3. Affective factors (e.g., emotional problems such as anxiety, boredom, and feelings of powerlessness)
4. Interpersonal factors (e.g., family problems, difficulties with fellow workers or colleagues)
5. Sociocultural factors (food selection, food preparation, and food consumption practices)
6. Environmental factors (e.g., salient cues for eating behavior and level of environmental sensitivity)

Although heredity plays a role in predisposition toward excessive weight gain, it is more important to focus on personal (cognitive, affective), interpersonal, sociocultural, and environmental influences.[55,56]

The primary goal of interventions for weight loss is the permanent alteration of eating patterns and physical activity, rather than weight loss only. Actually, adopting more healthful eating behaviors is directed toward increasing rather than decreasing the pleasures derived from eating. New awareness of taste, texture, and form of foods allows the individual to participate to the fullest in the eating experience, totally involving gustatory, visual, olfactory, and tactile senses. Eating that promotes optimum health can be fulfilling, self-actualizing, and totally enjoyable.

The individual who maintains desired weight has taken a major step toward decreasing risk for many chronic health problems. Average recommended caloric intake for men and women of different ages to maintain weight, assuming that they are moderately active, appears in Table 9–3. Not only does weight loss decrease the risk of chronic disease, it has been shown to increase self-esteem, perceptions of control, and feelings of social desirability

TABLE 9-3 Average Recommended Caloric Intake for Men and Women of Different Ages: Moderate Activity (in kilocalories)

| Age | Men | | Women | |
---	Mean	Range	Mean	Range
19–22	2,900	2,500–3,000	2,100	1,700–2,500
23–50	2,700	2,300–3,100	2,000	1,600–2,400
51–75	2,400	2,000–2,800	1,800	1,400–2,200
over 75	2,050	1,650–2,450	1,600	1,200–2,000

and acceptance. Individuals of normal weight are more active than their overweight counterparts, and this further promotes health and decreases risk for health problems. On the other hand, frequent bouts of weight loss may be detrimental to health, as serum cholesterol is elevated during weight loss. Adipocytes are the fat cells within the body that increase in lipid content with weight gain. Weight reduction is achieved through decrease in size of cells. As increased by-products of fat metabolism enter systemic circulation, precautions must be taken to prevent their deposit in the lining of vessels and their detrimental effects to internal organs such as liver and kidneys. Stability of weight can prevent many of these potential hazards.

Initiating a Weight-Reduction Program

The individual who desires to lose more than 20 pounds should obtain a health history, physical examination, blood lipid and glucose analysis, and electrocardiogram before beginning a weight-loss program. Also, careful assessment of current dietary habits is essential in order to develop an individualized, effective program.

Other points to consider include the following:

- Is the person strongly motivated to change?
- Are there health conditions that make weight reduction a high priority?
- If change is desired, are expectations realistic?
- Does the person have a support system within or outside of the family to facilitate weight loss?
- Has the person had past successes in weight loss? If so, what worked? What did not work?

The best weight-loss program will be one that closely mirrors the *Dietary Guidelines* described earlier. Caloric reduction while maintaining adequate nutrient levels, adequate vitamins and minerals, and adequate fiber is the best way to achieve and maintain desired weight. Thus radical changes in food consumption patterns are not recommended as a means of weight loss. The nurse can review the many weight-loss Web sites to help clients determine if a Web site program is a practical alternative to in-person diet counseling. One such site, Shape Up America, is operated by former Surgeon General C. Everett Koop, MD.[57]

A combination of dietary modifications that individuals find palatable and adequate exercise offer the best approach to achieving and maintaining recommended weight. Physical activity promotes expenditure of energy and can facilitate weight loss. Exercise is not only useful in burning excess calories; studies have suggested that it also prevents the loss of protein from muscle and minerals from bone that frequently occur when attempts at weight loss are accompanied by inactivity. Exercise in combination with restricted calories also assists in reducing undesirable lipoprotein lipids, increasing work capacity, lowering resting heart rate, and decreasing blood pressure. Increased physical activity generally decreases appetite and increases basal metabolism rate for several hours, offsetting the reduced metabolic rate that accompanies calorie restriction.[36]

Further, positive changes in affect and mood that often accompany exercise can improve the long-term compliance with newly acquired eating behaviors. Both exercise during leisure time and lifestyle exercise should be increased as a complement to healthy nutritional practices. The reader is referred to Chapter 8 for discussion of further benefits of exercise and how to facilitate exercise adherence.

 # Directions for Research in Nutrition and Health

Further research is needed to understand the links between nutrition and health. Studies on the effects of fats, fiber, and sodium on the development of cardiovascular disorders and cancer are only beginning. Further research is needed to explore the positive and negative effects of various food components on health as well as on specific disorders. A better understanding of factors related to undernutrition, particularly eating disorders in adolescents and young adults, and overnutrition is critically needed as a basis for effective nursing interventions.

To promote healthy eating habits across the life span, behavioral theories and models applicable to eating behavior should be tested predictively and, as warranted, incorporated into intervention studies. Existing theories in nursing, psychology, and public health can be used to design behavioral interventions that focus on the individual, the family, and the community. Studies should be conducted where assessments allow determination of the most appropriate behavioral model to employ to augment positive eating behaviors of a given client. The availability of new technology provides the base for developing powerful assessment tools to facilitate tailoring of nutrition interventions.

Further research will provide additional answers concerning the underlying mechanisms through which nutrition improves health and well-being.

 # Directions for Practice in Nutrition and Health

The responsibility for monitoring the nutritional health of individuals, families, and the community is shared among nurses, nutritionists, and other health professionals. There is a tremendous gap between the knowledge about nutrition and diet and the eating behaviors of the U.S. population. The lack of adoption of positive dietary habits and good nutrition has resulted in a population of children, adolescents, and adults who are overweight and/or obese. The chronic health problems that often follow are costly to the individual and family, as well as the national economy. Dietary counseling and education should be an integral part of nursing practice in all settings. Counseling and follow-up of each client whose BMI is outside the normal range is a challenge the nurse must accept.

Opportunities can be created to engage clients and others in dialogue about their dietary practices and modifications that would improve their health. Nurses are respected professionals who influence their communities and schools. School nurses and occupational health nurses must work with school and industry officials to improve the food choices in cafeterias and vending machines. Internet Web sites that focus on nutrition are a quick way to keep current on research findings and practice outcomes as well as to share with clients. Clients need to be encouraged to seek information from the Internet and discuss it with the nurse. One of the most important ways the nurse can influence others is to role model weight management and good dietary habits.

SUMMARY

Professional support of the client by the nurse and suggestions for constructively dealing with barriers to changing eating behaviors facilitates the client's efforts to eliminate or minimize obstacles that block attainment of desired nutritional goals. Promoting good nutrition is a critical concern in illness prevention and health promotion and an important dimension of competent self-care and dependent care. Cultural background influences eating behavior. The family and community should be considered as points for nutritional intervention that may, in the long run, be more productive than individual interventions. Because much is yet to be learned about nutrition and health, nurses and other health scientists should accept the challenge of exploring eating behavior as an important health promotion activity.

REFERENCES

1. U.S. Department of Health and Human Services. *Healthy People 2010* (Conference Edition, in Two Volumes). Washington, DC: U.S. Government Printing Office; January 2000.
2. U.S. Department of Agriculture and U.S. Department of Health and Human Services. *Dietary Guidelines for Americans.* 4th ed. Home and Garden Bulletin; 1995 Dec; no. 232.
3. Glanz, K. Progress in dietary behavior change. *Am J of Health Prom,* 1999 Nov–Dec;14(2): 112–117.
4. Goran, MI. Measurement issues related to studies of childhood obesity: Assessment of body comparison, body fat distribution, physical activity, and food intake. *Pediatrics.* 1998 Mar;101(3)(suppl):505–518.
5. National Cholesterol Education Program. *Report of the Expert Panel on Population Strategies for Blood Cholesterol Reduction: (Adult Treatment Panel II): Executive Summary. Cholesterol in Adults.* 1993.

6. Stewart KJ, Seemans CM, McFarland LD, Weinhufer JJ, Brown CS. Dietary fat and cholesterol intake in young children compared with recommended levels. *Journal of Cardiopulmonary Rehabilitation*. 1999 Mar–Apr;19(2):112–117.

7. Myers S, Vargas Z. Parental perceptions of the preschool obese child. *Ped. Nurs.* 2000 Jan–Feb;26(1):23–30.

8. Hernandez B, Uphold CR, Graham MV, Singer, L. Prevalence and correlates of obesity in pre-school children. *J of Ped Nurs.* 1998 Apr;13(2):68–76.

9. National Institutes of Health. *Clinical Guidelines on the Identification, Evaluation, and Treatment of Overweight and Obesity in Adults*. NIH Publication No. 98-4083;1998 Sep.

10. U.S. Department of Health and Human Services, Public Health Service, National Institutes of Health. *Second Report of the Expert Panel on Detection, Evaluation and Treatment of High Blood Cholesterol in Adults (Adult Treatment Panel II): Executive Summary*. 1993 Sep. NIH Publication No. 93-3096.

11. Ludwig DS, Pereira MA, Kroenke CH, Hilner JE, Van Horn L, Slattery ML, Jacobs DR. Dietary fiber, weight gain, and cardiovascular disease risk factors in young adults. *JAMA*. 1999 Oct;282(16):1539–1546.

12. U.S. Preventive Services Task Force. *Guide to Clinical Preventive Services*. 2nd ed. Washington, DC: U.S. Government Printing Office; 1996.

13. Robertson I, Bound R, Segal L. Colorectal cancer, diet and lifestyle factors: Opportunities for prevention. *Health Promotion International*. 1998 Jun;13(2):141–150.

14. Cox RH, Gonzales-Vigilar MCR, Novascone MA, Silva-Barbeau I. (July–Aug). Impact of a cancer intervention on diet-related cardiovascular disease risks of white and African-American EFNEP clients. *J Nut Educ*. 1996;28(4):209–218.

15. Crane NT, Hubbard VS, Lewis CJ. National nutrition objectives and the Dietary Guidelines for Americans. *Nutr Today*. 1998;33:49–58.

16. U.S. Department of Agriculture. *The Food Guide Pyramid: A Guide to Daily Food Choices*.

17. Rosenberg IH, ed. A healthful diet goes beyond this or that food. *Tufts University Health & Nutrition Letter*. 2000 Jun;18(4):8.

18. National Center for Health Statistics. *Healthy People 2000 Review 1998–1999*. DHHS Pub. No. (PHS) 99-1256. Hyattsville, MD: Public Health Service, U.S. Department of Health and Human Services; 1997.

19. Kayser-Jones J, Schell E. The effect of staffing on the quality of care at mealtime. *Nurs Outlook*. 1997 Mar–Apr;45(2):64–72.

20. Keller HH. Weight gain impacts morbidity and mortality in institutionalized older persons. *J Am Geriatrics Society*. 1995 Feb;43(2):165–169.

21. Bessesen DH. Obesity as a factor. *Nutr Rev*. 2000 Mar;58(3 Pt 2):S12–15.

22. Friedman MI. Fuel partitioning and food intake . . . proceedings of a symposium held at The University of Texas Southwestern Medical Center, Dallas. April 22–23, 1996. *Am J Clin Nutr*. 1998 Mar;67(3S):(suppl):513S–518S.

23. Duffy VB, Bartoshuk LM. Food acceptance and genetic variation in taste. *J Am Diet Assoc*. 2000 Jun;100(6):647–655.

24. Blundell JE, Cooling J. High-fat and low-fat (behavioral) phenotypes: Biology or environment? *Proc Nutr Soc*. 1999;58(4):773–777.

25. Heitmann BL, Harris JR, Lissner L, Pedersen NL. Genetic effects on weight change and food intake in Swedish adult twins. *Am J Clin Nutr*. 1999 Apr;69(4):597–602.

26. MacIntosh CG, Andrews JM, Jones KL, Wishart JM, Morris HA, Jansen JB, Morley JE, Horowitz M, Chapman IM. Effects of age on concentrations of plasma cholecystokinin,

glucagon-like peptide 1, and peptide YY and their relation to appetite and pyloric motility. *Am J Clin Nutr.* 69(5):999–1006.

27. Louis Harris Associates. *The Kellogg's Child Nutrition Survey.* New York: Louis Harris and Associates; 1989.

28. Martin RA, Poland EY. *Learning to Change: A Self-Management Approach to Adjustment.* New York: McGraw-Hill, Inc; 1980.

29. Brownell KD. The central role of lifestyle change in long-term weight management. *Clin Cornerstone.* 1999;2(3):43–51.

30. Shepherd R. Social determinants of food choice. *Proc Nutr Soc.* 1999 Nov;58(4):807–812.

31. Purcell AC, O'Brien E, Parks PL. Cholesterol levels in children: To screen or not to screen. *J Ped Nurs: Care of Children and Families.* 1996 Feb;11(1):40–44.

32. Guillen EO, Barr SI. Nutrition, dieting, and fitness messages in a magazine for adolescent women, 1970–1990. *J Adolesc Health.* 1994;15;464–472.

33. Choi ESK, McGandy RB, Dallal GE, et al. The prevalence of cardiovascular risk factors among elderly Chinese-Americans. *Arch Intern Med.* 1990;150:413–418.

34. Sun WY, Chen W. (1994). A preliminary study of potential dietary risk factors for coronary heart disease among Chinese-American adolescents. *J School Health.* 1994;64:368–371.

35. Story M, Harris LJ. Food preferences, beliefs, and practices of Southeast Asian refugee adolescents. *J School Health.* 1988;58:273–276.

36. Zephier EM, Ballew C, Mokdad A, Mendlein J, Smith C, Yeh JL, Lee E, Welty TK, Howard B. Intake of nutrients related to cardiovascular disease risk among three groups of American Indians: The strong heart dietary study. *Prev Med.* 1997 Jul–Aug;26(4):508–515.

37. Gutierrez YM. *Nutrition in Health Maintenance and Health Promotion for Primary Care Providers.* San Francisco: School of Nursing, University of California, San Francisco; 1994.

38. Wellman NS. Dietary guidelines and nutrient requirements of the elderly. *Prim Care.* 1994;21(1):1–18.

39. Morbidity and Mortality Weekly Report. *Recommendations to Prevent and Control Iron Deficiency in the United States.* Atlanta, GA: Centers for Disease Control; 1998 Apr.

40. U.S. Congress, Office of Technology Assessment. *Adolescent Health Volume II: Background and the Effectiveness of Selected Prevention and Treatment Services.* 1991 Washington, DC: US Government Printing Office. Publication OTA-H-466.

41. Morbidity and Mortality Weekly Report. *Guidelines for School Health Programs to Promote Lifelong Healthy Eating.* Atlanta, GA: Centers for Disease Control; 1996 Jun.

42. Ellison RC, Capper AL, Goldberg RJ, Witschi JC, Stare FJ. The environmental component: Changing school food service to promote cardiovascular health. *Health Educ Q.* 1989;16(2):285–297.

43. Blandford, G. Eating disorders. In: Tallis R, Fillit H, Brocklehurst JC, eds. *Brocklehurst's Textbook of Geriatric Medicine and Gerontology.* 5th ed. New York: Churchill Livingstone;1998:1413–1421.

44. Food and Drug Administration and National Institutes of Health. Nutrition and overweight (Chapter 19). In: *Healthy People 2010* (Conference Edition). Washington, DC: U.S. Government Printing Office; January 2000.

45. Gordon M. *Manual of Nursing Diagnosis:* 1998–1999 St. Louis: Mosby Year Book; 1999.

46. McCann BS, Bovbjerg VE. Promoting dietary change. In: Shumaker SA, Schron EB, Ockene JK, McBee WL, eds. *The Handbook of Health Behavior Change.* 2nd ed. New York: Springer;1998:166–188.

47. Kumanyika SK, Van Horn L, Bowen D, Perri MG, Rolls BJ, Czajkowski SM, Schron E. 2000; Maintenance of dietary behavior change. *Health Psychol.* 2000;19(1)(suppl):42–56.

48. Wing RR. Cross-cutting themes in maintenance of behavior change. *Health Psychol.* 2000 Jan;19(suppl 1):84–88.

49. Barnard ND, Akhtar A, Nicholson A. Factors that facilitate compliance to a low fat intake. *Archives of Family Medicine.* 1995;4:153–158.

50. Brunner E, White I, Thorogood M, Bristow A, Curle D, Marmot M. Can dietary interventions change diet and cardiovascular risk factors? A meta-analysis of randomized controlled trials. *Am J Public Health.* 1997;87:1415–1422.

51. Beresford SAA, Curry S, Kristal A, Lazovich D, Feng Z, Wagner EH. A low intensity dietary intervention in primary care practice: The eating patterns study. *Am J Public Health.* 1997;87:610–616.

52. Sorenson G, Stoddard A, Peterson K, Cohen N, Hunt MK, Stein E, Palombo R, Lederman R. Increasing fruit and vegetable consumption through worksites and families in the Treatwell 5-a-day study. *Am J of Public Health.* 1999 Jan;89(1):54–60.

53. Shintani T, Beckham S, Kanawaliwali H, et al. The Waianae Diet Program: A culturally sensitive, community-based obesity and clinical intervention program for the native Hawaiian population. *Hawaii Med J.* 1994;53:136–147.

54. Prochaska JA, DiClemente C, Norcross J. In search of how people change: Applications to addictive behaviors. *Am Psychol.* 1992;47:1102–1114.

55. Kikuchi Y, Watanabe S. Personality and dietary habits. *J Epidemiol.* 2000 May 10(3):191–198.

56. Ounpuu S, Woolcott DM, Greene GW. Defining stage of change for lower-fat eating. *J Am Diet Assoc.* 2000 Jun;100(6):674–679.

57. Rosenberg IH, ed. A guide to rating the weight-loss websites. *Tufts University Health & Nutrition Letter, Special Supplement;* 2000 Jun.

10

Stress Management and Health

Stress is of theoretical and practical interest to nurses. Nurse researchers have studied various aspects of stress in attempts to understand the stress–illness relationship as well as how to promote health through fostering stress resistance and overall resilience among individuals and families. It is estimated that 60% to 90% of visits to health care professionals are for stress-related disorders. With this high an incidence of stress-related health problems, strategies for promoting stress reduction among clients are of critical importance to minimize insults to well-being and maximize positive challenge and realization of personal potential.

Stress is an inevitable human experience in any modern society characterized by rapid and accelerating change. Selye, a pioneer in stress research, defined stress as "the nonspecific response of the body to any demand made on it."[1] Internal and external manifestations of stress are referred to as the General Adaptation Syndrome (GAS) or the "fight-or-flight" response. Specific physiologic or behavioral changes that occur in response to stressors include:

- Dilatation of pupils
- Increased respiratory rate
- Increased heart rate
- Peripheral vasoconstriction
- Increased perspiration
- Increased blood pressure
- Increased muscle tension
- Increased gastric motility
- Release of adrenalin
- Increased blood glucose level
- Raising of body hair
- Cold and clammy hands

The major sources of distress experienced by individuals in modern society originate in interpersonal relationships (communication) and performance demands (action) rather than from direct physical threat. Because communication and action represent two basic human processes, the potential for stress is always present.[1]

Stressors, the cause of stress, are defined by Lazarus and Folkman[2] as "environmental and internal demands and conflicts among them, which tax or exceed a person's resources." The body's response to stress involves the nervous, endocrine, and immunologic systems, which in turn affect all organ systems. Although all individuals experience stress, people interpret and react to it differently, resulting in differing vulnerabilities to the deleterious effects of stress. Some stressors are viewed as challenges, creating stimulation and excitement. Other stressors are viewed negatively, perhaps because they are considered undesirable, uncontrollable, or emotionally distressing. There is much scientific interest in the "resistance resources" that enable some individuals to successfully manage stressors and flourish whereas others find the same stressors debilitating.

Coping strategies assist individuals in dealing with stress and can be described as learned and purposeful cognitive, emotional, and behavioral responses to stressors used to adapt to the environment or to change it.[2] In the coping process, the ability to regulate emotions, behavior, and the environment are critical to successful adjustment. Cognitive appraisal and coping constitute the stress-coping process. Cognitive appraisal consists of two phases. In *primary appraisal*, the person evaluates whether he or she has anything at stake in the encounter. Is there potential harm or benefit to cherished commitments, values, goals, self-esteem, or the health and well-being of a significant other?[3] If an encounter is threatening, primary appraisal can serve to reduce its significance for the person experiencing it. For example, if a person receives notice that the results of a laboratory test are "abnormal," the person may discount the validity of the test.[3(p 133)] In *secondary appraisal*, the person evaluates what, if anything, can be done to overcome or prevent harm or to improve the prospects of benefit. Various coping options are evaluated, such as altering the situation, accepting it, seeking more information, or holding back from acting in an impulsive way. Primary and secondary appraisals converge to determine if the person–environment transaction is primarily threatening or challenging. Coping regulates stressful emotions (emotion-focused coping) and alters the person–environment relation that is causing the distress (problem-focused coping). Both forms of coping occur in stressful encounters. The success of problem-focused coping may in large part depend on the success of emotion-focused coping, because heightened emotions are likely to interfere with cognitive activity necessary to deal effectively with stressors. Problem-focused coping is likely to be dominant in encounters viewed as changeable, whereas emotion-focused coping often dominates in encounters viewed as unchangeable, with acceptance as the only recourse.[3] Encounters involving threat to self-esteem are often the most difficult to resolve. These threats include the possibility of losing the affection of someone one cares about, losing self-respect or the respect of others, and appearing to be unethical or incompetent.

It is estimated that disability, absenteeism, decreased productivity, and health-damaging effects of stress cost business and industry more than $150 billion annually.[4] Thus, there are considerable financial incentives to businesses and health maintenance organizations to help individuals manage stress and avoid its costly, health-impairing effects.

The goal of *Healthy People 2010*[4] related to mental health is to improve mental health and ensure access to appropriate, quality mental health services. One of the *Healthy People 2010 Mental Health and Mental Disorders* community-focused objectives is increasing the number of persons seen in primary health care settings who receive mental health screening. Adults who seek mental health care in primary care settings have fewer visits per year (4) than do those adults who are seen by specialists (14). Because approximately 6 % of the adult population in the United States use their primary care provider for mental health care, it is imperative that nurses and other providers ensure that all adults are screened and treated for mental health disorders.[4] Of the four *Healthy People 2000* objectives that focused on adults with mental health disorders, the least progress was made on controlling stress and seeking treatment for depression. Measures of progress on the objective related to mental health services showed that nurse practitioners inquired less about parent–child relationships and about their adult patients' cognitive, emotional, or behavioral functioning than when assessed at base line.[4] Professional nurses in community settings including schools, clinics, and work sites have a responsibility to promote and conduct early screening and intervention for stress-related problems.

Stress and Health

Stress is linked to decreased life satisfaction, the development of mental disorders, the occurrence of stress-related illnesses (such as cardiovascular disease, gastrointestinal disorders, low back pain, headaches), and decreased immunologic functioning, which has been implicated in cancer. In terms of heart disease, long-term stress is thought to sensitize arterioles to catecholamines, with even short-term stress responses causing overconstriction of the vessels and endothelial damage. Repetitive overconstriction can lead to hypertension, decreased myocardial perfusion, and arrhythmias.[5, 6]

Social factors are considered to be intimately related to the experience of stress and subsequently to health and disease. Social isolation increases a person's risk for heart disease and survival following a heart attack. Patients who have a heart attack and live alone are one and a half times more likely to have a second heart attack than are those who live with someone else.[7, 8] In other instances, the nature of interpersonal relationships may be detrimental to health. For example, elderly caregivers experienced chronic distress when caring for a family member with a chronic illness, resulting in impairment of their immune system.[9] Because both the absence of social relations and certain characteristics of social relations serve as stressors that can have an impact on health, understanding how social relationships affect the brain, physiologic processes, and health is of critical importance.[10, 3(p 136)]

Psychoneuroimmunology examines the effects of social and psychologic phenomena on the immune system as mediated by the nervous and endocrine systems. This arena of science is particularly important, because both acute and chronic infections as well as cancer have been linked to compromised immune functioning. In a series of studies, male undergraduate college students with high heart-rate reactivity to stressors (mental arithmetic test with noise superimposed) were compared to low heart-rate reactors on neuroendocrine and immune responses to stressors. High reactors compared to low showed higher stress-related levels of plasma cortisol and increased natural killer (NK) cell lysis. The finding that cortisol was elevated in high reactors is particularly interesting in view of the extensive literature linking cortisol with down-regulation of multiple aspects of cellular immune function. These findings suggest that individual variation in activation of the hypothalamic-pituitary-adrenocortical axis by brief psychologic stressors may explain why daily stressors have greater health consequences for some individuals than for others. Different mediating roles may be played by the hypothalamic-pituitary-adrenocortical axis and the sympathetic adrenomedullary systems. Evidence is growing that the immune system is influenced by central nervous system processes that are shaped by social psychologic factors.[10, 11]

The experience of stress can also influence the immune system. Berger and O'Brien[12] studied the effect of a cognitive-behavioral intervention on salivary immunoglobulin (sIgA) (a factor related to host defense), self-reported levels of stress, and the physical health of 57 undergraduate students. The students were randomly assigned to either the intervention or control group. Each group was divided into sections of 10 students. The five-week intervention period consisted of giving information about stress, the body's response to stress, immunity, relaxation techniques, cognitive restructuring, and assertiveness training. Pre-and postintervention measures included saliva testing, rating of physical symptoms of stress, and self-reported physical problems. Change was measured using the Undergraduate Stress Questionnaire, the Cohen-Hoberman Inventory of Physical Symptoms, the Daily Stress Inventory, and saliva cultures. Stress was reduced for both the control and intervention groups based on changes in the scores of the self-reported instruments. There was no change in the sIgA results. These findings suggest that the intervention reduced reported stress in the participants but did not have any immunoenhancing effect.[12] Another study reported different findings. The study found daily events to be associated with fluctuations in immune response. Immune response was measured by salivary immunoglobulin (sIgA). In a community-living sample of 96 men who completed daily event questionnaires, day-to-day reporting of more *desirable* events was related to more sIgA antibody. Reporting more *undesirable* events was related to less sIgA. *Positive affect* in relation to events was related to more sIgA and *negative affect* to less sIgA. Desirable events were more strongly related to secretory immune response than were undesirable events.[13] These studies validate that additional research should focus on identifying immune-enhancing interventions.

A number of physiologic systems seem to be highly responsive to life experiences and the psychologic states that accompany them. Further studies of varying human responses to stress are important as a basis for developing effective stress-management techniques, supporting healthy coping mechanisms, and restructuring faulty psychologic defenses.[14] A holistic approach that integrates the mind and body has long characterized nursing. Nurses understand the relationships between stress and health as well as stress and illness as a basis for client assessment and nursing care. Nurses are in a key position to identify individuals and families who are coping ineffectively. The nurse should assess coping strategies for stress reduction; perceived controllability, intensity, and duration of stressors; emotional and behavioral regulation skills; and perceived availability of social support. This assessment can assist the nurse in structuring appropriate interventions or in making referrals to assist clients in dealing with stressors before they exert health-damaging effects.

Stress Across the Life Span

Children experience stress and develop coping patterns early in life. Nurses are concerned with children's stress-coping processes because of the hazards imposed by prolonged stress. The potential to increase children's well-being and health through constructive stress management is another concern. Sources of stress are related to the child's age, gender, and developmental stage. Children and adults identify very different stressors. For example, children are mostly concerned about daily events that relate to school, peers, parents, and self. Environmental and social stressors that place children and adolescents at high risk for poor adjustment include personal safety concerns, community violence, prolonged poverty, increased availability of drugs, homelessness, and AIDS.[15] The majority of children, regardless of their environment, have a resiliency that allows them to function well in spite of major stressors. This type of competency develops over time.[16] Some children are more affected by stressful situations and need intervention. Personal resilience and environmental protective factors that mediate the relationship between risk factors and healthy development need to be identified and incorporated into family, community, and school interventions. Higher stress has been associated with a range of risk-taking behaviors such as smoking and alcohol use in early adolescence. On the other hand, use of behavioral coping (information gathering, decision making, problem solving), cognitive coping (minimizing distress, focusing on the positive), adult social support (talking with an adult), and relaxation were found to be inversely related to substance abuse.[17] Nurses and other health professionals may find that the best approach to avoidance of substance abuse and other risky behaviors is to assist children and adolescents in learning effective stress-coping processes to apply across a variety of life circumstances.

Most of the knowledge about stress has been gained from studies of adults. This information may or may not be directly applicable to children. Some factors that are known to be related to stress in children include self-esteem, personality characteristics (type A behavior and temperament), gender, locus of control, social support, parental child-rearing behavior, and previous stressful experiences. The five most frequently occurring stressors identified by children included feeling sick, having nothing to do, not having enough money to spend, being pressured to get good grades, and feeling left out of the group. These differed from parents' perceptions of the most distressing events. Research is needed on sources of stress for children, developmental changes in stressors, coping strategies across childhood and adolescence, and how challenging rather than stressful environments can be created for youth. Wagner and Compas[18] found developmental differences in the stressors most strongly related to psychologic symptoms: family stressors in junior high, peer stressors in high school, and academic stressors in college. Particularly important are studies of the coping strategies used by resilient children who, despite high levels of stress, appear to cope well with adversity. An excellent overview of instruments to measure stressors in children and physiologic and behavioral indicators of acute and chronic stress is provided by Ryan-Wenger and colleagues.[19]

The stresses often experienced in young and middle-age adulthood relate to establishing oneself in a productive career, nourishing enduring relationships in a dyadic unit, childbearing and child rearing, and creating a sense of self-identity as an independent yet interdependent adult. Work is often cited as a source of stress, and work site stress-management programs are increasingly offered by many employers. Sources of work stress include lack of control over job environment or production demands, being "caught in the middle" between supervisors and customers, being underprepared for the job, lack of clarity about job expectations, unexpected transfers across departments or company locations, feeling trapped in a particular job, and lack of positive relationships with coworkers. Stress often causes deterioration in performance, which can further escalate already existing causes of stress and tension.

Support at home can buffer work-related stressors, or the existence of additional stressors at home can have a cumulative effect with those at work and further threaten health. The Double ABCX[20] model of family stress and adaptation describes how families manage stressful events over a period of time. The family demands or accumulation of stressors are referred to as the A factor. Family changes and transitions as well as daily hassles among family members may cause stress. These demands on the family can produce internal tension that requires management. The B factor represents all the assets and resources that a family can draw upon in a time of stress. These can include strengths of individual members, strengths of the family unit (open communication, cohesion), and strengths of the community (helpful agencies, supportive social networks). The third factor, C, includes the family's definition and perception of all the demands, the family's stress-meeting resources, and actions that need to be taken to resolve the stress. The result of the interaction between a family's demands and capabilities is its state of adaptation, X. This model is useful to nurses in primary care settings in helping them to conceptualize the stressors and coping capabilities of families as a basis for assessment and intervention.

Constrained finances or arguments between spouses about how to spend limited income can markedly increase tension in the home. Single parents are particularly vulnerable to stress, as they may lack social support and also find that job demands leave them little time for parenting responsibilities. In the absence of authoritative parenting, children may get into difficulties that further stretch limited psychologic resources of parents. Stress-management programs that address changing work and home environments to minimize stress and developing effective coping strategies best meet the needs of young and middle-age adults.

Although some sources of stress may abate in older adulthood, other stressors, particularly those resulting from loss, are more prevalent. The elderly are particularly vulnerable to negative life events such as death of a spouse, death of a close family member, personal injury or illness, health change of a family member, and retirement. Hassles of daily living may increase as a result of diminished sensory acuity, decreased dexterity and strength, loss of flexibility, and increased fatigue. The elderly may neglect health behaviors that augment their strength and resilience such as proper nutrition, adequate exercise, proper rest, and sleep. Cumulative stress along with depression can compromise immune function, leaving the elderly more vulnerable to acute and chronic infections and chronic disease.[21, 22]

It is in old age when we begin to see the increased morbidity and mortality associated with years of daily hassles and cumulative major life events, particularly where coping strategies have been ineffective. Systemic effects on the cardiovascular, gastrointestinal, neurologic, endocrine, and immune systems may become increasingly apparent. Because of decreased resistance to disease, helping elderly adults to use existing coping techniques productively or learn new ones is of great importance. Nurses familiar with the problems of aging and the capabilities of older adults can equip them to manage the stressors that they encounter more effectively and efficiently, thus conserving valuable personal resources.

Approaches to Stress Management

At any point in time, an individual or family may be subjected to many sources of potential stress. Multiple stressors can combine synergistically, resulting in cumulative stress. A number of nursing diagnoses specific to problems in stress management (defensive coping, ineffective family coping, etc.) are described by Gordon in the functional health pattern category of Coping-Stress Tolerance Pattern.[23] The reader is referred to the *Manual of Nursing Diagnosis: 1998–1999* for further diagnostic information. The nurse and client together must assess the level of existing stress and the sources of stress and then determine the appropriate point(s) for intervention to achieve stress reduction.

The primary modes of intervention for stress management consist of the following:

- Minimize the frequency of stress-inducing situations.
- Increase resistance to stress.
- Countercondition to avoid physiologic arousal resulting from stress.

In general, changing the environment to decrease the incidence of stressors should be the "first line of defense." When that is not possible, individual and family coping resources need to come into play to reinterpret stress as a challenge, increase resilience against stress, or decrease the health-threatening effects of stressors.

Minimizing the Frequency of Stress-Inducing Situations

In a technologic society, the need for adjustment to externally imposed change is continuous. Approaches to assisting clients in preventing stressful situations include (1) changing the environment, (2) avoiding excessive change, (3) time control, and (4) time management.

CHANGING THE ENVIRONMENT

Widely held values and beliefs shape the environment in any society. Changing the environment, when it is possible, is the most proactive approach to minimizing the frequency of stress-inducing situations. Major changes in societal beliefs, values, and actions are necessary if stress is to be reduced for some vulnerable populations. Sexism, racism, and ageism create stress for selected groups as a result of devaluation of their status and lack of acknowledgment of their contributions to society. Discrimination directed at any group can result in decreased educational and employment opportunities, poverty, and personal devaluation. Kessler argued that the primary causes of racial disparities in disease rates are rooted in differences between races in exposure or vulnerability to pathogenic factors in the physical, social, economic, and cultural environment. The association between perceived discrimination and mental health confirmed that perceived discrimination was a stressor that did not vary on the basis of social status of the minority person.[24]

Racial discrimination and blood pressure of young black and white adults showed that differences in blood pressure of the two groups were reduced when the reported experiences of racial discrimination and unfair treatment were accounted for in the blood pressure readings.[25] Attempts to improve social environments for low-income African Americans requires changes in policies, values, and belief systems.

The work environment is frequently identified as a major source of stress. Changes in the work environment itself can reduce the incidence of stressful events. For example, instituting policies that provide flextime, job sharing, or child-care benefits or facilities can ease the stress on parents who must both maintain a job and care for young children. Protecting workers from job-related hazards, redesigning work assignments, creating pleasant work stations, instituting quality circles, or employing more participatory management styles also can foster lower levels of stress at work. Job-related stresses may also be avoided by becoming more aware of those persons or experiences that create personal stress and minimizing contact to the extent possible. Committee membership in groups that are stress inducing might be better delegated to someone else who experiences less stress from the activity or who obtains actual enjoyment from participation.

If a job change is required by the client to decrease stress, new employment possibilities should be analyzed to make sure that stress phenomena similar to those already encountered are not an inherent part of the new employment setting. Protective factors in the broader environment that can further decrease stress include family characterized by warmth and cohesion, culture and ethnic events and customs that promote identity, supportive relationships with others outside the family, and involvement in community structures such as churches and neighborhood organizations that promote competence and support.[26]

AVOIDING EXCESSIVE CHANGE

When children as young as 8 to 12 years of age were asked to report the coping strategies that they used in anticipation of stressful events, they reported avoidance of the situation, distracting behaviors, and some reported using relaxation behaviors.[19(p 272)] Teaching children when and how to avoid excessive change is important, as coping strategies developed early in childhood often continue into adulthood and affect patterns of behavior throughout the life span.

During periods of high life change and resulting negative tension states, any unnecessary changes should be avoided. For example, if a family is experiencing the illness of one of its family members and a subsequent job loss, this may not be the time to consider geographic relocation, pregnancy, or any other change in lifestyle. Negative tension created by multiple changes is synergistic. Each time a distressing change occurs, the potency of previous changes for upsetting stability is increased. Deliberately postponing changes that result in negative tension assists clients in dealing more constructively with unavoidable change and prevents the need for multiple adjustments all at one point in time.

Any changes that are made in lifestyle during periods of high or moderate stress should be self-initiated and provide challenge to the client rather than threat. Increasing positive sources of tension that promote growth and self-actualization can offset the deleterious effects of negative tension. For instance, learning to play tennis, to swim, or to dance may provide an enjoyable challenge to counterbalance potentially debilitating stress.

TIME CONTROL

Alec Mackenzie has suggested time control as a technique to set aside specific time for adaptation to various stressors.[27] This period of personal time may be daily, weekly, or monthly. It offers clients time to focus on a specific change and develop strategies for adjustment. The major advantage of time control is that it ensures that important goals or concerns will be addressed and critical tasks accomplished. Mackenzie encourages individuals to focus on managing time more effectively in order to prevent most of the stress that time shortages can produce.[27(p 241)] This can reduce the sense of urgency and lack of time, the level of anxiety, and associated feelings of frustration and failure.

TIME MANAGEMENT

This approach to stress management actually refers to organizing oneself to accomplish those goals most important in life within the time available. Because lack of time is often given by individuals and families as a reason for not participating in health-promoting activities, assisting clients to manage time better can make a major contribution to their health and fitness. Time-pressured, type A clients with high risk for cardiovascular disease may be particularly in need of time-management skills.

Identifying values and goals and prioritizing goals can serve as a framework for time management. Identifying time wasted on activities unrelated to personal goals can permit the client to restructure how time is spent. Overcommitment to others or unrealistic expectations of oneself is a frequent source of stress. Time overload can be avoided by learning to say "no" to demands of others that are unrealistic or of low personal or family priority. Overload results in frustration and loss of satisfaction from the work accomplished, because one can seldom expend one's best efforts under strain and pressure.

An important approach to time management is the reduction of a task into smaller parts. A task as a whole may appear as an overload; however, if the task is broken down into smaller segments, accomplishment becomes feasible. An example of this for a client may be learning several effective conditioning exercises before learning a complete conditioning routine, or developing skill with a conditioning routine before beginning a walk-jog activity. To take the whole health-promoting behavior as one task may be overwhelming. Breaking it down into component parts allows mastery and feelings of competence.

Avoiding overload by delegating responsibilities to others and enlisting their assistance is also important. Making use of the skills of others and recognizing their ability to perform assigned tasks provides freedom from the expectation of having to be "all things to all people."

Another important aspect of time management is to reduce the perception of time pressure and urgency. Not all perceptions of time urgency are warranted; some are needlessly self-imposed. The client should differentiate between time urgencies that are valid and others that are needlessly created. Time urgency can also be minimized by avoiding procrastination. Leaving tasks that need to be completed until the last minute can result in needless pressure and stress.[28]

Increasing Resistance to Stress

Resistance to stress is achieved through either physical or psychologic conditioning. Physical conditioning for stress resistance focuses on exercise. Psychologic conditioning to increase resistance resources focuses on (1) enhancing self-esteem, (2) enhancing self-efficacy, (3) increasing assertiveness, (4) setting realistic goals, and (5) building coping resources.

Promoting Exercise

Exercise is discussed at length in Chapter 8. However, the relationship between exercise and stress is addressed here briefly. Four processes have been suggested in accounting for the positive effects of exercise on responses to mental stress. The first is that psychologic changes are the by-product of cardiorespiratory fitness. However, this explanation is weakened by the fact that psychologic responses and fitness are frequently not correlated. A second possibility is that changes in exercise-related self-efficacy and mastery generalize to other situations, resulting in improvements in self-concept and coping ability. A third process that may underlie decreased stress responses following periods of exercise is a blunting of the psychophysiologic responsiveness to stressors.[29] The third process suggests that exercise might help the brain deal better with stress by enhancing the body's response. Long-term exercise may increase the efficiency of the body's stress reaction system. Exercise is thought to require that all of the body systems (e.g., cardiovascular, muscular, and kidney) communicate with each other giving the systems practice in dealing with stress. This "workout" of the body's systems may make communication between the systems more efficient and be the significance of exercise.[30] Epidemiologic research suggests that physical activity is positively related to good mental health. In general, people who are inactive are twice as likely to be depressed whereas people who exercise regularly report feelings of well-being. However, increased fatigue, anxiety, and decreased vigor can occur with overtraining. Regular physical exercise contributes to good mental health.[31(p 136–140),32,33]

Enhancing Self-Esteem

Self-esteem is the value attributed to self or how the person feels about self. This valuation is based on a person's concept of his or her desirable and undesirable attributes, strengths and weaknesses, achievements, and success in interpersonal relationships. Research is limited on the relationship between exercise and self-esteem in older adults.[34(pp 151–154)] Research on self-esteem indicates that it is associated with a history of an active physical lifestyle. However, most studies recruit persons who already have a positive self-esteem so one would expect change to be minimal. Exercise is more likely to increase the self-esteem of persons who have low self-esteem before the intervention and that of women more so than men. Cousins and Horn summarized intervention and comparison studies and correlational and epidemiological studies of self-esteem and exercise in older people.[34(pp 155–156)] Felton and colleagues[35] studied self-image in 128 adolescent girls ages 16 to 19 years. Self-image related significantly to positive health-promoting behaviors including exercise. Hoffman and colleagues[36] found that adolescents who have parents and friends who are very supportive tend to achieve higher levels of self-esteem. Nurse practitioners and school nurses have excellent opportunities to promote positive self-concepts and healthy levels of self-esteem for adolescents as a basis for healthy functioning throughout life.

Although self-esteem is developed over time, studies have shown that the level of self-esteem can be changed. One approach is positive verbalization. In using this technique, clients identify positive aspects of self or personal characteristics that they value highly. They should also ask significant others to comment on their positive attributes. Each characteristic, one per day, is placed on a 3 × 5 index card, and the cards placed in a conspicuous place. Each card should be read several times a day. This technique helps clients to spend more time thinking positively about themselves and decreases the amount of time spent in self-devaluation. Increased self-awareness of positive characteristics and their presence in conscious thought will result in more frequent behavior that reflects these attributes and more positive responses from significant others.

ENHANCING SELF-EFFICACY

Mastery experiences also appear to positively build a sense of competence to perform effectively and overcome obstacles. Experiencing successful performance of a particular, valued behavior provides positive messages concerning personal skills and abilities. Counseling clients to undertake tasks that are challenging but from which they can experience success rather than failure can build a sense of efficacy in a particular domain. Self-beliefs about personal efficacy have wide-ranging ramifications affecting level of motivation, affect, thought, and action. Perceiving oneself to be efficacious has been shown to predict performance better than actual ability. In other words, if people's beliefs in their efficacy are strengthened, they approach situations more assuredly and make better use of the skills that they have.[37 (pp 1–45)]

Persons with high levels of efficacy, compared to low levels, mentally rehearse success rather than failure at a task, set high goals and make a firm commitment to attain them, perceive more control over personal threats, and are less anxious in the face of day-to-day challenges. Highly efficacious persons also tend to be more assertive in accessing the support they need to optimize their chances of success.[38 (p 495)] The nurse can help clients to identify areas of skill most important to them and then help them plan to augment their efficacy in these highly valued areas.

INCREASING ASSERTIVENESS

Substituting positive, assertive behaviors for negative, passive ones can increase personal capacity for psychologic resistance to stress. Assertiveness is the appropriate expression of oneself, one's thoughts, and one's feelings and can result in greater personal satisfaction in living. Assertiveness is more constructive than aggression and deals more effectively than aggression with most problems encountered in the course of living. Many books and articles have been written on assertiveness training. Assertiveness allows individuals to share their perceptions and feelings with others in a way that facilitates rather than inhibits personal or group productivity. Several suggestions for becoming more assertive that clients ought to be encouraged to use include the following:

- Making a deliberate effort to greet others and call them by name
- Maintaining eye contact during conversations
- Commenting on the positive characteristics of others
- Initiating conversation
- Expressing opinions
- Expressing feelings
- Disagreeing with others when holding opposing viewpoints
- Taking initiative to engage in a new behavior or learn a new activity

The webs and constraints that entangle human beings are frequently self-constructed and disappear easily when efforts are made to become more open, assertive, and self-fulfilling. Although it is possible for clients through use of simple techniques to become more assertive, very passive and reserved clients might well benefit from more comprehensive assertiveness training by a competent instructor or counselor. The nurse can assist clients in locating such resources for personal development.

SETTING REALISTIC GOALS

Clients must be aware not only of the goals that they have set but why accomplishment of those goals is rewarding. Long- and short-term goals will help the client stay on course. Reward or reinforcement may be possible through accomplishment of alternative goals. Long-term goals set the direction for change and short-term goals allow for immediate successes. Goals should be set that can be attained within a reasonable time frame. If goals are met, it may reinforce the client's desire to continue to set health-promoting goals. Another useful rule is to plan to change only one behavior at a time. Flexibility on the part of the client permits achievement of desired outcomes through several approaches. As a result, lack of success in initial attempts to reach goals becomes much less ominous because of the probability of success in achieving alternative goals that bring similar rewards.[39] (pp 73–75)

BUILDING COPING RESOURCES

Stress results when there is an imbalance between appraised demands and appraised coping capabilities. Hobfoll[40] suggests that more attention be directed to the resource side of the equation rather than the demand side. He maintains that coping resources are more predictive of reactions to stressors than the actual demands. General coping resources that have been identified for development to enhance stress resistance include:

- Self-disclosure: predisposition to share one's feelings, troubles, thoughts, and opinions with others
- Self-directedness: degree to which a person respects his or her own judgment for decision making and, therefore, demonstrates assertiveness in interpersonal relationships
- Confidence: ability to gain mastery over one's environment and to control one's emotions in the interest of reaching personal goals
- Acceptance: degree to which persons accept their shortcomings and imperfections and maintain a positive and tolerant attitude toward others and the world at large

- Social support: availability and use of network of caring others
- Financial freedom: extent to which persons are free of financial constraints on their lifestyles
- Physical health: overall health condition including absence of chronic disease and disabilities
- Physical fitness: conditioning resulting from personal exercise practices
- Stress monitoring: awareness of tension buildup and situations that are likely to prove stressful
- Tension control: ability to lower arousal through relaxation and thought control
- Structuring: ability to organize and manage resources such as time and energy
- Problem solving: ability to resolve personal problems

The Coping Resources Inventory for Stress measures these stress-coping resources of older adolescents and adults.[41,42] After assessing the extent to which the various coping resources are present, nurses should assist clients in maximizing existing strengths and in developing additional resistance resources.

Counterconditioning to Avoid Physiologic Arousal

Research findings have substantiated the ability of individuals to intentionally control auto-nomic nervous system functions such as respiratory rate, heart rate, heart rhythm, blood pressure, and temperature in the extremities, functions previously thought to be under unconscious control. Training aimed at assisting clients to attain conscious control of physiologic responses to stressful events provides an important set of strategies for the management of stress. The goal of counterconditioning is to replace muscle tension and heightened sympathetic nervous system activity produced by stress with muscle relaxation and increased parasympathetic functioning. The two interventions most frequently used to assist the client in accomplishing this are relaxation training and imagery.

PROGRESSIVE RELAXATION THROUGH TENSION-RELAXATION TECHNIQUES

Progressive Muscle Relaxation (PMR), developed by Edmund Jacobson in 1938, involves decreasing voluntary muscle activity and activity within the sympathetic nervous system while increasing parasympathetic functioning.[43(p 74)] There has been increasing accumulation of evidence in the scientific literature that supports Jacobson's findings that tension levels can be reduced through use of relaxation skills. Relaxation appears to be a way of turning off the body's response to the sympathetic nervous system and of actually decreasing neurohormonal changes that take place in reaction to the experience of negative tension states.[44(p 1),45]

Relaxation is thought to result in the following changes:

- Decrease in the body's oxygen consumption
- Lowered metabolism
- Decreased respiration rate
- Decreased heart rate
- Decreased muscle tension
- Decreased premature ventricular contractions
- Decreased systolic and diastolic blood pressures

- Increased alpha brain waves
- Enhanced immune function

Stress can cause changes in the body's immune system. The overreaction or underreaction of the immune system to stress can result in disease or illness. Research is mixed on whether PRM has any positive effect on the body's immune system.[46(143–150),44,47] However, positive outcomes have been documented when PMR is used for stress reduction either as the prescribed therapy or as an adjunct therapy. Whitman and colleagues[48] reported a 54% decrease in patients' stress levels (using stress assessment instruments) when PMR was used with their prescribed anticonvulsant.[47] Snyder[49] also reported changes in blood pressure and anxiety levels after PRM. Although PRM has not been shown to reduce blood pressure in healthy persons, PRM is a valuable tool to use to maintain health. The reader is referred to *Complementary Alternative Therapies in Nursing*[44] for further information and precautions in the use of PMR.

A very pleasant, quiet, soundproof room in which lighting can be dimmed, with reclining lawn or lounge chairs for clients, provides an optimum setting for relaxation training. Tight clothing should be loosened, glasses removed, shoes removed, and a comfortable position assumed in the chair. Relaxation should never be taught with clients lying flat. Although this is a common position assumed for rest and sleep, it often results in muscle strain in the upper back and neck along with drowsiness, which interferes with training. A reclining position or sitting position is most appropriate.

At the beginning of each session, clients should be encouraged to focus on their own breathing as the air moves gently in and out. The purpose of this focusing activity is to increase awareness of self and the often imperceptible functions of the human body. Following the focusing activity, clients are moved slowly through tension and relaxation cycles for each of the major muscle groups listed in Table 10–1, maintaining tension for 8 to 10 seconds and releasing tension instantaneously on cue. The entire tension–relaxation cycle should be repeated twice during the first session to increase clients' awareness of the differences in body sensations during tensed and relaxed periods. The tension–relaxation instructions should be given very slowly, allowing clients to enjoy the feelings of relaxation they are experiencing. The guidance provided by the nurse is critical for successful relaxation.

Training tapes can be used by clients at home to facilitate daily practice of relaxation techniques. Clients should keep a schedule of the frequency and length of time that relaxation is practiced. Clients are encouraged to "think through" the relaxation procedure and do their own coaching. A "prompt sheet" on the sequence of the muscle groups should be sent home with them for easy reference. This is intended to move clients toward independent practice of relaxation rather than encouraging reliance on the nurse or the coaching tape as a means of providing relaxation cues.

Some common problems that clients report include:

- Overly rapid self-pacing through the relaxation sequence
- Distraction by environmental noise
- Difficulty keeping attention on own monologue
- Interruption of distracting thoughts during relaxation
- Residual tension in some muscles after tension–relaxation

The problem of overly rapid self-pacing can usually be solved by encouraging clients to slow down internal speech or coaching pace. Autogenic phrases such as "I feel calm," "I feel very

TABLE 10-1 Fifteen-Muscle Group Sequence for Tension–Relaxation Cycle

Muscle Group	Abbreviated Instructions
1. Right hand and forearm	Make a fist.
2. Right upper arm	Pull elbow tightly into side.
3. Left hand and forearm	Make a fist.
4. Left upper arm	Pull elbow tightly into side.
5. Forehead	Wrinkle brow.
6. Upper cheeks and nose	Squint eyes and wrinkle nose.
7. Lower cheeks and jaws	Place teeth together and make a "forced" smile.
8. Neck and throat	Pull chin toward chest.
9. Chest, shoulders, and upper back	Take a deep breath. Push shoulder blades toward each other.
10. Upper abdomen	Pull stomach in and hold.
11. Lower abdomen	Bear down against the seat of the chair.
12. Right upper leg	Push down against the foot of the chair.
13. Right lower leg and foot	Point toes toward head and body.
14. Left upper leg	Push down against the foot of the chair.
15. Left lower leg and foot	Point toes toward head and body.

relaxed," and "my arms and legs feel heavy" can be interspersed throughout self-instruction. Encouraging family members to join in the relaxation practice sessions can foster stress-management skills among the entire family unit.

PROGRESSIVE RELAXATION WITHOUT TENSION

While tension–relaxation techniques result in high levels of voluntary muscle relaxation, clients can be taught how to relax without first tensing muscles. Relaxation through counting down and relaxation through imagery are strategies frequently used. The major advantage of these techniques is that tension is no longer required. This is particularly important for clients with hypertension or coronary heart disease, because elevations in blood pressure caused by prolonged or extensive muscle tensing may be contraindicated. Deep relaxation without tension is the goal. Phrases that might be repeated to facilitate relaxation include:

- I feel quiet.
- I am beginning to feel quite relaxed.
- My feet feel heavy and relaxed.
- My ankles, my knees, and my hips feel heavy.
- My solar plexus and the whole central portion of my body feel relaxed and quiet.
- My hands, my arms, and my shoulders feel heavy, relaxed, and comfortable.
- My neck, my jaws, and my forehead feel relaxed. They feel comfortable and smooth.
- My whole body feels quite heavy, comfortable, and relaxed.
- I am quite relaxed.
- My arms and hands are heavy and warm.

- My whole body is relaxed and my hands are warm—relaxed and warm.
- My hands are warm.
- Warmth is flowing into my hands. They are warm, warm.
- I can feel the warmth flowing down my arms into my hands.
- My hands are warm, relaxed, and warm.
- My whole body feels quiet, comfortable, and relaxed.
- My mind is quiet.
- I withdraw my thoughts from the surroundings and I feel serene and still.
- My thoughts are turned inward and I am at ease.
- Deep within my mind, I can visualize and experience myself as relaxed, comfortable, and still.
- I am alert, but in an easy, quiet, inward-turned way.
- My mind is calm and quiet.
- I feel an inward quietness.

These phrases have been suggested by Elmer and Alyce Green as a result of work in biofeedback at the Menninger Foundation. Such phrases result in physiologic imagery that can decrease both sympathetic nervous system activity and tension in voluntary muscles.

Relaxation through the countdown procedure initially focuses on each of the muscle groups used previously. The client is encouraged to relax each muscle group progressively as the count proceeds from 10 down to 1. When the client has practiced and becomes skilled with this procedure, total body countdown can be used: relaxing the entire body while silently counting down from 10 to 1. This is a particularly useful procedure for the office or when facing stressful social situations. In two to three minutes, the skilled client can achieve total body relaxation while in a sitting position with eyes open and focused on a specific object. This is one of the shortest procedures through which relaxation can be accomplished. Minirelaxation sessions several times throughout the day can promote generalization of relaxation training to everyday life.

RELAXATION THROUGH IMAGERY

Imagery is an intervention in which the interrelationship of the body and mind is used to influence physiologic responses. Many of the benefits of imagery are thought to be its influence on physiological and immunological responses of the autonomic nervous system that results in stress reduction. Research supports imagery as an effective intervention for reduction in stress in many situations including the birth process, pain management, and changing of health behaviors. However, it is difficult to determine if the outcomes are directly related to imagery or a combination of interventions. The reader is referred to *Complementary Alternative Therapies in Nursing*[44] for further information and precautions in the use of imagery.

Using imagery to relax requires that the client passively concentrate on pleasant scenes or experiences from the past to facilitate relaxation. Recalling the warmth of the sun, the feeling of warm sand, the sensations of a gentle breeze, the vision of palm trees swaying, or the sounds of ocean waves may be comfortable and pleasant for clients. Such recall can promote muscle relaxation.

Each client will vary in those scenes or images that result in actual changes in muscle tension. For some clients, visualizing specific colors, shapes, or patterns will be as effective as visualizing landscapes or scenes. If clients initially have difficulty in using imagery or visualization for relaxation, the nurse may use one of the following techniques:

- Have the client, with eyes closed, visualize a particular room of his or her house (living room, bedroom, kitchen), focusing on colors, shapes, and specific objects. The client's mind should wander about the room, with the client describing verbally what is seen in as much detail as possible.
- Have the client focus on a particular piece of clothing that is a personal favorite. The client should describe the color, texture, design, and trim of the clothing and how it feels when worn (e.g., soft, loose, fitted, light, warm).

As individuals become more vivid in descriptions of concrete objects, their ability to use less concrete imagery for purposes of relaxation increases. Imagery is a highly useful relaxation technique in many settings in which muscle tension or biofeedback equipment would be obtrusive.

 # Directions for Research on Stress Management

The ability to regulate processes previously considered to be under autonomic rather than voluntary control has been one of the most exciting research discoveries during the last several decades. In addition, major advances toward understanding the effects of stressors on the neuroendocrine and immune systems has offered new possibilities for managing the brain–body interface to promote health. A number of coping strategies have been tested. More research is needed concerning the profile of stressors most likely to occur at different developmental stages and the best way to match stressors with targeted coping processes. A research challenge is discovering how to build coping resources, resilience, and personal competence in the early childhood years so that patterns of successfully coping manifest themselves throughout adolescence and adulthood.

Research that suggests how to decrease environmental and family stressors for vulnerable populations is a priority. Human tolerance for stress is finite—with the best of coping strategies, people can manage only so much stress. What are the changes in social policies, social structures, and relationships across cultures that need to be addressed to get at the root of the problem: the social injustice, discrimination, and inequity that are the unfortunate experience of many? Through the efforts of scientists from multiple disciplines, the phenomenon of stress pervasive in our society can be addressed. Results of the research can be applied to create a better world for all.

Directions for Practice in Stress Management

Everyone experiences stressors and yet individuals who experience the same stressors often respond differently. Stress-related illnesses are very common and require appropriate interventions or referrals to assist the client in dealing with stress before negative outcomes present. The promotion and conduct of early screenings and developmentally-specific interventions are necessary because children, adolescents, young adults, and older adults develop and use different coping strategies. Awareness of these differences will ensure that the nurse intervenes at the appropriate time and with the appropriate strategy to achieve stress reduction. While the techniques of stress management discussed in this chapter are within the nurse's scope of practice, one should gain expertise in the use of them by working with an experienced provider. Research into the relationship between stress and health is offering new insights into the causes and treatments of stress-related illnesses. This rapidly growing field of research in nursing and other disciplines mandates that each practitioner stays abreast of advances in practice.

SUMMARY

A number of different approaches for assisting individuals and families in managing stress have been presented in order to familiarize the reader with the range of strategies available. Some approaches suggested are relatively unstructured, whereas others are more formally defined and require instrumentation. The decision regarding which strategies to use must be made collaboratively by the client and the nurse. This decision should be based on the characteristics of the client, sources of stress experienced by the client, and general patterns of response to stressful events.[50] The reader is encouraged to consult references at the end of this chapter for further information on use of stress-management strategies as nursing interventions.

REFERENCES

1. Selye H. Introduction. In: Wheetley D, ed. *Stress and the Heart.* New York: Raven Press; 1977.
2. Lazarus RS, Folkman S. *Stress, Appraisal and Coping.* New York: Springer; 1984:293.
3. Lerman C, Glanz K. *Health Behavior and Health Education. Stress, Coping, and Health Behavior.* 2nd ed. San Francisco:Jossey-Bass Publishers; 1996.
4. *Healthy People 2010* (Conference Edition). *Mental Health and Mental Disorders.* Washington DC: U.S. Public Health and Human Services publications PHS 91-50212.
5. Engler MB, Engler MM. Assessment of the cardiovascular effects of stress. *J Cardiovasc Nurs.* 1995 Oct;10(1):51–63.
6. Castillo RA, Schneider RH, Alexander CN, Cook R, Myers H, Nidich S, Haney C, Rainforth M, Salerno J. Effects of stress reduction on cartoid atherosclerosis in hypertensive African Americans. *Stroke.* 2000 Mar; 31(3):568–573.
7. Underwood PA. Social support: The promise and the reality. In: *Handbook of Stress, Coping, and Health: Implications for Nursing Research, Theory, and Practice.* Thousand Oaks: Sage Publications; 2000.
8. American Psychological Association. *Psychology Helps After a Heart Attack;* 1997.
9. Bauer ME, Vedhara K, Perks P, Wilcock GK, Lightman SL, Shanks N. *J Neuro-immunal.* 2000 Feb 1;103(1):84–92. Name: Chronic stress in caregivers of dementia patients is associated with reduced lymphocyte sensitivity to glucocorticoids.
10. Cacioppo JT. Social neuroscience: Autonoimic, neurendocrine, and immune response to stress. *Psychophysiology.* 1994;31:113–128.

11. Witek-Janusek L, Mathews HL. Stress, immunity, and health outcomes. In: *Handbook of Stress, Coping, Health: Implications for Nursing Research, Theory, and Practice.* Thousand Oaks: Sage Publications; 2000.

12. Berger JA, O'Brien WH. Effect of a cognitive-behavioral stress management intervention on salivary IgA, self-reported levels of stress, and physical health complaints in an undergraduate population. *Int J Rehabil Health.* 1998 Jul;4(3):129–152.

13. Stone AA, Neale JM, Cox DS, et al. Daily events are associated with a secretory immuneresponse to an oral antigen in men. *Health Psychol.* 1994;13:440–446.

14. Werner JS, Frost MH. Major life stressors and health outcomes. In: *Handbook of Stress, Coping, Health: Implications of Nursing Research Theory and Practice.* Thousand Oaks: Sage Publications; 2000:97–124.

15. Carroll MK, Ryan-Wenger NA. School age children's fears, anxiety, and human figure drawings. *J Ped Health Care.* 1999;13:24–31.

16. Masten AS, Coatsworth JD. The development of competence in favorable and unfavorable environments: Lessons from research on successful children. *Am Psychol,* 1998;53:205–220.

17. Millstein SG, Petersen AC, Nightingale EO, eds. *Promoting the Health of Adolescents: New Directions for the Twenty-first Century.* New York: Oxford University Press;1993: 261.

18. Wagner BM, Compas BE. Gender, instrumentality, and expressivity: Moderators of the relation between stress and psychological symptoms during adolescence. *Am J Community Psychol.* 1990;(18):383–406.

19. Ryan-Wenger, NA, Sharrer VW, Wynd CA. Stress, coping and health in children. In: *Handbook of Stress, Coping, Health: Implications of Nursing Research Theory and Practice.* Thousand Oaks: Sage Publications; 2000:265–294.

20. Demarco R, Ford-Gilboe M, Friedmann ML, McCubbin HI, McCubbin MA. *Handbook of Stress, Coping, Health: Implications of Nursing Research Theory and Practice.* Thousand Oaks: Sage Publications; 2000:295–333.

21. Ferraro KF, Su Y. Financial strain, social relations, and psychological distress among older people: A cross-cultural analysis. *J Gerontol B Psychol Sci Soc Sci.* 1999 Jan;54(1):53–55.

22. Lenze EJ, Mulsant BH, Shear MK, Schulberg HC, Dew MA, Begley AE, Pollock BG, Reynolds CF. 3rd ed. Comorbid anxiety disorders in depressed elderly patients. *Am J Psychiatry.* 2000 May;157(5):722–728.

23. Gordon M. *Manual of Nursing Diagnosis:* 1998–1999. St. Louis: Mosby Year Book; 1998.

24. Kessler RC, Mickelson KD, Williams DR. The prevalence, distribution, and mental health correlates of perceived discrimination in the United States. *J Health Soc Behav.* 1999 Sep; 40(3):208–230.

25. Krieger N, Sidney S. Racial discrimination and blood pressure: the CARDIA Study of young black and white adults. *Am J Public Health.* 1996 Oct;86(10):1370–1378.

26. Friedman MN. *Family Nursing: Research Theory and Practice.* 4th ed. New York: Appleton-Century-Crofts; 1998.

27. MacKenzie A. *The Time Trap.* 3rd ed. New York: AMACOM; 1997.

28. Davis M, McKay M, Eshelman E. *The Relaxation and Stress Reduction Workload.* 2nd ed. Oakland, CA: New Harbinger; 1995.

29. Roy M, Steptoe A. The inhibition of cardiovascular responses to mental stress following aerobic exercise. *Psychopophysiology.* 1991;28:689–700.

30. Sothman M, Kastello GK. Simulated weightlessness to induce chronic hypoactivity of brain norepinephrine for exercise and stress studies. *Med Sci Sports Exerc.* 1997 Jan;29(1):39–44.

31. Physical Activity and Health: A Report of the Surgeon General. U. S. Department of Health and Human Services. Atlanta, GA: U.S. Department of Health and Human Services, Centers for

Disease Control and Prevention, National Center for Chronic Disease Prevention and Health Promotion. 1996:31–32,136–140.

32. Hassman P, Koivula N, Uutela A. Physical exercise and psychological well-being: A population study in Finland. *Prev Med.* 2000:Jan;30(1):17–25.

33. Sothern MS, Loftin M, Suskind RM, Udall JN, Blecker U. The health benefits of physical activity in children and adolescents; implications for chronic disease prevention. *Eur J Pediatr.* 1999 Apr;158(4):271–274.

34. Cousins SO, et al. (This is a team made up of 11 people noted in the beginning of the textbook) *Active Living Among Older Adults: Health Benefits and Outcomes.* (Faculty of Physical Education and Recreation, University of Alberta, Edmonton, AB, Canada, and Well Quest Consulting, LTD in Canada.) Taylor & Francis; 1999:151–154.

35. Felton GM, Liu Q, Parsons MA, Geslani GP. Health promoting behaviors of rural adolescent women. *Women and Health.* 1998; 27(4)67–77.

36. Hoffman MA, Levy-Shiff R, Ushpiz V. Moderating effects of adolescent social orientation on the relation between social support and self esteem. *Journal of Youth and Adolescents.* 1993; 22(1),23–31.

37. Bandura A. Exercise of personal and collective efficacy in changing societies. In: Bandura A, ed. *Self-Efficacy in Changing Societies.* New York: Cambridge University Press; 1995.

38. Seila D, Wieiseke AW. Stress, self-efficacy, and health. In: *Handbook of Stress, Coping, Health: Implications of Nursing Research Theory and Practice.* Thousand Oaks: Sage Publications; 2000:495–516.

39. Upson JG, Steiger NH. *Self-Care Nursing in a Multi-Cultural Context.* Thousand Oaks: Sage Publications; 1996.

40. Hobfoll SE. *The Etiology of Stress.* Washington, DC: Hemisphere Publishing Cor.; 1988.

41. Matheny KB, Aycock DW, Curlette WL, Junker GN. The coping resources inventory for stress: A measure of perceived resourcefulness. *J Clin Psychol.* 1993 Nov;49(6):815–830.

42. Ingledew DK, Hardy L, Cooper CL. Do resources bolster coping and does coping buffer stress? An organizational study with longitudinal aspect and control for negative affectivity. *J Occup Health Psychol.* 1997 Apr;2(2):118–133.

43. Clark CC. *Wellness Practitioner: Concepts, Research and Strategies.* 2nd ed. New York: Springer; 1996.

44. Snyder M, Lindquist R. *Complementary Alternative Therapies in Nursing.* 3rd ed. New York: Springer; 1998.

45. Hahn YB, Ro YJ, Song HH, Kim NC, Sim HS, Yang SY. The effect of thermal biofeedback and progressive muscle relaxation training in reducing blood pressure of patients with essential hypertension. *Image: Journal of Nursing Scholarship.* 25:204–207.(1993)

46. Wimbush FB, Nelson ML. *Handbook of Stress, Coping, Health: Implications of Nursing Research Theory and Practice.* Thousand Oaks: Sage Publications, 2000:143–150.

47. Lekander M, Furst CJ, Rotstein S, Hursti TJ, Frederickson M. Immune effects of relaxation during chemotherapy for ovarian cancer. *Psychother Psychosom.* 1977;66(4):185–191.

48. Whitman S, Dell J, Legion V, Eibhyln A, Staatsinger J. Progressive relaxation for seizure reduction. *Journal of Epilepsy.* 1990; 3:17–22.

49. Snyder M. The influence of interventions on the stress-coping linkage. In: Barnfather J.; Lyon B, eds. *Stress and Coping: State of the Science and Implications for Nursing Theory, Research, and Practice.* Indianapolis, IN: Sigma Theta Tau International; 1993.

50. Weinberger R. Teaching the elderly stress reduction. *J Gerontol Nurse.* 1991;17(10):23–27.

11

Social Support and Health

Understanding the social context in which individuals live and work is critically important in health promotion. In human interactions, individuals and groups both give and receive social support, a reciprocal process and interactive resource that provides comfort, assistance, encouragement, and information. Social support fosters successful coping and promotes satisfying and effective living. The amount and type(s) of social support needed fluctuates across the life span and across varying situations. Individuals and families usually call on internal resources first to cope with unanticipated, difficult, or threatening circumstances. Contacts with others in the support system may then be initiated only when self-reliance fails. All individuals need a system of sustaining support to realize their full potential. Given that social support is a basic human need, researchers have explored its multiple dimensions, defined it operationally in various ways, and studied the relationship between social support and health. Social support is considered to be a person–environment interaction that decreases the occurrence of stressors, buffers the impact of stress, and decreases physiologic reactivity to stress.

Much of our understanding of the effects of social support on health has come from mental health. Results of research in this discipline indicate that social support is related to decreased stress during times of life crisis. Advances in our understanding of how social support actually affects mental and physical health are essential to be able to design interventions to promote mental, social, and physical well-being.[1] Relationships among social support, health behaviors, and health are addressed in this chapter. In addition, the role of the nurse in assisting clients to assess, modify, and develop effective social support systems that meet their needs is described.

 # Social Networks

The collective social relationships of a client are referred to as the social network.[2] Social networks are defined as the objective, structural components of support, whereas social support is considered the perceived or functional component.[3] A *social network* is made up of persons an individual or family knows and with whom they interact. These interactions may occur frequently or infrequently and may include a large number of individuals. *Social support* refers to the social interactions within the network that are sensed as being available and supportive (perceived) or that actually provide support (received). The social support system for any given individual or family is usually much smaller than the social network or array of contacts. Focusing on the individual for purposes of illustration, each individual is a node in the social network and each exchange is a link. An individual influences the environment at any point in time through network links, and links provide pathways through which the environment influences the individual. Social networks can be defined with the following terms.[4]

- Size: the actual number of individuals
- Composition: types of persons within the network, such as friends or relatives
- Geographic dispersion: distances separating network members
- Homogeneity: similarity of network members on various characteristics
- Intensity: frequency and extent of contact, or extent of emotional closeness
- Density: extent to which people know and interact with each other

Social network has been considered a static concept, as it refers to relationships across the life span. Social convoy, a term suggested by Antonucci,[5] is considered a more dynamic concept to describe an individual's social network. Three progressively enlarging concentric circles around an inner circle designating the individual depict the social convoy model. The inner circle consists of close, intimate relationships such as family and long-time friends. Individuals in the middle layer may be relatives, friends, and neighbors. The outer circle reflects contacts as a result of social roles, such as coworkers. This convoy, or set of relationships that provides support, moves with the individual throughout life. Middle and outer layers are more likely to change, whereas the inner layer tends to be more stable. Inner circle members are difficult to replace and when they are no longer available, there is a sense of grief and loss.

Networks are important to individuals and families to the extent that they fulfill members' needs. In addition, knowledge of the interactions of network characteristics shed light on how they influence the quantity and quality of social support. The size of the network is the major component in social support.[6] However, the types of persons in the network who provide the support, not the network size, have been associated with satisfaction. For example, in certain situations, support from a family member may be more valued than support from friends.

Social Support

It is well known that the extent and nature of one's social relationships affect one's health. Social support can be defined as a network of interpersonal relationships that provide companionship, assistance, and emotional nourishment.[7] Social support is an interpersonal transaction involving emotional concern (expressions of caring, encouragement, empathy), aid (services, money, or information), and affirmation (constructive feedback, acknowledgment).[5,8] The type of support that is beneficial at any given time may differ, depending on the nature and stage of the confronting situation. Emotional support may help in a crisis circumstance, whereas informational support may be more useful in assisting individuals to understand how to relate effectively with their peers. Assistance, also called instrumental or tangible aid, provides help with specific tasks, such as the preparation of nutritious meals or the transport of children to recreational activities. Affirmation helps individuals to realize their own strengths and potential.

Understanding social support within the context of culture requires knowledge of cultural characteristics that shape receiving and giving support. Cultural boundaries define the various subgroups of American society, such as African Americans, Asian Americans, Hispanic–Latinos, American Indians, and Native Americans. Within these cultural boundaries, social support operates uniquely within their social context. For example, based on the history of slavery in the African American community and group effort needed for survival, the family and church have been the major providers of social support.[9] Hispanic–Latino Americans and Asian Americans are similar in that the core of their social support systems is familism or the family that reflects close and distant kin. Asian Americans have rules regulating gender hierarchies (patrilineage) and respect for older adults, and use shame and harmony in giving and receiving support. In the American Indian culture, social support is less well understood, as the term is not defined in many tribal languages. However, American Indians live in relational networks that foster mutual assistance and support, and the extended family is a core feature of their network. Opportunities for affiliation and attachment enables support to be provided within cultures in spite of transitions or disruptions such as migration.

Although many similarities in social support exist among the various American cultures, the influence of the sociohistorical context differs greatly across the different populations.[9] More culturally sensitive theoretical views need to be formulated to understand the role of social support as well as gender and life-span differences in these populations.

Several social support systems relevant to health have been identified and described in the literature: natural support systems, peer support systems, organized religious support systems, organized support systems of caregiving or helping professionals, and organized support groups not directed by health professionals. Peer, professional and volunteer support can now be provided through computer-based systems. In most instances, the family (natural support system) constitutes the primary support group. Families, in order to provide appropriate support, must be sensitive to the needs of their members, establish effective communication, respect the unique needs of members, and establish expectations of mutual help and assistance.

Peer support systems consist of people who function informally to meet the needs of others. These persons maintain a reputation of helpfulness because of the support they provide. Many of these individuals have encountered an experience that has had a major influence in their own life and achieved successful adjustment and growth. Because of personal insight, their advice is sought primarily in relation to resolving a problem of immediate concern with which they are familiar. Examples include the avid runner, the health-food enthusiast, the widow, or the parents of a retarded child. Successful coping is the primary credential of an individual credible as a source of peer support.

Organized religious support systems such as churches or other religious meeting places constitute a support system for individuals because the congregation share a similar value system, a common set of beliefs about the purpose of life, traditions of worship, and a set of guidelines for living. Even highly mobile individuals may find a support system in the local church or synagogue. The church takes primary responsibility for support to enhance the spiritual dimension of health, which has been defined as the ability to develop one's spiritual nature to its fullest potential.[10] This includes the ability to discover and articulate one's basic purpose in life, to learn how to experience love, joy, peace, and fulfillment, and how to help oneself and others achieve full personal potential.

A third type of support system is composed of professional helpers with a specific set of skills and services to offer clients. Interestingly, many questions have been raised about the effectiveness of their role in social support.[4] Although professionals have access to information and resources that might not otherwise be available, they are seldom the first source of help for an individual. Family and close friends or peers are sought for advice and support initially. Health professionals are rarely included as members of an individual's social network in an assessment and become the support system only when other sources of help are unavailable, interrupted, or exhausted. Professionals are rarely able to provide support over long periods of time. In addition, these relationships are not characterized by reciprocity, usually involve a power differential, and offer limited empathic understanding due to lack of intimacy. In spite of these limitations, professional helpers have a role to play in offering support over the short term as well as in playing a major role in informational support.

Organized support systems not directed by health professionals include voluntary service groups and mutual help groups. These are also called self-help groups, as they do not have an expert leader, as distinguished from support groups, which are led by a trained facilitator.[11] Voluntary service groups provide assistance to individuals who are in need or for some reason are unable to provide services for themselves. Mutual help groups (e.g., Alcoholics Anonymous, Take Off Pounds Sensibly [TOPS], and Recovery, Inc.) attempt to change behavior of members or promote adaptation to a life change such as chronic illness, or disabled family member. The number of self-help groups continues to increase in the United States. Some have sprung up because of disenchantment with the health care system. Others are a result of attempts to manage problems uncommon in the general society. Service groups and mutual help groups play a significant role in social support relevant to health.

All support systems of a given individual or family are synergistic. In combination, they represent the social resources available to the client to facilitate stability and actualization. Various systems will be dominant at different points in the life cycle, depending on stage of development and the stressors or challenges at hand. For example, in preadolescence and early adolescence, parents are the greatest source of support. The network shifts to a greater reliance on peers for lifestyle choices during middle adolescence with a decreased perception of parental support.[12,13] Friends remain dominant in young adults, whereas the family network as well as friends are important sources of support for the elderly.

Functions of Social Support Groups

The primary functions of social support groups are to augment personal strengths of members and promote achievement of life goals. The functions of social support groups in promoting and protecting health can be conceptualized in four ways, as depicted in Figure 11–1. Social groups can contribute to health by (1) creating a growth-promoting environment that supports health-promoting behaviors, self-esteem, and high-level wellness;

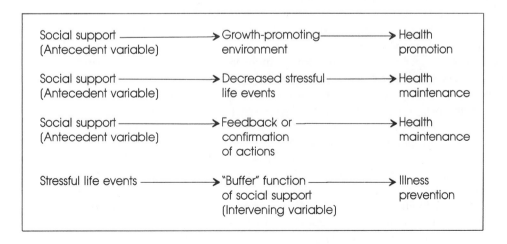

FIGURE 11-1 Possible impact of social support on health status

(2) decreasing the likelihood of threatening or stressful life events; (3) providing feedback or confirmation that actions are leading to anticipated and socially desirable consequences; and (4) buffering or mediating the negative effects of stressful events through influencing interpretation of events and emotional responses to them, thus decreasing their illness-producing potential. Support groups can be characterized as sharing common social concerns, providing intimacy, preventing isolation, respecting mutual competencies, offering dependable assistance in crises, serving as a referral agent, and providing mutual challenge.

Computer-based support groups are increasing in popularity because of their ability to be a resource for ongoing information, emotional support, and encouragement.[14] Computer-based systems have been found to improve quality of life and self-care through the provision of information, support in decision making, and connections to experts as well as peers.[15] This technology has been shown to be acceptable across ethnically diverse groups.[16] Many elders have a strong aversion to computers, pointing to the need to improve user interface in this group.[17] This is significant, as computer-based social support among the elderly has the potential to overcome many of the barriers that prevent elders from participating in groups, such as mobility changes, lack of available transportation, and finances.[18]

Family as the Primary Support Group

The family is the primary context for learning about giving and receiving social support. Family cohesion, expressiveness, and lack of conflict are reflected in the supportive behaviors that family members provide to one another. Studies indicate that low family support and poor child–parent interactions influence a child's cognitive, emotional, and social development.[19] In addition, family stressors, such as loss of a job or divorce, may decrease family cohesion and increase conflict. In a sample of single- and two-parent families, family cohesion was the most consistent predictor of health-related problem solving and goal attainment behaviors.[20]

In a longitudinal study of children of Kauai raised in adverse conditions (poverty, perinatal stress, parental substance abuse, and family discord), competent parenting styles that were supportive and enhanced self-esteem fostered resilience.[21] The results of this 40-year study suggest that the effects of risk factors on children can be buffered by the existence of protective factors such as social competencies, communication skills, and social support. Those who grew to be competent, caring adults were more likely to have had a supportive caregiving environment with more parental attention and less parental conflict. Other studies attribute resilience to the presence of a family environment that provides cohesion, encourages positive coping, and helps children develop feelings of competence and self-efficacy.

Family social support exerts complex effects on the physical and mental health of its members. The well-known Alameda County, California, study provided the initial findings on the association of social networks and support and mortality.[22] Men who are single or widowed have consistently shown higher mortality rates than married men. However, the mechanisms underlying this relationship are not well understood. Depressive symptoms have been associated with an adverse family environment that offers low levels of social support. Men who remain alone after losing their partners are at higher risk of developing symptoms of chronic depression,[23] and having a supportive spouse and relatives has been associated with a decreased risk for major depression.[24] Having a marital partner, or if unmarried having social support, significantly reduces the incidence of depression in community living elders.[25] Using the convoy model,[5] two aspects of social support networks—a greater proportion of kin and the presence of family members in the inner circle—significantly reduce distress, especially in young adults.[26] The interplay between family stressors and family support is depicted in Figure 11–2.

Within families, both positive and negative interactions occur. Negative interactions can be viewed as stressors, whereas positive, helpful interactions constitute support. A family's ability to foster positive interactive styles among its members may also relate to the extent to which the family has its own social network of long-term supportive relationships, and the extent to which the family is accorded respect within the community. Positive emotional bonds of the family with its social network buttress the family's competence and effective functioning.

Community Organizations as Support Groups

The characteristics of a community and its organizations have a direct bearing on the level of well-being of individuals and families that reside in it. The quality of social interaction and the life experiences of residents can contribute positively to health or negatively, resulting in social disorganization and overt illness. Stability within a community tends to promote close-knit ties among residents that mitigate the effects of crises on community members. Stable communities are characterized by value similarity, mutual assistance, shared trust, and concern for members.

Organizations, particularly churches, are viewed as a source of support in the community for health and healing. This is especially true for African Americans for reasons mentioned earlier. Churches represent miniature, dynamic communities that may provide assistance for the development and implementation of supportive programs through provision of child care, meals, transportation, and other resources. In addition, volunteer helpers

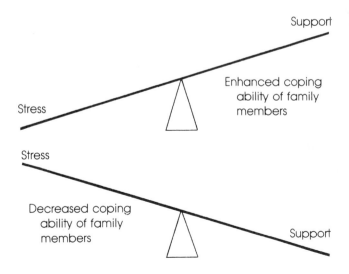

FIGURE 11-2 Family as a source of support or stress

are readily available. For this reason, church peer workers play an important role in many health promotion projects.[27] Nurses are also beginning to volunteer in churches to support health promotion and well-being through telephone calls and home visits.[28]

Self-Help Groups

Whereas family and friends generally serve as primary sources of support, self-help groups are an important source of assistance within most communities. Examples of self-help groups include Mended Hearts, Compassionate Friends, Weight Watchers, and physical fitness clubs. Characteristics of self-help groups include a critical mass sufficient to form a group, a form of publicity or recruitment to attract members, and a central goal or activity that gives the group purpose and sustains the investment of its members. The question has been raised as to why individuals use self-help groups rather than other resources, such as professional services. Two possible reasons are offered: (1) Self-help groups arise to fulfill a need for services not being offered, or (2) self-help groups arise because of disappointment with inadequate or lack of meaningful resources within the community.

Self-help groups are an important resource, as they enable group members to expand their social networks as well as receive informational, instrumental, and emotional support from others. Self-help groups as well as lay health promotion programs empower individuals by increasing hope, support, and affirmation.[29,30] The helping transactions that occur in these groups are thought to be an important therapeutic mechanism.[31] Self-help groups are considered beneficial because they compensate for deficits in one's naturally occurring network.[11] Intensive support by lay volunteers was shown to help women in a barrio of San Antonio, Texas, keep their appointments for screening examinations.[32] In women with breast cancer, a self-help group helped bridge the isolation gap experienced by those in rural areas and improved life quality and well-being.[33] A cancer prevention intervention for Hispanic–Latinos used layworkers to conduct group sessions, resulting in an increased use of cancer screening tests.[34]

Self-help groups are a valuable source of support within many communities. Their records of success in assisting millions of individuals cope with a variety of different life experiences attest to their continuing viability as an integral part of community health resources. However, few support groups that have been conducted have targeted men, so the role of self-help groups to provide support for men needs exploration.

Reviewing Social Support Systems

It is important for both clients and health care providers to be aware of sources of social support available. Two approaches for reviewing the social support networks of clients are suggested. These approaches can be useful in giving both client and nurse increased insight into existing support resources. When assessing the adequacy of a client's support systems, it is important to be cognizant of factors that may cause the assessments to vary. Such things as the client's culture, stage of life-span development, social context (school, home, work), and role context (parent, student, professional) need to be considered for their influence on perceived and received support.

Support Systems Review

One straightforward, useful approach asks the client to list individuals who provide personal support (financial, emotional, or instrumental).[35] The client is then asked to indicate whether the individuals listed are family members, fellow workers, or social acquaintances. By next identifying persons who have been sources of support for five years or more, the client becomes aware of the stability of personal support systems. Examining current sources of support enables the client and the nurse mutually to assess the adequacy of support. If it is inadequate, strategies are generated about what can be done to enhance existing social support networks. Figure 11–3 provides a sample support system review for a hypothetical client. After a review of the client's social support systems, the following questions can be explored:

- In what areas do you need more support: financial, emotional, instrumental?
- Who within your present support system might provide the additional needed support?
- Who else can become a part of your support system?
- What can you do to add the people you believe you need to your support system?

Answers to these questions suggest actions the client can take to expand sources of personal support.

List those individuals below who provide financial, emotional, or instrumental support (assistance with tasks) to you. Indicate the type of support provided by placing the appropriate letter next to each name. *F* = financial support, *E* = emotional support, and *I* = instrumental support. Any individual may provide more than one type of support. Next, indicate whether the supportive other is a family member (*FM*), fellow worker (*FW*), or social acquaintance (*A*). Finally, after each person who has been a source of support for 5 years or more, place the number 5.

John	F, E, I, FM (husband), 5	Nancy	E, A
Peter	E, FM (son), 5	Larry	E, I, A
Carmen	E, FM (daughter), 5	Arlene	E, I, A
Helen	E, FM (mother), 5	Duane	I, A, 5
Ted	E, FM (father), 5	Elaine	I, A, 5
Audrey	E, FM (cousin), 5	Margaret	E, I, FW
Andrew	E, I, FM (cousin), 5	Marlene	E, I, FW
Jane	E, I, A	Frances	I, FW
David	E, I, A	Rose	I, FW
Tom	I, A, 5	Karen	I, FW
Elsa	E, I, A, 5	Theresa	I, FW
Jack	E, A	Diane	I, FW

continued

FIGURE 11-3 Support systems review

The individuals identified on the previous page should be grouped in the following way:

Sources of Emotional Support

FAMILY	WORK	SOCIAL GROUP
John	Margaret	Jane
Peter	Marlene	David
Carmen		Elsa
Helen		Jack
Ted		Nancy
Audrey		Larry
Andrew		Arlene

Sources of Instrumental Support

FAMILY	WORK	SOCIAL GROUP
John	Margaret	Jane
Audrey	Marlene	David
Andrew	Frances	Tom
	Rose	Elsa
	Karen	Larry
	Theresa	Arlene
	Diane	Duane
		Elaine

Sources of Financial Support

FAMILY	WORK	SOCIAL GROUP
John		

Sources of Support for More than 5 Years

FAMILY	WORK	SOCIAL GROUP
John		Tom
Peter		Elsa
Carmen		Duane
Helen		Elaine
Ted		
Audrey		
Andrew		

FIGURE 11-3 Support systems review *(continued)*

Emotional Support Diagram

Sources of emotional support can also be diagrammed in such a way that strength of support is readily apparent. Figure 11–4 presents a sample emotional support diagram that is coded to indicate strong, moderate, and weak sources of support, as well as current conflicts with supportive individuals. The length of each line is used to indicate geographical proximity to the client. This approach is particularly appropriate for clients who need a more visual presentation of their emotional support system in order to take action effectively to sustain or enhance emotionally satisfying relationships.

Review of sources of social support is an integral part of the decision-making phase of health behavior. Through review, the client is able to recognize current sources of support and identify barriers in social relationships that may thwart desirable health actions. The nurse must always be alert to client situations where social support is minimal or nonexistent. Extensive review of support systems may cause anxiety and depression for the client. In this case, a more informal, nonthreatening approach should be used.

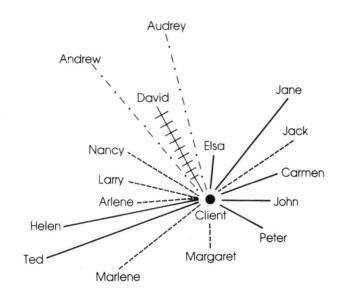

FIGURE 11-4 Emotional support for client

Social Support and Health

The importance of social support to mental and physical health is now well established. Lower levels of support are consistently linked to higher rates of morbidity and mortality. However, the actual mechanisms linking social support to health are still not well understood. Several different processes have been proposed. Social support may directly link to health by promoting healthy or unhealthy behaviors, by supplying information, or by making available tangible resources (child care, opportunities for work). Psychologically, social support may foster a sense of meaning in life or be associated with more positive affective states, such as enhanced sense of self-worth and increased sense of control. Individuals may appraise events as less threatening, resulting in less physiologic arousal. Biologically, social support may intensify positive neuroendocrine and immunologic responses despite the presence of stressors.[36,37] All of these possible mechanisms present challenging topics for social support research.

Although the relationship between social support and health is well known, a review of research in which interventions have been tested to improve some type of social support reveals varying long-term results.[38] Numerous studies have been conducted. However, many suffer from conceptual and methodological flaws, limiting the ability to generalize the findings.[6] In addition, studies that were well designed showed no intervention effects or an improvement in support was not measured as an outcome. In other words, while the intervention may have improved health or well-being, if the client's naturally occurring social support did not change, the desired outcomes would not last when the intervention was completed. The research suggests that social support is complex and includes characteristics of the person who needs or desires support (perceiver), characteristics of the person who gives the support (supporter), characteristics of the situation, and the interaction of these factors. All of these factors need to be taken into consideration when designing interventions to improve social support.

The positive effects of providing support to others is a relatively new area of social support research. Most studies have focused on the positive effects of receiving support. Giving help may have positive effects on well-being for at least three different reasons: The realization that one has helped an individual in need is a self-validating experience that can bolster feelings of psychological well-being; giving aid to others fosters intimacy and trust, thereby strengthening existing social bonds; and giving support to significant others increases the probability that one's own need for assistance will be met in the future. Helping others informally has a greater impact on well-being than does helping others through formal organizational structures.[39] This contrast between providing informal and formal support and its relationship to health needs further exploration.

Social Networks and Social Support and Use of Prevention Services

The role of social networks and social support in promoting use of prevention services has been demonstrated in a number of studies. It is widely accepted that social networks function as conduits for information and as links to broader societal contacts, such as health care providers. In a multiethnic Asian population, women who reported ever having Pap screening were more likely to have close friends with whom they could discuss their health and have a regular physician.[40] A cancer prevention intervention for Hispanics–Latinos indicates that peers recruited from the community to deliver the intervention were effective in increasing cancer screening tests in comparison to the control group.[34]

The mechanisms linking social support and use of preventive services need to be better understood. Particularly important is understanding how beliefs about personal vulnerability to disease or illness and cultural beliefs interact with the level and type of social support necessary to motivate use of screening services for early detection.

Social Support and Health Behavior

Research also indicates that social support systems influence health behavior. It is well known that significant others function as an important lay referral system for individuals in making decisions to seek professional care for health promotion, illness prevention, or care in illness. The resultant effects can be negative or positive. When a client is a member of a culture that differs markedly from that of health professionals, an extended lay-consultant structure may be available, which delays seeking professional care. In contrast, when the client's culture is similar to that of health professionals, the lay system is usually bypassed, and contact with health providers is made early in the course of a problem or concern. Individuals use their lay referral system not only during the decision phase, when deciding whether to seek care, but also during the action phase to make decisions about adherence. Diagnostic decisions, prescriptions for medication, and life changes recommended by health professionals frequently are discussed with significant others who constitute the individual's lay referral system. Concurrence by the lay referral system often determines the extent to which advice from health professionals is actually followed.

Social support from spouses is related to health behaviors. This relationship may be due to the encouragement and support of the health behavior, including giving approval and disapproval, having control over aspects of the proposed change such as food shopping and preparation, and participating in the behavior change, such as joining the exercise program. High levels of warmth, encouragement, and assistance occur in spousal support.[41] In a two-year study examining the association of spousal support with maintenance of a low-fat diet in men with hypercholersterolemia, men who had spouses who supported maintenance of the lipid-lowering diets attained their dietary goals sooner and maintained the diet change for two years.[42]

Social support has been correlated with adoption of other health behaviors or cessation of negative behaviors. The effectiveness of a work site nutrition intervention to increase fruit and vegetable consumption found that being in the preparation stage of the Transtheoretical Stage of Change Model was related to coworker support.[43] In a work site smoking intervention, social support had a direct effect on smoking cessation. The interventions tested were (1) self-help manuals; (2) self-help manuals and incentives; or (3) self-help manuals, incentives, and support groups.[44] The group intervention increased partner support, which facilitated quitting smoking. In addition, higher levels of perceived support facilitated successful quitting. In the Women's Determinants Study, women who reported high levels of support for physical activity were less likely to be sedentary.[45] Hispanic women reported a higher level of support for physical activity than did other racial–ethnic groups. No differences in support were found between friends and family.

Adoption and maintenance of health-behavior change over time is difficult unless the behavior is encouraged through support from family members and friends. This points to the importance of naturally occurring support and connectedness or long-term formal or informal support systems if natural ones are not available. Although many retrospective studies have described the effect of social support on health behavior, prospective studies are needed to identify networks of social support that promote health promotion and illness prevention behaviors.

Identifying Social Support Strengths and Needs

Functional health patterns relevant to the area of social support include self-perception–self-concept pattern, role–relationship pattern, and coping–stress tolerance pattern. Each functional health pattern contains a number of diagnoses relevant to social support problems or needs such as altered family processes, hopelessness, self-esteem disturbance, and chronic low self-esteem.[46] The diagnostic taxonomy, while facilitating problem identification, does not allow clear specification of social support assets and resources. Houldin and colleagues[47] have attempted to address this gap by proposing that nurses diagnose for wellness to clearly identify and support client strengths. Inclusion of assets and strengths of clients as phenomena relevant to nursing care is extremely important if nurses are to provide leadership in developing positive strategies for enhancing the health of populations.

Enhancing Social Support Systems

Support-enhancing strategies have three goals: assisting individuals and families to strengthen existing supportive relationships, helping individuals and families to establish satisfying interpersonal ties, and preventing disruption of ties from evolving into mental or physical illness.

Facilitating Social Bonding

Social skills training represents one approach to changing the characteristics of clients to enable them to develop supportive interpersonal relationships with others. Training can be carried out with individual clients or with groups of people who have similar skill deficits, such as dysfunctional families.[38] Social skills training is based on the belief that socially competent responses can be learned just like other behaviors. Initially, training is directed toward assessing and modifying perceptions of appropriate behavior in social situations. In addition, persons are taught to reevaluate their thoughts about themselves in a more positive manner. Attempts are made to improve social interaction patterns through modeling, role playing, performance feedback, coaching, and homework assignments. Skills to be taught might include initiating conversations, giving and receiving compliments, handling periods of silence, enhancing physical attractiveness, nonverbal methods of communication, and handling criticism and conflict.[38] Within the school setting, training in social skills and problem solving can be provided in the classroom as an approach to preventing the acquisition of socially alienating behaviors. To complement such work, the broader aspects of the school environment should be assessed to determine the extent to which they facilitate or inhibit students' opportunities for and skills in developing social ties.[48]

Enhancing Coping

Preventing the lack of social ties from resulting in serious psychologic and physical problems is particularly important during developmental or situational transition periods. Support seminars or groups for widows, children of separated or divorced parents, parents who have lost a child, or relatives of persons imprisoned can assist such persons to learn to cope effectively with life stress. Benefits from such programs include help in understanding puzzling and disturbing emotional reactions, reducing feelings of alienation, and assisting people to move ahead into the future. It is important that programs be tailored to the unique needs of individuals, as clients desire different types of support from different members in their networks.[49,50]

Preventing Loss of Support and Loneliness

Preventing loneliness is a more desirable approach than treatment of loneliness and isolation after it has occurred. Two approaches to prevention include the identification of high-risk groups and educational interventions for persons of all ages focused on developing social support ties.[51,52] Young, unmarried, unemployed, and low-income persons appear particularly vulnerable to lack of support and loneliness. Obstacles to social participation, such as lack of transportation for the elderly or constant caretaking responsibilities for middle-age women with elderly parents, create populations at risk for loneliness. When such groups are identified, programs can be planned to decrease aloneness and isolation. Possible programs include transportation vehicles staffed by volunteers for those in need, respite programs to provide relief for caretakers, community support groups for families with disabled or impaired members, and teleconference or computer-mediated support groups that can be accessed at home.

Educational approaches to prevent loss of social support and subsequent loneliness include classroom experiences for schoolchildren that help them gain experience in making friends, working cooperatively with others, and resolving differences or conflict. Over the past 30 years there is a growing body of evidence that poor social functioning of children often leads to serious personal adjustment problems in later life. Most experts would agree that children require the security of positive reciprocal relationships with their peers, parents, and teachers for maximum growth and development.[13]

For older adults, media campaigns, such as public service announcements about resources for formal support or the health benefits of staying connected with relatives and friends, may be cues needed to initiate support-enhancing behaviors. In addition, pamphlets, community programs, and neighborhood activities can be designed to help persons build relationships or to reach out to others who may need emotional or instrumental support.

Other general suggestions for enhancing social support include:

- Mutual goal setting with significant others to achieve common directions in actions and efforts
- Constructively resolving conflict between oneself and support network members
- Frequently offering assistance to individuals within social network to show concern and promote trust
- Seeking counseling, if needed, to enhance marital and/or family adjustment
- Making use of the nurse and other health professionals as community support resources
- Increasing ties to social groups to expand growth opportunities

Clients should be encouraged to identify specific goals to be achieved when counseling to enhance personal support networks. By focusing on one or two realistic changes relevant to goals of highest priority, clients can alter the breadth and depth of social support available to them.

Directions for Research in Social Support

A convincing number of studies have demonstrated the relationship between social networks and social support and health. However, there are inconsistencies in this body of research and many questions remain to be answered. For example, because social support is a concept and not a theory, theory development is needed to guide research, which adequately tests antecedents and consequences of social support. The specific functions of social support in enhancing health is not known and needs further investigation. Interventions need to be refined and tested that enhance social support as well as develop long-term support systems. The "dosage" of social support necessary to promote health also needs to be explored. Culturally sensitive interventions as well as interventions across the life span to enhance support need to be developed and tested in subgroups of the population. Additionally, culturally sensitive, reliable, and valid measures need further development and testing. Immune function and its relationship to social support also need further exploration. Outcomes of social support interventions need to include changes in the support system as well as health behaviors. Nurse scientists play a major role in social support research and should lead interdisciplinary teams to investigate these issues.

Directions for Practice in Social Support

Although research findings are available that provide important information about social support and health, many of these findings have not been incorporated into practice. Utilization of research findings should become part of the nurses' practice to learn better ways to intervene to enhance social networks and social support. Assessment of social support systems should be a component of the initial nursing assessment, using strategies such as those described in this chapter. In these assessments, nurses should be knowledgeable of strategies to obtain culturally sensitive information from diverse populations. Finally, nurses need to incorporate sources of social support such as families, self-help groups, and community organizations in their interventions to increase the potential for success in health promotion and lifestyle change.

SUMMARY

Social support plays an important role in the health and well-being of clients. To be able to provide comprehensive health protection and health promotion care, the nurse must consider the client as well as the social context. Social support groups are instrumental in assisting clients to cope with everyday hassles and major stressful life experiences and in enhancing emotional and physical well-being. The extent to which stressful events threaten health may well depend on the support available from core (family) or extended (community and professional) social networks. The design and evaluation of nursing interventions to enhance social support is critical. These studies will contribute to the development of scientifically sound nursing care interventions directed toward enhancing the quality of human social transactions across the life span.

REFERENCES

1. Langford CP, Bowsher J, Maloney JP, Lillis PP. Social support: A conceptual analysis. *J Adv Nurs.*1997 Jan; 25(1):95–100.
2. Kane, R. Social assessment of geriatric patients. In: Tallis R, Fillit H, Brocklehurst JC, eds., *Brocklehurst's Textbook of Geriatric Medicine and Gerontology.* 5th ed., New York: Churchill Livingstone; 1998:227–234.
3. Roberts JE, Gotlib IH. Social support and personality in depression: implications from quantitative genetics. In: Pierce GR, Lakey B, Sarason IG, Sarason BR, eds. *Handbook of Social Support and Personality.* New York: Plenum Press; 1997:187–214.
4. Heaney CA, Israel BA. (1997). Social networks and social support. In: Glanz K, Lewis FM, Rimer BK, eds. *Health Behavior and Health Education.* 2nd ed. 1997:179–205, San Francisco: Jossey-Bass.
5. Antonucci TC, Kahn RL, Akiyama H. Psychological factors and the response to cancer symptoms. In: Yancik R, Yates JW, eds. *Cancer in the Elderly: Approaches to Early Detection and Treatment* New York: Springer; 1989:40–52.
6. Underwood, P. Social support: The promise and the reality. In: Rice VH, ed., *Handbook of Stress, Coping and Health: Implications for Nursing Research, Theory, and Practice.* Thousand Oaks: Sage Publications; 2000:367–391.
7. Newcomb MD, Bentler PM. Loneliness and social support: A confirmatory hierarchical analysis. *Personality and Social Psychology Bulletin.* 1986;12:520–535.
8. House JS. *Work, Stress, and Social Support.* Reading, MA: Addison-Wesley Publishing Co., Inc.; 1981.
9. Dilworth-Anderson P, Marshall S. Social support in its cultural context. In: Pierce GR, Sarason BR, Sarason IG, eds. *Handbook of Social Support and the Family,* New York: Plenum Press, 1996:67–79.
10. Chapman LS. Developing a useful perspective on spiritual health: Love, joy, peace and fulfillment. *Am J Health Prom.* 1987;2:12–17.
11. Helgeson VS, Cohen S, Schulz R, Yasko J. Group support interventions for women with breast cancer: Who benefits from what? *Health Psychol.* 2000; 19(2):107–114.
12. West P, Sweeting H, Ecob R. Family and friends' influences on the uptake of regular smoking from mid-adolescence to early adulthood. *Addiction.* 1999 Sep;94(9):1397–1411.
13. Barrera M Jr., Li SA. The relation of family support to adolescents' psychological distress and behavior problems. In: Pierce GR, Sarason BR, Sarason, eds. *Handbook of Social Support and the Family.* New York: Plenum Press; 1996:313–343.
14. Fernsler JI, Manchester LJ. Evaluation of a computer-based cancer support network. *Cancer Pract.* 1997 Jan–Feb; 5(1):46–51.
15. Gustafson DH, Hawkins R, Boberg E, Pingree S, Serlin RE, Graziano F, Chan CL. Impact of a patient-centered, computer-based health information/support system. *Am J Prev Med.* 1999 Jan; 16(1):1–9.

16. Bock B, Niaura R, Fontes A, Bock F. Acceptability of computer assessments among ethnically diverse, low-income smokers. *Am J Health Prom.* 1999 May–Jun;13(5):299–304.

17. Inoue M, Seam A, Takeuchi Y, Meshitsuka S. Application of a computer based education system for aged persons and issues arising during the field test. *Comput Methods Programs Biomed.* 1999 Apr; 59(1):55–60.

18. Hendrix CC. Computer use among elderly people. *Comput Nurs.* 2000 Mar–Apr; 18(2):62–68.

19. Timko C, Moos RH. The mutual influence of family support and youth adaptation. In: Pierce GR, Sarason BR, Sarason IG, eds. *Handbook of Social Support and the Family.* New York: Plenum Press;1996:289–310.

20. Ford-Gilboe M. Family strengths, motivation, and resources as predictors of health promotion behavior in single-parent and two-parent families. *Res Nurs Health.* 1997 Jun; 20(3):205–217.

21. Werner EE. Vulnerable but invincible: High-risk children from birth to adulthood. *Acta Paediatr Suppl.* 1997 Jul;422:103–105.

22. Berkman L, Syme SL. Social networks, host resistance, and mortality: A nine-year follow-up study of Alameda County residents. Am J Epidemiology. 1979;115:684–694.

23. van Grootheest DS, Beekman AT, Broese van Groenou MI, Deeg DJ. Sex differences in depression after widowhood. Do men suffer more? *Soc Psychiatry Psychiatr Epidemiol.* 1999. Jul;34 (7):391–398.

24. Wade TD, Kendler KS. The relationship between social support and major depression: Cross-sectional, longitudinal, and genetic perspectives. *J Nerv Ment Dis.* 2000 May;188(5):251–258.

25. Schoevers RA, Beekman AT, Deeg DJ, Geerling MI, Jonke C, Van Tilbur W. Risk factors for depression in later life; results of a prospective community based study (AMSTEL). *J Affect Disord.* 2000 Aug;59(2):127–137.

26. Peek MK, Lin N. Age differences in the effects of network composition on psychological distress. *Soc Sci Med.* 1999 Sep;49(5):621–636.

27. Castro FG, Elder J, Coe K, Tafoya-Barraza HM, Moratto S, Campbell N, Talavera G. Mobilizing churches for health promotion in Latino communities: Companeros en la Salud. *J Natl Cancer Inst Monogr.* 1995(18):127–135.

28. Chase-Ziolek M, Striepe J. A comparison of urban versus rural experiences of nurses volunteering to promote health in churches. *Public Health Nurs.* 1999 Aug;16(4):270–279.

29. Mok E, Martinson I. Empowerment of Chinese patients with cancer through self-help groups in Hong Kong. *Cancer Nurs.* 2000 Jun;23(3):206–213.

30. Booker VK, Robinson JG, Kay BJ, Najera LG, Stewart G. Changes in empowerment: Effects of participation in a lay health promotion program. *Health Educ Behav.* 1997 Aug;24(4):452–464.

31. Roberts LJ, Salem D, Rappaport J, Toro PA, Luke DA, Seidman E. Giving and receiving help: Interpersonal transactions of members. *Am J Community Psychol.* 1999 Dec;27(6):841–868.

32. Ramirez AG, McAlister A, Gallion KJ, Ramirez V, Garza IR, Stamm K, de la Torre J, Chalela P. Community level cancer control in a Texas barrio: Part I—Theoretical basis, implementation, and process evaluation. *J Natl Cancer Inst Monogr.* 1995;(18):117–122.

33. Curran VR, Church JG. A study of rural women's satisfaction with a breast cancer self-help network. *J Telemed Telecare.* 1999;5(1):47–54.

34. Navarro AM, Senn KL, Kaplan RM, McNicholas L, Campo MC, Roppe B. Por La Vida intervention model for cancer prevention in Latinas. *J Natl Cancer Inst Monogr.* 1995;(18):137–145.

35. Glaser B, Kirschenbaum H. Using values clarification in a counseling setting. *Personnel and Guidance Journal.* 1980;59:569–575.

36. Lekander M, Furst CJ, Rotstein S, Blongren H, Fredrikson M. Social support and immune status during and after chemotherapy for breast cancer. *Acta Oncol.* 1996;35(1):31–37.

37. Nunes JA, Raymond SJ, Nicholas PK, Leuner JD, Webster A. Social support, quality of life, immune function, and health in persons living with HIV. *J Holis Nurs.* 1995 Jun;13(2):174–198.

38. Lakey B, Lutz CJ. Social support and preventive and therapeutic interventions. In: Pierce GR, Sarason BR, Sarason IG, eds. *Handbook of Social Support and the Family.* New York: Plenum Press; 1996:435–465.

39. Krause N, Ingersoll-Dayton B, Liang J, Sugisawa H. Religion, social support, and health among the Japanese elderly. *J Health Soc Behav.* 1999 Dec;40(4):405–421.

40. Seow A, Huang J, Straughan PT. Effects of social support, regular physician and health-related attitudes on cervical cancer screening in an Asian population. *Cancer Causes Control.* 2000 Mar;11(3):223–230.

41. Simons RL, Johnson C. The impact of marital and social network support on quality of parenting. In: Pierce GR, Sarason BR, and Sarason IG, eds. *Handbook of Social Support and the Family.* New York: Plenum Press; 1996:269–287.

42. Bovbjerg VE, McCann BS, Brief DJ, Follette WC, Retzlaff BM, Dowdy AA, Walden CE, Knopp RH. Spouse support and long-term adherence to lipid-lowering diets. *Am J Epidemiol.* 1995 Mar;141(5):451–460.

43. Sorensen G, Stoddard A, Macario E. Social support and readiness to make dietary changes. *Health Educ Behav.* 1998 Oct;25(5):586–598.

44. McMahon SD, Jason LA. Social support in a worksite smoking intervention. A test of theoretical models. *Behav Modif.* 2000 Apr;24(2):184–201.

45. Eyler AA, Brownson RC, Donatelle RJ, King AC, Brown D, Sallis JF. Physical activity social support and middle- and older-aged minority women: Results from a U. S. survey. *Soc Sci Med.* 1999 Sep;49(6):781–789.

46. Gordon M. *Manual of Nursing Diagnosis, 1993–1994.* St. Louis: Mosby Year Book; 1999.

47. Houldin AD, Salstein SW, Ganley KM. *Nursing Diagnosis for Wellness: Supporting Strengths.* New York: J. B. Lippincott Co.; 1987.

48. Thompson EA, Horn M, Herting JR, Eggert LL. Enhancing outcomes in an indicated drug prevention program for high-risk youth. *J Drug Educ.* 1997;27(1):19–41.

49. Orleans CT, Boyd NR, Bingler R, Sutton C, Fairclaugh D, Heller D, McClatchey M, Ward JA, Graves C, Fleisher L, Baum S. A self-help intervention for African American smokers: tailoring cancer information service counseling for a special population. *Prev Med.* 1998 Sep–Oct;27(5 Pt 2):S61–S70.

50. Carpenter BD, Van Haitsma K, Ruckdeschel K, Lawton MP. The psychosocial preferences of older adults: A pilot examination of content and structure. *Gerontologist.* 2000 Jun;40(3):335–348.

51. Hagerty BM, Williams RA. The effects of sense of belonging, social support, conflict, and loneliness on depression. *Nurs Res.* 1999 Jul–Aug;48(4):215–219.

52. Bonin MF, McCreary DR, Sadava SW. Problem drinking behavior in two community-based samples of adults: Influence of gender, coping, loneliness, and depression. *Psychol Addict Behav.* 2000 Jun;14(2):151–161.

Part V

Evaluating the Effectiveness of Health Promotion

12

Measuring Outcomes of Health Promotion and Prevention Interventions

The goal of nursing in health promotion is to maintain or enhance the client's health status and well-being. Nurses throughout the world have accepted the call to be leaders in health promotion. Nurses in all types of settings have implemented interventions that promote health and prevent disease. However, until recently, assessment of the outcomes of health promotion has received less attention by most practicing nurses. Today's emphasis on the use of outcomes measures to demonstrate the effectiveness of health promotion interventions challenges nurses in all settings to describe the effects of their practice on client–patient outcomes.

Florence Nightingale is recognized as the first person who used outcomes measures in health care.[1] Nightingale used morbidity and mortality statistics to measure the quality of care for British soldiers during the Crimean War. These traditional outcomes have continued to be used in medicine and epidemiology. In today's health care environment, outcome measurement is much more comprehensive and complex and takes into account all factors that influence health outcomes, including client, provider, and system characteristics, as well as the process of delivering the health promotion interventions.

The increased emphasis on outcomes measurement in this country has occurred as a result of the need to determine the most appropriate and cost-effective interventions in the current competitive health care market with its fiscal restraints. Substantial variations in practice exist in different settings, irrespective of the same organizational and financial arrangements, with resulting variations in outcomes.[2] This lack of uniformity has prompted questions about the relation of the use of clinical services (process) and their end results (outcomes). Policy makers and purchasers of health care are also interested in sources of costs that do not result in a benefit to enable clinicians to select effective interventions and to provide informed choices for clients. All of these factors have resulted in an emphasis on the measurement, monitoring, and management of outcomes to improve the quality of care. Nurses are responding by beginning to evaluate their contribution to the outcomes of health care and health-related interventions.

Defining Health Outcomes

Outcomes or patient–client outcomes refer to the consequences of a treatment or intervention.[3] In this definition, the consequences or results of care may be intended or unintended changes in individuals and populations. Intended changes are desired results of interventions, whereas unintended changes are unanticipated outcomes that may occur as a result of the intervention. Outcomes are the results obtained from interventions directed toward accomplishing a goal. Health outcomes are the effects of interventions manifested by changes in any dimension of health or resolution of the problem targeted by the intervention.[4] Health outcomes focus on the health status of individuals, families, or communities. The health outcomes of health promotion interventions will vary with the purpose, complexity, and strength of the intervention.[5] For example, a physical activity intervention that involves weekly monitoring and supervision over a six-month time period is anticipated to result in significant changes in the client's level of activity, as compared to a physical activity intervention that provides minimal monitoring and supervision over a three-month period of time. Thus, outcomes differ according to the structure of the intervention, as well as the process of implementing the intervention.

Over 30 years ago, Donabedian[6] proposed structure, process, and outcome indicators or measures to assess the quality of health care. Although his model has mainly been applied to acute care organizations, it is relevant for all health care settings. Structure, process, and outcomes are three characteristics that are used to measure health care quality. Structure refers to characteristics of the environment in which nurses practice, and process is what the nurse actually does. For example, structure measures might include the number of nurses in a community health clinic who are available to educate clients about their health. Process refers to the amount and nature of care provided by the nurse in any setting, such as the type, intensity, and length of educational interventions implemented by the nurse. Knowledge of process is important in health promotion, as outcomes may not occur for a long period of time. Knowledge of the educational process may shed light on what really happened, to whom, and why. For example, which interventions attracted the targeted group? Why did some groups, such as minorities, not participate? The actual questionnaires or tools used to measure these three characteristics of health care quality are called performance measures by the Joint Commission on Accreditation of Healthcare Organizations (JCAHO).[7]

Client choice is important when defining outcomes of health promotion interventions. The client's view, as well as the health care provider's view, is needed to determine appropriate outcomes. Clients may have very different preferences for outcomes, depending on factors such as health status or age, or where there are important trade-offs between survival and quality of life. The nurse needs to know what the client wants and expects from the intervention in order to define achievable and acceptable health outcomes.

Health outcomes have traditionally included the five "Ds": death, disease, disability, discomfort, and dissatisfaction.[8] In the past, patient preferences were seldom used to evaluate health services. They were considered important, but subjective and unreliable. However, this has changed as individuals have become active participants in decision making related to their care. Health outcomes have now been expanded to include subjective health perceptions and appraisals, functional measures, preferences, and satisfaction with services.[2] Many consider these outcomes broad measures of health-related quality of life.

Sidani and Braden [5] categorize health outcomes into four major categories: clinical endpoints related to the client's response to health interventions; functional status related to the maintenance or improvement in physical, mental, and social functioning; perceptual outcomes related to clients' well-being and life satisfaction with the care received; and financial outcomes related to the use of resources and costs.

Two additional terms that need to be understood are outcomes monitoring and outcomes management. *Outcomes monitoring* is the repeated observation, description, and quantification of outcome measures for the purpose of improving care or practice.[9] Outcomes may be monitored intermittently or continuously during a health promotion intervention to make needed changes in the intervention. *Outcomes management* refers to all activities in which nurses use data collected from measuring and monitoring outcomes to continuously improve nursing practice. In outcomes management, costs and quality are concurrently and retrospectively measured and examined to improve the quality of care and health status of clients. Information is used to continuously reexamine practice in outcomes management.

Nurses need to demonstrate the effectiveness of their practice in achieving desired health outcomes by individuals, families, and communities.[9] However, assessment of outcomes that result from nursing treatments and interventions is considered rudimentary in most health care settings. Although quality of care has always been a concern for nursing, quality improvement programs have focused on structure and process outcomes. The shift to outcomes poses a major issue for nursing, because nurses often practice in an interdisciplinary role, whereby health outcomes are influenced by more than one discipline. For example, in many health promotion programs nurses, along with nutritionists, psychologists, and exercise physiologists, may be involved. The challenge is to identify and measure nursing-sensitive outcomes, or those outcomes that are influenced by nursing activities, to document nursing's contributions. Dependent, independent, and interdependent nursing activities need to be differentiated in order to determine outcomes that nurses are accountable for in their practice.

Several sources are available to assist in identifying health outcomes. For example, the Agency for Healthcare Research and Quality (AHRQ), a federal agency which funds research on health care outcomes, provides information on outcomes that have been documented across populations. Its Web site is listed at the end of this chapter. Specialty organizations have also begun to publish outcomes relevant to specific populations.

Nursing-Sensitive Outcomes

The American Nurses Association as well as several nurse authors have identified nursing-sensitive outcomes.[10,11,12] Categories of these outcomes are summarized in Table 12–1. Physiological outcomes are the most commonly used and include such things as weight, skinfold thickness, blood pressure, and cholesterol values. Psychosocial outcomes measure patterns of behavior, communication, and relationships. Psychosocial measures may include attitude, mood, emotions, coping, and social functioning. Functional measures include activities of daily living, mobility, and self-care ability. Behavioral outcomes are concerned with the client's activities and actions. For example, the behavioral outcome may be regular physical activity. Knowledge, the cognitive level of understanding, is a common nursing-sensitive outcome, because teaching is a major component of nursing practice.

Home functioning outcomes focus on the performance of the client and family in the home environment. Measures of this outcome may include family support, family functioning, and role function. Safety is a nursing-sensitive outcome, as nurses implement interventions to promote safe home environments. For example, the nurse may work with clients in work sites to promote safe work environments that prevent hearing loss.

Symptom control outcomes are concerned with the nursing management of symptoms. For example, health promotion interventions for smoking cessation may need to manage symptoms associated with smoking withdrawal. Or, symptoms of low self-esteem or depression as a result of unsuccessful health behavior change may need attention.

Goal attainment outcomes refer to the accomplishment of goals at designated intervals. Client satisfaction, as an outcome, is a global measure of contentment with the services provided to the client. For example, measures of satisfaction or dissatisfaction with health promotion programs provide valuable information for potentially needed changes in the program.

Cost outcomes are also considered sensitive to nursing practice. However, nursing is in its infancy in measuring the cost effectiveness of nursing interventions. Health promotion and risk reduction interventions offer an exciting opportunity to assess the cost effectiveness of their counseling and teaching activities.

TABLE 12-1 Categories of Nursing-Sensitive Interventions

Category	Examples
Physiological	Blood Pressure
	Weight
	Laboratory Values
Psychosocial	Attitudes
	Emotions
	Moods
	Social Functioning
Functional	Activities of daily living
	Mobility
	Self-care
Behavioral	Actions
	Activities
Cognitive	Knowledge
Home functioning	Family support
	Family roles
Safety	Noise-free environment
Symptom control	Smoking withdrawal
Goal Attainment	Behavior change
Satisfaction	Program/Service Contentment
Costs	Cost effectiveness

The Nursing Outcomes Classification (NOC) is a standardized classification of patient–client outcomes developed at the University of Iowa College of Nursing to evaluate the effects of nursing interventions.[13] The NOC system defines an outcome as a variable representing an individual, family, or community condition that is measurable along a continuum and responsive to nursing intervention. The standardized outcomes are developed to use in all settings and with all patient populations. Each outcome has a definition and a list of indicators that can be used to measure the client's status. Currently a total of 260 outcomes have been coded in the taxonomy, which include 247 individual-level outcomes, 7 family outcomes, and 6 community-level outcomes. Seven domains or categories have also been identified. These domains are physiological health, functional health, psychosocial health, family health, health knowledge and behavior, perceived health, and community health. The classification is continually being updated and revised based on user feedback and new research.

The NOC system has been linked to the North American Diagnosis Association (NANDA) diagnoses, to Gordon's functional patterns, to Omaha System problems, to resident admission protocols used in nursing homes, and to Nursing Intervention Classification (NIC) interventions.[13] NOC is also one of the standardized languages recognized by the

American Nurses Association (ANA). Information about the nursing outcome classification system is available on its Web site (see end of chapter). In addition, a newsletter and numerous publications and a book containing the 260 NOC outcomes are available to learn more about this proposed nursing-sensitive outcome system.

The ANA has also published a list of nursing-sensitive outcomes.[14] Its report has enabled nurse researchers to begin documentation of these outcomes following interventions. The report card has identified outcomes for acute care. However, many of the outcomes are relevant across settings. In addition, the ANA's project, the National Database of Nursing Quality Indicators (NDNQI), is developing an information resource to quantify the specific role of nursing interventions in patient outcomes.[15] Within this project the Center for Nursing Quality has been created to promote and facilitate the standardization of information on nursing quality and patient outcomes. Currently, the focus is also on acute care settings. However, it is anticipated that health promotion outcomes will be added as the project continues.

Health outcomes that reflect nursing's contribution to health promotion and risk reduction need to be identified and measured. Some of these include lifestyle behaviors (e.g., dietary and physical activity behaviors), knowledge, attitudes, values, coping behaviors, physiological changes (e.g., weight, blood cholesterol values, blood pressure), self-esteem, self-efficacy, and empowerment. Nursing's focus on positive lifestyle change and wellness places an emphasis on positive health-promoting behaviors. In addition, nurses create environments conducive to health, which presents a challenge in identifying and measuring community health outcomes.

After appropriate health promotion outcomes have been identified, accurate and reliable instruments need to be developed to measure these outcomes. Although measures are available, many do not fully capture the effects of nursing practice. Nurse researchers have begun developing measures. The Health Promoting Lifestyle Profile[16] developed by Pender and colleagues is an example. However, scale development to measure health promotion outcomes is still in its infancy.

Significance of Nursing-Sensitive Outcomes

All health care providers are being pressured to demonstrate their contributions to patient outcomes as a result of the high costs of health care, increasing health care competition, and the need to balance quality and costs.[17] Nursing has been challenged to provide information about which nursing interventions are the most effective and efficient. Although it is known that clients benefit from nursing actions, nursing's effectiveness must be demonstrated to employers, consumers, and health policy makers. Health outcomes that occur as a result of nursing interventions are a measure of nursing's contribution. Documentation of nursing's contribution enhances our visibility and insures that we are not overlooked by health care organizations, health care purchasers, consumers, and health policy makers.[9,17] Nurses are key players in implementing health promotion interventions and measuring their effectiveness. Our view of the total situation and the holistic view of the individual and family is unique, and this contribution needs to be made explicit.

Deciding Which Health Outcomes to Measure

Choice of which health promotion outcomes to measure is dependent on the goals to be attained, the purpose and type of intervention, and the ability to access the information needed to measure the results of care. The challenge is to select health outcomes that are comprehensive, comparable, meaningful, and accurate in reflecting the effects of the health promotion intervention.

Client, Provider, and Community Outcomes

Three categories help to organize outcomes: Client-focused, provider-focused, and community-focused outcomes are described in Table 12–2.[18,19]

Client-focused outcomes measure the end results of health care interventions. These outcomes have been further classified into diagnostic specific and holistic.[18] Diagnostic-specific outcomes focus on a specific client problem and are measured as a subelement within the patient, such as laboratory values or other physiologic measures. These outcomes are discrete and limited in scope. However, they are necessary to measure the physiologic effects of health promotion or risk reduction interventions. For example, health promotion outcomes as a result of a nutritional intervention for weight reduction might include weight or body mass index, blood pressure, and triglycerides.

Holistic outcomes extend beyond the diagnosis or client problem to measure the overall functioning and health of the individual, family, or community.[18] Holistic outcomes include knowledge, lifestyle change, functional status, psychosocial functioning, perceptions, self-care, and health-related quality of life. A major issue in measuring these types of outcomes is lack of clarity in the definitions, which results in lack of clarity in measures of the

TABLE 12-2 General Classification of Outcomes

Category	Types of Outcomes
Client Focused	
Diagnostic specific	Physiologic measures
	Weight
	Body mass index
Holistic	Lifestyle change
	Functional status
	Perceptions
	Self-care
	Quality of life
Provider Focused	
Health care provider	Appropriate interventions
	Expertise
	Client outcomes
Family	Support
Community Focused	
	Costs
	Service use
	Health of community

outcomes. For example, quality of life has been defined and measured differently in many studies. Consistent definitions are needed in health promotion outcomes with measures that accurately reflect the definitions. Monitoring holistic outcomes is important in health promotion efforts, as these outcomes may detect change before physiologic effects are measurable. When measuring client-focused outcomes, both problem-specific and holistic measures may be needed to capture effects of the interventions.

Provider-focused outcomes address aspects of practice that affect client outcomes. Provider may refer to the health care professional or family member. Outcome measures in this category may include the appropriateness of the intervention, technical expertise of the provider, such as the number of physical activity programs that have been conducted. Negative outcomes may also be measured, such as the number of persons who continued to smoke after a smoking cessation program. Provider-focused outcomes are an issue as many nurses practice in teams or groups. However, work to classify nursing interventions and link outcomes to these interventions is ongoing to solve this problem. More work is needed to identify the contributions of nurses in health promotion at the individual, family, and community levels.

Community outcomes are the most global types of measures in health promotion, as they focus on results of community- or organizational-level interventions and the quality of services and care delivered by community organizations as entities.[18,19] Community outcomes include costs of care and use of services as well as other measures to evaluate the services provided by the community organizations. These outcomes also measure aggregates or groups of clients rather than individual clients. This type of measurement poses multiple challenges, but has great potential for communities and community-based systems.

Short-Term, Intermediate, and Long-Term Outcomes

The lack of effectiveness of health promotion interventions may be due to inappropriate timing of outcome measures. The timing of measurement of outcomes is critical to the result obtained.[20] If information is collected immediately following the intervention, it may be too soon to capture the change in lifestyle behaviors. If the nurse waits too long, other factors may have intervened to influence the expected results. Therefore, the timing of measurement of health outcomes is critical and needs to be planned carefully to capture the anticipated effects. Measurement at multiple time points is usually necessary. Short-term outcomes are measured immediately following the intervention. Appropriate short-term outcomes are knowledge, coping behaviors, readiness to change, and so forth. Intermediate outcomes are those targeted at a period of time following the intervention when a change is expected to have occurred. Intermediate outcomes are measured soon enough following the intervention so that its effects can be accurately isolated from other possible reasons. Intermediate interventions may be useful in reflecting attitude changes or attempts to change, although lifestyle change has not yet occurred. Long-term outcomes are the ultimate outcomes, as they are the final or end results of the health promotion intervention.[21] Long-term outcomes include lifestyle change, longevity, and improved quality of life. These long-term outcome measures may also be used to measure intermediate outcomes. When measured at a longer distance from the intervention, the nurse is able to document long-term change. However, the intervening factors mentioned earlier must be considered when interpreting the results of long-term measurement.

Economic Outcomes

The role of economic outcomes in health promotion is becoming increasingly important because of the increased attention on the costs of health care in this country. Several types of analyses currently exist, including cost of illness, cost effectiveness, cost utility, and cost benefit.[22]

A simple way to describe the different types of analyses is by the questions they answer. Cost of illness outcomes answer the question What is the cost of the illness of interest? Cost-effective analysis answers the question What is the most inexpensive way to achieve a given outcome? In cost–utility analysis, the question answered is What is the cost per quality-adjusted life years? Finally, in cost–benefit analysis, the question answered is What is the net benefit of a given alternative? Cost of illness outcomes were the initial cost outcomes reported.[23] This led to cost–benefit analysis, which placed a monetary value on a health outcome. However, this was not readily accepted, so cost-effective analysis emerged as an alternative. Currently research on cost-effective analysis (CEA) is in great demand.

Cost-effective analysis reflects the amount of benefit a treatment or intervention provides relative to alternatives.[24] CEA does not determine whether an intervention is worth its cost in some absolute sense. It provides a relative measure of which services afford the highest health benefit per dollar. The cost-effective ratio (C/E) the central measure used in CEA, is the incremental price of obtaining a unit of health effect from a given health intervention when compared to an alternative intervention. Implicit in the C/E ratio is a comparison between alternatives: the intervention under study with another intervention or no intervention. CEA is meant to be informative and provide additional information for a decision. It is not meant to be the sole determinant of the decision to use or eliminate the intervention.

Examples of CEA studies are available in the literature. For example, Eddy[25] showed that the incremental cost effectiveness of screening for Pap smears more often than every three years for some age ranges was questionable. His recommendations were adopted by the American Cancer Society. In another CEA study, the cost effectiveness of the use of cholesterol-modifying agents for primary and secondary prevention for heart disease was analyzed.[26] Findings showed that primary prevention using these agents was not cost effective unless the person had three or more risk factors. For secondary prevention, the agents were very cost effective. The authors concluded that emphasis should be placed on the use of these agents in secondary prevention with persons who have had heart attacks or angina. In a more recent nutritional counseling intervention, results indicated a counseling group headed by a dietitian was more cost effective than the group co-led by a physician and dietitian.[27]

Cost-effective analysis and other economic evaluations are increasingly assuming an important role in health care policy decisions. Regulatory bodies are considering cost effectiveness in the approval process for new medications and technologies.[28] However, the technique has many methodological pitfalls and should be used only by those who have the background to do so. In addition, consensus-based recommendations to guide CEA to improve the comparability and quality of studies and a standard set of methods has only recently been developed.[29] Nurse researchers need to develop expertise in CEA and other types of economic analyses, as these methods have important implications for nursing practice.

Developing a Plan to Measure Health Outcomes

Developing a plan to measure health outcomes begins with thinking about health promotion interventions in terms of outcomes.[17] Nurses and all health care providers continually need to ask if their interventions are achieving the most effective outcomes. First select the specific health promotion intervention. The choice is based on the client's lifestyle area that either is of interest for change or one in which change is needed. Decide what needs to be achieved with the intervention and how these outcomes can be most effectively attained. Next identify the most effective way to manage the problem or the most effective method to implement the intervention by reviewing the literature. A literature search will shed light on how the problem has been approached successfully by others. For example, if planning to intervene with a client to improve nutrition, a literature review of nutritional programs will help to identify aspects that work and aspects that should be avoided. Findings from the literature facilitate tailoring the intervention to the specific needs of the client or family. In the outcomes literature, this step is also known as identifying best practices, or the most effective way to solve the problem.

The next step is to identify the factors that could affect the client's response to the intervention.[30] For example, characteristics of the client, such as weight, the values placed on foods, eating habits, any symptoms that are occurring as a result of poor nutrition, and motivation to change eating behaviors will affect the success of the intervention. Demographic characteristics that may influence the outcomes also need to be identified, as factors such as age, education, socioeconomic status may be significant. Family characteristics might also play a role. For example, if others in the home practice unhealthy nutritional behaviors, it may be more difficult to get support to change. Environmental factors may also influence the outcomes and need to be identified as well. All factors that may potentially influence the outcomes need to be specified and addressed before the intervention begins.

Next, select the outcomes that will be used to measure the success of the intervention and decide how and when they will be measured. For example, in the nutrition program, although the long-term outcome may be sustained weight loss or normal blood sugar or cholesterol, short-term outcomes may be a change in attitude toward eating and significant other support to change dietary behaviors. Intermediate outcomes might be a decrease in the number of high-fat foods consumed per day. The client needs to be involved to establish realistic outcomes that will enable success. Identification of reliable and valid measures of selected health outcomes is critical to insure accurate results. Measures that have been tested beforehand should be used whenever possible.

Additional resources may be needed to measure outcomes and analyze the data for complex interventions with groups of clients, families, or communities. Costs, time, and effort must always be considered when deciding which outcomes to measure, as well as the number of outcomes to measure. Attention also needs to be given to the burden placed on clients when measuring outcomes. Too many measures at multiple time points may result in a low participation rate. The earlier steps are easy to follow when planning to measure outcomes. Each step should be carefully considered and completed before moving to the next one. By following this type of plan, information about the outcomes of health promotion

TABLE 12-3 Steps in Developing A Plan to Measure Outcomes

1. Select health protection–health promotion area of interest.
2. Identify most effective intervention for defined area.
3. Tailor intervention to client.
4. Identify potential factors that may influence outcomes.
   - Client characteristics
   - Demographic factors
   - Family characteristics
5. Select outcomes to measure effects of intervention.
   - Short term
   - Intermediate
   - Long term

interventions implemented by nurses will begin to accumulate. Table 12–3 reviews the steps in developing a plan to measure outcomes of health promotion interventions.

Challenges in Measuring Health Outcomes

Many challenges confront health care providers in the measurement of health outcomes. Several of these have already been described. For example, separating the contribution of nursing from other health care providers remains a task. This challenge has increased with the proliferation of paraprofessional groups in school settings, the workplace, and the community, as many of these groups focus on health promotion and health education in their practice.[20] The interdisciplinary emphasis is expected to continue, so it is more critical than ever to clearly define nursing's role in health promotion and identify health outcomes that measure the contribution of nursing.

Sensitivity of measures of outcomes is a challenge when measuring many of the health promotion outcomes.[31] Sensitivity of outcomes measures refers to the ability to detect small differences in behaviors, attitudes and values, and outcomes of interest in health promotion. For example, many quality-of-life measures are not sensitive enough to detect changes in life quality at multiple time points. Lack of sensitivity means that important changes that occur are missed or thought to be insignificant. The challenge is to find measures that are sensitive to the anticipated change and to measure outcomes at multiple time points to be able to detect the change.

The choice of measures for holistic-focused outcomes is another challenge.[32] Although these types of measures enable comparison of clients across interventions and populations, they often lack the sensitivity to detect clinically important changes. On the other hand, measures that are specific to a particular problem may be more sensitive but may not be usable across groups of clients or settings. The challenge is to decide if it is important to compare across populations or focus on a specific group or problem.

Another challenge is the measurement of community- or organizational-focused outcomes, when the data are aggregated instead of reported for individual clients. Because most measures have been developed to measure individual outcomes, few aggregate measures are available. Measurement of community-focused outcomes means that more attention is needed to develop instruments to assess community outcomes accurately.

Directions for Nursing Research in Outcome Measurement

The science related to the measurement of outcomes sensitive to health promotion nursing interventions is limited due to several factors. First, because the emphasis on outcomes research began in the 1990s, nurse scientists have only recently begun to implement studies to identify and evaluate health promotion outcomes. Second, the challenges that have been discussed in this chapter pose issues for research as well as practice. All of these challenges create many opportunities for research in health promotion. Exploratory studies are needed to identify holistic outcomes that reflect nursing's contribution as a member of the health care team. Exploratory studies are also needed to learn patient preferences. Experimental research needs to be designed to test health promotion interventions and evaluate client outcomes at multiple points in time. Sensitive measures of health promotion outcomes that reflect nursing's influence need to be developed and tested. Measures of community-level outcomes also need to be designed and tested for use in community interventions. Nurse scientists need to learn how to measure economic outcomes, such as cost-effective outcomes, and implement studies to evaluate the costs of health promotion and risk reduction interventions. The science of outcomes for health promotion is in its infancy in nursing as well as other disciplines, creating opportunities for collaboration in research endeavors across disciplines. Nurse scientists have opportunities to work with other disciplines on research projects to understand how clients change their lifestyle practices as well as how to measure these changes effectively.

Directions for Nursing Practice in Achieving Health Outcomes

The outcomes movement in health care has forced nurses to reflect on the value of their practice. The mandate of health care environments to deliver the most effective, cost-efficient care means that nursing must delineate its contribution to health outcomes. Plans of care should continually be assessed to identify the most effective approaches for quality care. Identification of best approaches means that familiarity with the current literature will become more and more important for nurses in practice. Prior to implementing health promotion interventions, detailed assessments need to be conducted that take into account client, family, and environmental factors that may influence the outcomes of the intervention. It is also important to learn about the standardized outcome taxonomies that are available to be able to choose appropriate outcomes for health promotion and risk reduction interventions. In addition nurses are being called upon to identify specific health outcomes that are relevant for their practice and to document these outcomes. Documentation of interventions and outcomes is critical to assess nursing's contribution to health care. Measuring outcomes that are sensitive to change is often a challenge. However, nurses can seek expertise to assist in identifying accurate and sensitive outcomes that are easily implemented in practice. Last, nurses need to play a major role as members of interdisciplinary health care teams, as they view the totality of factors that influence the client's health. These teams are expected to continue to play a major role in health care delivery to enhance client outcomes. The nurse needs to be a contributing member of the team by being credible and competent in outcomes measurement, monitoring, and management.

SUMMARY

Changes in health care have resulted in a mandate to measure the outcomes of health promotion interventions. In the current competitive, cost-conscious environment, nurses and other health care providers are documenting the effectiveness and efficiency of their care. Payers of health care are demanding accurate information about the costs of provider services and the effects of these services on the quality and costs of care. Nurses are challenged to document the value of their practice to health care for payers and consumers of care. Nurses are key players in health promotion and are now validating their contribution by identifying outcomes of their interventions that are sensitive to the holistic wellness perspective. Although much work remains for both practicing nurses and nurse scientists, evidence of nursing's contribution is being documented as health outcomes sensitive to nursing interventions are identified, refined, and measured.

SELECTED WEB SITES RELEVANT TO OUTCOMES MEASUREMENT

Agency for Healthcare Research and Quality (AHRQ)
www.ahrq.gov

American Nurses Association
www.nursingworld.org

Joint Commission on Accreditation of Healthcare Organizations
jcaho.org

National Commission for Quality Assurance
www.ncqa.org

National Database of Nursing Quality Indicators
www.mriresearch.org/health/ndnqi/html

University of Iowa Nursing Outcome Classification System
www.uiowa.edu/noc

REFERENCES

1. Nightingale F. *Notes on Matters Affecting the Health, Efficiency, and Hospital Administration of the British Army.* London: Harrison & Sons Nightingale; 1858.

2. Clancy CM, Eisenberg JM. Outcomes research: Measuring the end results of health care. *American Association for the Advancement of Science.* 1998 Oct; 282: 245–246.

3. Huber DL, Oermann MH. The evolution of outcomes management. In: Blancett SS, Flarey DL, eds. *Health Care Outcomes: Collaborative Path-Based Approaches.* Gaithersburg, MD: Aspen; 1998: 3–12.

4. Hegyvary ST. Patient care outcomes related to management of symptoms. *Annual Review of Nursing Research.* 1993: 11:145–168.

5. Sidani S, Braden CJ. (1996). Outcomes-related factors. In: *Evaluating Nursing Interventions: A Theory-Driven Approach.* Thousand Oaks: Sage Publications; 1998:138–160.

6. Donabedian A. Evaluating the quality of medical care. *Milbank Memorial Fund Quarterly.* 1966. 44(part 2): 166–206.

7. Joint Commission on Accreditation of Healthcare Organizations. *Glossary of Terms for Performance Measurement Systems.* Available from: www.jcaho.org/prefmeas/glossry.html.

8. Lohr KN. Outcome measurement: Concepts and questions. *Inquiry.* 1988; 25(1):37–50.

9. Oermann M, Huber D. New Horizons (Editorial). *Outcomes Management for Nursing Practice.* 1997 1(1):1–2.

10. Lewin-VHI, Inc. Nursing Report Card for Acute Care. Pub. No. NP-101, Washington, DC: American Nurses Association; 1995.

11. Irvine D, Sidani S, Hall LM. Finding value in nursing care: a framework for quality improvement and clinical evaluation. *Nurs Econ.* 1998 May–Jun; 16(3):110–116, 131.

12. Marek KD. Measuring the effectiveness of nursing care. *Outcomes Management for Nursing Practice.* 1997; 1(1):8–12.

13. Johnson M, Maas M, eds. Iowa Outcomes Project. *Nursing Outcomes Classification (NOC).* 2nd ed. St. Louis: Mosby Year Book; 2000.

14. Pollard PB, et al. *Nursing Quality Indicators: Definitions and Implications.* Washington, DC: American Nurses Association; 1996.

15. Midwest Research Institute. Available from: http://www.mriresearch.org/health/ndnqi.html; 1999.

16. Pender NJ. Motivation for physical activity among children and adolescents. *Annu Rev Nurs Res.* 1998; 16:139–172.

17. Oermann MH, Huber D. Patient outcomes. *American Journal of Nursing.* 1999 Sep; 99(9):40–47.

18. Jennings BM, Staggers N, Brosch LR. A classification scheme for outcome indicators. *Image: Journal of Nursing Scholarship.* 1999; 31(4):381–388.

19. Kleinpell RM. Whose outcomes patients, providers, or payers? *Nursing Clinics of North America.* 1997 Sep; 32(3):513–521.

20. Gillis A. Exploring nursing outcomes for health promotion. *Nursing Forum.* 1995 Apr–Jun; 30(2):5–12.

21. Wojner AW, MacCutcheon MA. Longitudinal outcomes measurement and management. *Critical Care Nursing Clinics of North America.* 1998 Mar; 10(1):33–40.

22. Max W. Economic analysis in health care. In: Harrington C, Estes C, eds. *Health Policy and Nursing.* 2nd ed., Basten: Jones & Bartlett 1997; 283–298.

23. Buerhaus PI. Milton Weinstein's insights on the development, use and methodologic problems in cost-effectiveness anaylsis. *Image: Journal of Nursing Scholarship*. 1998; 30(3):223–227.

24. Siegel JE. Cost-effectiveness analysis and nursing research—Is there a fit? *Image: Journal of Nursing Scholarship*. 1998; 30(3):221–222.

25. Eddy DM. Screening for cervical cancer. *Annals of Internal Medicine*. 1990; 113:214–226.

26. Goldman L, Weinstein MC, Goldman PA, Williams LW. Cost-effectiveness of HMG-CoA reductase inhibition for primary and secondary prevention of coronary heart disease. *JAMA*. 1991; 265:1145–1151.

27. Pritchard DA, Hyndman J, Taba F. Nutritional counseling in general practice: A cost effective analysis. *J Epidemiol Community Health*. 1999 May; 53(5):311–316.

28. Finlayson SRG, Birkmeyer JD. Cost-effectiveness analysis in surgery. *Surgery*. 1998, Feb; 123(2):151–156.

29. Russell LB, Gold MR, Siegel JE, Daniels N. The role of cost-effectiveness analysis in health and medicine. *JAMA*. 1996 Oct; 276(14):1172–1177.

30. Cassidy CA. Want to know how you're doing? *American Journal of Nursing*. 1999 Sep; 99(9):51–59.

31. Strickland OL. Challenges in measuring patient outcomes. *Nursing Clinics of North America*. 1997 Sep; 32(3):495–511.

32. Murdaugh CL. Outcome measurement and clinical resource management. In: Parsons ML, Murdaugh CL, Purdon TF, Jarrell BE. *Guide to Clinical Resource Management*. Gaithersburg, MD: Aspen; 1997:212–218.

13

Evaluating Individual and Community Interventions

A scientific knowledge base to guide health promotion interventions is established by evaluating the accumulating results of research. Improvements are made in the quality of health promotion interventions when their effectiveness is carefully evaluated. Evaluation information can then be used to select and implement health promotion activities that provide the most favorable outcomes for clients. Our knowledge of the effectiveness of health promotion interventions is based on research that has been conducted and published and the scientific rigor of this research. Nurses and other health care providers are continually being asked about the effectiveness of their health promotion and risk reduction efforts. This question can be answered only by carefully examining the research and evaluation evidence that has accumulated about a specific type of intervention.

Deciding How to Evaluate Health Promotion Interventions

A growing body of evidence supports the belief that health promotion programs have a positive effect on health and health care costs.[1] Identifying and evaluating the evidence can be a challenge for clinicians. Several components of evaluation need to be understood before collecting information to evaluate health promotion interventions. Knowledge of differences in efficacy and effectiveness of interventions and differences in process and outcome evaluations is needed to develop a plan to evaluate evidence for one's practice.

Efficacy or Effectiveness of Interventions

Efficacy refers to the improvements in health outcomes of interventions achieved in a research setting, under ideal circumstances, by expert researchers.[2] In other words, the intervention is studied and evaluated under controlled or ideal conditions to demonstrate that the outcomes are due to the intervention and not to chance or other factors unrelated to the intervention. Efficacy is best demonstrated by randomized clinical trials, when clients are randomly assigned to the intervention or a comparison condition. The *effectiveness* of an intervention is the effect it achieves in the real world, with limited resources, in entire populations or specified subgroups of a population. In other words, effectiveness addresses the clinical usefulness of the intervention, as the intervention is implemented and evaluated in a typical community setting, where it will eventually be applied. Effectiveness studies have also been called large sample trials and public health trials, because they are implemented in large populations and are expected to have an immediate effect on clinical practice.[3] Both types of studies are useful in developing and testing interventions and disseminating their results. Efficacy studies are considered less applicable to the general population because they are tested under ideal circumstances with a targeted group of clients. However, both types of evidence need to be evaluated. Efficacy studies are often the first phase to test the usefulness of interventions, followed by effectiveness studies in which the findings are applied to real-life settings for feasibility, cost utility, effectiveness of the intervention in actual practice, and acceptance of the intervention by differing groups of clients. For example, if the efficacy of a health promotion intervention has been scientifically tested, clinicians can take the evidence and evaluate its effectiveness in their client population or clinical setting. In the practice setting, it is difficult to control implementation of the intervention, which often leads to inconsistent delivery across clients. Some clients may receive all of the intervention, whereas others may receive less of the intervention, leading to inaccurate evaluation results. Strategies to avoid misleading results have been described elsewhere.[4,5] It is important for the nurse to implement the intervention as faithfully as possible and keep good records of the extent to which the intervention reached the intended audience.

Process or Outcome Evaluation

Process and outcome measures were described briefly in Chapter 12. Process evaluations of health promotion interventions refer to verifying the content of the intervention and whether it was delivered as intended, whereas outcome evaluations focus on the results, intended or unintended, of the intervention. Process evaluations provide information to help refine the intervention and define the needs and preferences of the targeted group. Evaluation of the health outcomes of interventions is critical. However, process evaluations provide valuable information about how the program is being implemented. Variations in delivery among sites and clients are identified as well as "breakdowns" between what was intended and what was actually delivered. Process evaluations also provide feedback on the quality of delivery of the intervention, who received the intended intervention, and whether the intervention was implemented as planned. In other words, process evaluation answers the questions: Is the intervention being implemented as planned? Is the intervention reaching its target audience? And are the participants satisfied with the intervention? Process evaluations may help understand how interventions achieve their effects and how to best conduct interventions to maximize health outcomes.[6] Process evaluations should involve a feedback loop, so that the intervention can be revised based on the information obtained.[7]

Collecting Evidence for Practice

In the current health care environment, health care practitioners can no longer rely solely on their clinical experiences, tradition, and opinion-based processes to guide their health promotion interventions.[8] They must also use the current best evidence in making decisions about their clients and interventions. Current best evidence is obtained from many sources: a synthesis of relevant research, international, national, and local standards of practice, cost-effectiveness analysis, clinical expertise, and patient preferences. A search of the literature is necessary to see first if an adequate research base is available. The research findings then need to be critically evaluated and the evidence synthesized. This process has given rise to a new term in health care, *evidence-based practice.*

Evidence-based practice is defined as the integration of clinical expertise with the best available clinical research findings.[9] The aim of evidence-based practice is to reduce wide variations in practice, eliminating worst practices and enhancing best practices to improve quality and decrease costs. Evidence-based clinical practice builds on research utilization as research results, along with other evidence mentioned above, are transformed into practice.

Evidence-based practice involves assessing the need for a change in practice, identifying the needed information, conducting a literature search, critically appraising the literature using the principles of evidence-based practice, identifying clinically applicable results, designing a practice change, and applying the change to one's practice.[10] Table 13–1 reviews the steps in establishing evidence for a practice intervention. After an evidence-based practice

TABLE 13-1 Steps in Evidence-Based Practice

Identify What Evidence is Needed

   1. Assess the Need for Change in Practice.

Retrieve and Evaluate the Evidence

   2. Conduct Literature Search.

   3. Critically Evaluate Literature.

Decide and Design What to Implement

   4. Identify Results Applicable to Practice.

   5. Develop Practice Change to Implement Results.

Implement

   6. Apply Change to Practice.

Evaluate

   7. Evaluate Outcomes of New Change.

change is implemented, plans are made to evaluate both the process for carrying out the change as well as the expected outcomes.

The process to examine the evidence does not replace clinical expertise, as the nurse has to evaluate new knowledge in light of its applicability to the target population. Although intuition and unsystematic clinical experiences are deemphasized, the process is not meant to be seen as a cookbook approach to nursing and health care. For example, the clinical problem might be the inability to promote physical activity interventions in a rural setting and the potential of using a telephone intervention to promote physical activity in adults in this setting. The literature related to telephone interventions for the promotion of physical activity is reviewed and critically evaluated for applicability to clients in rural settings. In addition, the sociocultural environment of the targeted population is considered, as well as prior experiences with health promotion in the target population in rural settings and available resources. If it is determined that the evidence is applicable and relevant, based on all of the factors considered, the intervention is adopted.

The results of an analysis to evaluate the evidence for health interventions may be useful to policy makers and payers, as well as practitioners.[11] Policy makers can use the information in more rational resource allocations or development of priorities for health promotion and risk reduction. Payers will use the information to eliminate interventions that are not effective, and practitioners will be able to use the results to make informed decisions for their clients.

The use of evidence to guide health promotion is the ideal. When evidence is available and evaluated, health promotion practices can be planned and evaluated systematically. However, community-based programs place a high value on the role of the community in defining the health problem and participating in the solution. In this case, the research evidence is only one component in the decision-making process to define the intervention. Therefore, the intervention chosen may not be the most effective even though it is strongly supported by the community. Last, a rapid response to a problem may be needed, or the government may take the opportunity to pursue a policy when time does not allow the establishment of evidence. For example, public education has been implemented to promote abstinence from drug use, without evidence of the effectiveness of media campaigns in promoting abstinence. These cases point to how research can be applied in varying ways, despite the availability or lack of evidence.[12] This points to the need for flexibility in order to match the evidence with the type of approach needed.

Evaluation of Interventions with Individuals and Communities

Changes in the conceptualization of health have resulted in different approaches to promoting and evaluating wellness. One difference focuses on whether health promotion strategies concentrate on individual lifestyle changes or community-wide changes.[13] Individual approaches identify a finite number of lifestyle areas that can be targeted for intervention. McKinlay[14] coined the term *downstream* to describe interventions that are aimed at individuals. *Midstream* interventions describe community-based interventions and are aimed at schools, work sites, health plans, and other organizational channels, as well as entire communities or specific populations. *Upstream* health behavior interventions are those that address policy and environmental changes. For example, upstream strategies may include protection from environmental hazards such as asbestos in old buildings or nuclear wastes, changes in advertising of unhealthy behaviors such as antismoking campaigns, food labeling, and economic incentives such as excise taxes on liquor and cigarettes. Table 13–2 describes the three levels of interventions adapted from McKinlay and suggested activities and outcomes for the three levels. Wellness behaviors are a result of individual attitudes, beliefs, and

TABLE 13-2 Levels and Types of Interventions

Level	Target	Types: Examples of Interventions
Downstream	Individuals	Education
		Counseling
		Support
Midstream	Communities	Work site programs
		School programs
		Community-based programs
Upstream	Public policy	Tax incentives or Deterrents
	Environment	Policy changes
		Local ordinances
		Laws
		Media campaigns

Based on McKinlay's[33] model for Health Behavior Change.

values as well conditions in the community. Because the three types of interventions are interrelated, success is more likely to be achieved if all are taken into consideration when planning health promotion programs to identify the major factors that are influencing behaviors of the target group.

Individual-level strategies provide clients with strategies for wellness and/or lifestyle change. These individuals must then maintain the new behaviors in the larger social environment that often rewards at-risk behaviors or provides barriers to the maintenance of healthy behaviors.[15] Low-income and disadvantaged individuals are at greatest risk because of their social and physical environments.[16,17] A challenge for health care professionals as well as researchers is to develop, test, evaluate, and implement models of health promotion that incorporate the influences of community factors (work sites, schools, etc.), environmental factors, and sociocultural factors with individual behaviors to promote wellness.

Individual models of health behavior were described in Chapters 2 and 3. These models focus on attitudes, beliefs, or other characteristics within the individual that are amenable to change. Interventions promote knowledge and skills needed to change individual behaviors. During the past 20 years, impressive gains have been made in the science and practice of health behavior change at the individual level.[15] Bandura's social learning theory [18] and Prochaska and DiClemente's stages of change model[19] have had major effects on the design and delivery of individual health promotion interventions. Effective short-term changes (6 to 24 months) have occurred as a result of cognitive–behavioral interventions.

Individual strategies for health promotion that warrant continued use based on evaluation results are contests and competition to recruit and maintain participants in programs.[20] Contests promote attention and excitement and the costs are modest, so they are recommended to promote awareness and participation. Self-help and minimal, but repeated, contact programs for individuals are also effective, relatively easy to implement, inexpensive, and they may reach persons who are not easily accessed by other means.

Media campaigns have also been found to be useful as an adjunct to both individual- and community-based interventions.[20,21] Message repetition is important and presentations must be of high quality, which means that media campaigns can be expensive. However, some media programs are inexpensive, such as bill inserts, grocery bag flyers, television feature news stories, and community newspapers. Modern technology has resulted in media-based interventions that are delivered in personalized, interactive formats. Media campaigns that use print and/or telephone have been found to be effective in changing short-term behavior.[22] Repeated contact media tailored to target audiences have also been found to be more effective than one shot, broad messages.

Screening for health education, rather than case finding, has also been found to be a successful intervention at the individual level. Health education provided to every person who is screened, regardless of risk, to improve lifestyle has been shown to change lifestyle patterns. However, screening is expensive and requires a high level of professional competence.

Community-based interventions build on existing community structures to promote wellness and behavior change. These types of interventions consider broader factors that influence health other than individual beliefs and attitudes. Instead, the system in which the individual lives and works is targeted. This approach necessitates the collaboration of individuals and organizations within the community and often demands considerable resources, including time and money.

Community settings that have most commonly been the site of health promotion programs include the workplace, churches, and schools. The work site is appealing because of the ability to implement comprehensive programs that may result in cost savings. The work site interventions reported in the literature vary in comprehensiveness, intensity, and duration in providing health education to employees. However, results from well-conducted studies suggest that providing opportunities for counseling employees within the context of a comprehensive program may be the critical component.[23] Work site programs for smoking cessation consistently show economic benefits.[24] Organizational factors have been shown to either facilitate or hinder the implementation of work site health promotion programs.[25] Specifically, leadership characteristics are key to acceptance and implementation.

Churches and other places of worship have been used as sites for health promotion in many large studies.[20,26] The main finding is there is a higher level of volunteer involvement to assist with program implementation, which then requires less professional involvement. Religious organizations have access to large numbers of people, effective communication channels, and adequate meeting facilities, all factors that have been shown to facilitate successful delivery of health education.

Another popular site for health promotion is the school, where the focus is on children and adolescents. Schools are appealing because of the amount of time students spend in this environment, and it is possible to involve the parents in health promotion activities. This social influence approach is based on the premise that the family, as well as peers, plays an important role in the adoption and maintenance of healthy behaviors.[27] A comprehensive school-based health promotion program consists of health instruction, health services, social support services, health education curricula, extracurricular activities that meet the needs and interests of the students, and involvement of the family. Additional program components have focused on specific behaviors, such as food service changes to promote a healthy diet, or physical activity instruction and programs.

Community health promotion relies on coalitions to address the targeted health behaviors, so community activation is a critical component in implementing community programs.[28] Activation of the community is also very difficult because of the need to coordinate many agencies and develop actions that will not reflect the interests of a particular group or agency. Because of the difficulty, successful, sustained community activation to promote health has been a commonly unfulfilled goal in community-based health promotion interventions. Factors that facilitate community activation include the ability of the community coalition to provide its own vision, members who have the skills and time to work together, frequent and productive communication, and a sense of cohesion.[29] Barriers to communication and coalition building include staff who lack organizational skills, staff turnover, difficulty recruiting members, and reluctance of community members to conduct activities.

In summary, intervention approaches at the individual and community levels have resulted in behavior change, which is cause for optimism in health promotion. Effective individual-based programs have mainly used cognitive–behavioral theories to guide the interventions. Growing awareness of the role of the context in which the individual works and lives points to the need for an approach that balances individual and community strategies. Community health promotion programs have potential to improve health because of their ability to target large segments of the population through broad-based interventions. Because of the broad base, community health promotion also offers many challenges in implementation and evaluation of these programs. Evaluation of policy-level interventions is complex and resource intensive. Policy-level interventions are described in Chapter 15.

Lessons Learned from Evaluation of Health Promotion Interventions

What lessons can be taken from the results of evaluations of major health promotion programs? The information gained from these evaluations can be categorized into those that focus on the program or intervention and its results, and those that address the individual who receives the intervention. Program components that facilitate success include the design of the intervention, selection of outcomes to measure the intervention and time frame for implementing the intervention and evaluating the results. Current knowledge about long-term maintenance of behavior change, the last step in the change process of health promotion, is also reviewed. In addition, the role of collaborative partnerships as well as the concept of sustainability of community-based programs is summarized.

Designing the Intervention

Health promotion interventions are complex and usually involve multiple components. When designing programs, one needs to assess the appropriateness of the intervention or intervention components for the target population. This can be accomplished by applying specific criteria.[30,31] First the intervention has to be affordable to individuals, agencies, or communities. Needless to say, a program that is too expensive will result in poor participation. If the intervention is too expensive or resource intensive for community-based systems, commitment by the agency will be lacking and participation will be poor. The intervention must also be manageable and compatible with existing programs in community agencies. In other words, the less complex the program and the greater likelihood of fit with existing programs, the more successful the implementation. Evidence should exist for the effectiveness of the intervention in the targeted setting and population. If the effectiveness of the intervention has not been tested with different sociocultural groups, results of implementing the intervention in the new group needs to be evaluated carefully.

Selecting Outcomes

Realistic outcomes need to be chosen when designing the evaluation phase of health promotion interventions.[7] The outcomes of many health promotion interventions may not be known for many years. In addition, community-level outcomes are complex and often very expensive, so the decision of which endpoints and outcomes are realistic is a critical one. Short-term, intermediate, and long-range outcomes need to be considered in the decision for their usefulness in measuring the anticipated results. The outcome evaluation component needs careful planning so that the results, while realistic and affordable, are meaningful. Choice of measurement of the outcomes is also an important consideration. Self-report measures are used in many health promotion programs.[32] However, objective measures need to be used whenever possible, as they are more precise and sensitive to change for many health promotion interventions, such as physical activity and dietary changes. Last, measurement of community-level outcomes has not received as much attention as individual outcomes as they are less well developed than individual outcomes because of their complexity. This issue also needs to be considered when deciding on outcome measures. One recommendation is to also measure improvements in the community, such as the number of new public physical activity facilities or the number of restaurants that provide healthy choices.[33] These broader outcomes measure how the outcome has improved the community, independent of behavior change of community members.

Potential outcomes that can be measured when behavioral long-term outcomes may not be realistic include program participation rates. Although participation does not measure effectiveness, it provides information about the acceptance of the intervention and its implementation, as the intervention cannot be successful if it is not well attended. Process measures are also potentially useful measures to assess the effectiveness of implementing the intervention and provide useful information to help refine the intervention. Measurement of program exposure has been conceptualized as "delivered dose," or an assessment of the aspects of the program that were delivered, and "received dose," which is the number of people who participated in the program.[7]

Deciding Time Frame

A realistic time frame is necessary to properly conduct the program and evaluate the results. What is realistic depends on the type, comprehensiveness, and complexity of the intervention and the target population. In a straightforward, individual-focused intervention targeted to a small group, six months may be a realistic period to implement and evaluate short-term results. However, five years may be needed to implement and evaluate a complex community-based program targeted to primary schools. The time frame for a community-based program is related to acceptance and action by the community and may backfire if it is rushed.

Maintaining Behavior Change

Most of the progress in health promotion research has been in promoting health-behavior change, while less progress has been seen in promoting maintenance of these changes. Maintenance of healthy behaviors is now seen as a process itself that needs exploration, rather than an end state.[34] Psychological processes that underlie the decision to adopt health behaviors have, until recently, been assumed to generalize to decisions to maintain a behavior.[35] This is evident in most of the current models of health behavior which stress how people decide to adopt health behaviors. Two exceptions are Bandura's cognitive theory, which states that self-efficacy beliefs are a critical determinant of both the initiation and maintenance of behavior change, and Prochaska and DiClemente's transtheoretical model, which includes maintenance as a stage in the model. However, neither of these theories offers guidance about the process of maintenance and how it differs from initiation and adoption of behaviors.[35] The distinction between initiation and maintenance of behavior change has opened new challenges for health promotion practice and research because the process is not well understood. Understanding the theoretical and behavioral processes that guide successful behavioral maintenance will enable interventions to be developed to address long-term behavior change.

Collaboration is a key to the success of maintenance of health promotion programs in the community. Models have been developed to link schools of nursing to communities to provide culturally competent, evidenced-based health promotion interventions.[36,37] A holistic approach that continually assesses community needs, nurtures collegial relationships, and supports the health of community residents has been shown to be effective.[37] Maintenance of these collaborations is a challenge, as they are dependent on funding and the ability to balance multiple agendas and missions. However, barriers need to be confronted as community collaborative partnerships are essential in promoting the health of the community.

Sustainability or institutionalization of community-based programs is determined by many factors. Empirical knowledge about the determinants of sustainability is at an early stage of development.[38] The intervention program needs to be transferred from outside agencies to the community to have a sustained effect. Sustainability is influenced by the design of the intervention and implementation factors, facilitators and barriers within the targeted community setting, and factors in the broader community environment. Sustainability is more likely to be successful when capacity building has occurred in the community and program strategies have included long-term maintenance. Sustainability needs to be conceptualized as an ongoing process that is ever changing as new knowledge is gained. An infrastructure that integrates resources needs to be established to support the program. For example, these resources might include state health department units, universities, professional societies, and federal organizations. Attention to sustainability is important for the program to continue to promote health behaviors.

Directions for Research in Evaluating Health Promotion

The results of health promotion research that have been summarized in this chapter offer many avenues for research. First, it is evident that our current theories of health promotion need to be expanded and tested, as most theories are not adequate for long-term behavior change. In addition, new innovative models of health promotion that identify determinants of behavior maintenance also need to be developed and tested. Socio-ecological models of health promotion, which integrate strategies of behavior change with social and physical environmental enhancements, need further exploration and testing.

Second, accurate measures of behavior change need attention. Self-report measures of behavior change need to be developed that are reliable and valid and sensitive to both short-term and long-term change. New objective measures of change also need to be developed to more precisely measure changes, such as dietary behaviors and physical activity. Outcome measures also need to be standardized across studies of health behaviors, such as physical activity, and dietary practices to enable researchers and practitioners to compare findings.

Evidence indicates that research to describe, predict, and intervene to promote long term maintenance has been limited. This opens possibilities for all types of research. Exploratory studies are needed to answer such questions as What factors promote successful maintenance of healthy behaviors? What factors promote relapse? What are the greatest difficulties encountered in maintenance? Descriptive studies are necessary to describe factors associated with maintenance of behaviors over long periods of time as well as differences in factors that predict success in various age groups. For example, what role do parents play in the maintenance of physical activity by children? Experimental studies that evaluate interventions to promote long-term maintenance are also needed. These studies need to be implemented for individuals as well as in schools and work sites in the community. Research also needs to evaluate the cost effectiveness of health promotion in behavior change. For example, what factors will increase the effectiveness of minimal contact self-care interventions?

As can be seen from this brief discussion, opportunities for research to evaluate individual- and community-based interventions are not lacking. Interdisciplinary teams, which capitalize on the expertise of all members, are encouraged to insure successful funding and rigorous studies that address the issues.

Directions for Practice in Evaluating Health Promotion

Evaluation of health promotion interventions provides nurses and other health care providers evidence on which to base their practice. As health care professionals are mandated to base their practice on current research findings, as well as other factors, it will become critical to understand criteria used to evaluate the evidence. Courses that teach theses skills should be offered in the clinical setting or through collaboration with local chapters of professional organizations or schools of nursing in university settings. Knowledge of evaluation criteria is critical to be able to accurately review the literature and make informed decisions about the research reviewed.

Knowledge of effective health promotion interventions and programs provide the nurse with information to refer clients to successful programs. In addition, the information will enable the nurse to deliver aspects of either individual- or community-based interventions that have been successful. As in research, an interdisciplinary approach has been shown to be more effective in the delivery of complex or community-based interventions.

Cost effectiveness also needs to be considered when intervening for health promotion. Telephone counseling and follow-up is a relatively low-cost intervention that can be effectively used by the nurse to provide ongoing contact, social support, and expertise to answer questions. Telephone interventions need to become a standard component of self-help interventions and follow-up, especially for elderly and rural populations.

Because maintenance is a major problem in health-behavior change, nurses need to follow up on clients carefully to identify early relapse and provide these individuals with ongoing interventions. Counseling to identify problems related to relapse is critical. Although little is known about successful strategies to promote maintenance, nurses can identify individual strategies based on counseling and discussions with clients and their families. New strategies should be implemented and evaluated with realistic outcomes and follow-up as long as feasible.

SUMMARY

Evaluation of health promotion enables us to learn what is most effective in promoting wellness and behavior change as well as what does not work. Evaluating health promotion interventions facilitates the development of a scientific knowledge base on which to make decisions that influence the health behaviors of our clients and communities. The evaluation process is complex and time-consuming, and requires advanced knowledge not previously applied in practice. However, the information gained by critically evaluating the literature provides valuable information about the usefulness of individual- and community-based interventions.

REFERENCES

1. U.S. Department of Health and Human Services. *Healthy People 2010* (Conference Edition, in Two Volumes). Washington, DC: U.S. Government Printing Office; January 2000.
2. Aral SO, Peterman TA. Do we know the effectiveness of behavioral interventions? *The Lancet.* 1998; 351: 33–36.
3. Piantadosi S. *Clinical Trials: A Methodologic Perspective.* New York: John Wiley & Sons; 1997.
4. Sidani S. Measuring the intervention in effectiveness research. *Western Journal of Nursing Research.* 1998; 20(5):621–635.
5. Lipsey MW. *Design Sensitivity: Statistical Power for Experimental Research.* Newbury Park, CA: Sage Publications; 1990.
6. Baranowski T, Stables G. Process evaluations of the 5-a-day projects. *Health Educ Behav.* 2000 Apr; 27(2):157–166.
7. Pirie PL. Evaluating community health promotion programs. In: Brach N., ed., *Health Promotion at the Community Level.* 2nd ed. Newbury Park, CA: Sage Publications; 1999:127–134.
8. Feinstein AR, Horwitz RI. Problems in the "evidence" of "evidence-based medicine." *American Journal of Medicine.* 1997; 103(6):529–535.
9. Sackett DL, Rosenberg WM, Gray JA, Haynes RB, Richardson WS. Evidence based medicine: What it is and what it isn't. *British Medical Journal.* 1996; 312(7023):71–72.
10. Rosswurm MA, Larrabee JH. A model for change to evidence-based practice. *Image: Journal of Nursing Scholarship.* 1999; 31(4): 317–322.
11. Woolf SH. The need for perspective in evidence-based medicine. *JAMA.* 1999 Dec; 282(24):2358–2365.
12. Nutbeam D. Achieving "best practice" in health promotion: Improving the fit between research and practice. *Health Education Research.* 1996; 11(3):317–326.
13. Murdaugh CL, Vanderboom C. Individual and community models for promoting wellness. *Journal of Cardiovascular Nursing.* 1997; 11(3):1–14.
14. McKinlay JB. A case for re-focusing upstream: The political economy of illness. In Enelow AJ, Henderson JB, eds., *Applying Behavioral Science to Cardiovascular Risk.* Seattle, WA: American Heart Association; 1975: 7–18.
15. Orleans CT. Promoting the maintenance of health behavior change: Recommendations for the next generation of research and practice. *Health Psychol.* 2000; 19(1)(Suppl):76–83.

16. Jeffery RW, Drewnowski A, Epstein LH, Stunkard AJ, Wilson GT, Wing RR, Hill DR. Long-term maintenance of weight loss: Current status. *Health Psychol.* 2000; 19(1)(Suppl):5–16.

17. Ockene JK, Emmons KM, Mermelstein RJ, Perkins KA, Bonollo DS, Voorhees CC, Hollis JF. Relapse and maintenance issues for smoking cessation. *Health Psychol.* 2000; 19(1)(Suppl.):17–31.

18. Bandura A. *Social Foundations of Thoughts and Actions.* Upper Saddle River, NJ: Prentice Hall, Inc.; 1986.

19. Prochaska JO, DiClemente CC. Stages and processes of self-change of smoking: Toward an integrative model of change. *Journal of Consulting and Clinical Psychology.* 1983; 51: 390–395.

20. Mittlemark MB, Hunt MK, Heath GW, Schmid TL. Realistic outcomes: Lessons from community-based research and demonstration programs for the prevention of cardiovascular diseases. *Journal of Public Health Policy.* 1993 Winter; 437–462.

21. Marcus BH, Owen N, Forsyth LH, Cavill NA, Fridinger F. Physical activity interventions using mass media, print media, and information technology. *Am J Prev Med.* 1998 Nov; 15(4):362–378.

22. Marcus BH, Dubbert PM, Forsyth LH, McKenzie TL, Stone EJ, Dunn AL, Blair SN. Physical activity behavior change: Issues in adoption and maintenance. *Health Psychol.* 2000; 19(1)(Suppl):32–41.

23. Heaney CA, Goetzel RZ. A review of health-related outcomes of multi-component worksite health promotion programs. *Am J Health Promo.* 1997 Mar–Apr; 11(4):290–307.

24. Warner KE, Smith RJ, Smith DG, Fries BE. Health and economic implications of a work-site smoking-cessation program: A simulation analysis. *JOEM.* 1996 Oct; 38(10):981–992.

25. Emmons KM, Thompson B, McLerran D, Sorensen G, Linnan L, Basen-Enquist K, Biener, L. The relationship between organizational characteristics and the adoption of workplace smoking policies. *Health Education and Behavior.* 2000 Aug; 27(4):483–501.

26. Campbell MK, Motsinger BM, Jewell D, Makarushka C, Beatty B, McClelland J, Demessie S., Demark-Wahnefried W. The North Carolina Black Churches United for Better Health Project: Intervention and process evaluation. *Health Educ Behav.* 2000; 27(2): 241–253.

27. Ross C, Richard L, Potvin L. One year outcome evaluation of an alcohol and drug abuse prevention program in a Québec high school. *Can J Public Health.* 1998 May–Jun; 89(3):166–170.

28. Wickizer TM, Wagner E, Cheadle A, Pearson D, Beery W, Maeser J, Psaty B, VonKorff M, Koepsell T, Diehr P, Perrin EB. Implementation of the Henry J. Kaiser family foundation's community health promotion grants program: A process evaluation. *The Millbank Quarterly.* 1998; 76(1):121–147.

29. Kegler MC, Steckler A, Malek SH, McLeroy K. A multiple case study of implementation in 10 local Project ASSIST coalitions in North Carolina. *Health Educ Res.* 1998 Jun; 13(2):225–238.

30. King AC. How to promote physical activity in a community: Research experiences from the U.S. highlighting different community approaches. *Patient Educ Couns.* 1998 Apr; 33(1 Suppl):S3–S12.

31. Steckler A, Allegrante JP, Altman D, Brown R, Burdine JN, Goodman RM, Jorgensen C. Health education intervention strategies: Recommendations for future research. *Health Educ Q.* 1995 Aug; 22(3):307–328.

32. Hardeman W, Griffin S, Johnston M, Kinmonth AL, Wareham NJ. Interventions to prevent weight gain: A systematic review of psychological models and behaviour change methods. *Int J Obes Relat Metab Disord.* 2000 Feb; 24(2):131–143.

33. McKinlay JB. The new public health approach to improving physical activity and autonomy in older populations. In: Heikkinen E, ed. *Preparation for Aging.* New York: Plenum Press; 1995:87–103.

34. Wing R. Cross-cutting themes in maintenance of behavior change. *Health Psychol.* 2000; 19(1)(Suppl):84–88.

35. Rothman AJ. Toward a theory-based analysis of behavioral maintenance. *Health Psychol.* 2000; 19(1)(Suppl):64–69.

36. Marcus T. An interdisciplinary team model for substance abuse prevention in communities. *J Prof Nurs.* 2000 May–Jun; 16(3):158–168.

37. Lundeen SP. An alternative paradigm for promoting health in communities: The Lundeen community nursing center model. *Fam Community Health.* 1999; 21(4):15–28.

38. Shediac-Rizkallah MC, Bone LR. Planning for the sustainability of community-based health programs: Conceptual frameworks and future directions for research, practice and policy. *Health Educ Res.* 1998 Mar; 13(1):87–108.

Part VI

Approaches for Promoting a Healthier Society

14

Health Promotion in Community Settings

- Health Promotion in Families
- Health Promotion in Schools
- Health Promotion at the Work Site
- Health Promotion in Nurse-Managed Community Health Centers
- The Community at Large as a Setting for Health Promotion
- Creating Health Partnerships
- The Role of Partnerships in Education, Research, and Practice
- Directions for Research in Multi-Level Health Promotion Strategies
- Directions for Practice to Promote Health in Diverse Settings
- Summary

More than ever before, the value of health promotion services for improving the health of populations is recognized worldwide. Increasingly, third-party payers are including health promotion benefits in their plans as reimbursable services. The many settings in which health promotion is now delivered offer the possibility for achieving an integration of effort across sites and among health professionals that has never been achieved before. If people of all ages are to benefit from quality health-promotive care, gender-and culture-sensitive services should be delivered at sites where people are, where they spend many of their waking hours. The purpose of this chapter is to provide an overview of health promotion settings from families and schools to the community at large. Partnerships for health promotion among groups and organizations in the community also will be discussed as multi-agency collaboration is the key to fostering healthy lifestyles as the norm within diverse populations.

 # Health Promotion in Families

Health values, attitudes, and behaviors are learned in the family context. Just as individuals must assume responsibility for their own health status, so families must assume similar responsibilities for the health of the family as a unit. Structural and functional features of the family that must be considered when attempting to influence health practices include value structure, role structure, power structure (decision-making patterns), communication patterns, affective function, socialization function, health care function, and coping function. Specific questions that should be explored in relation to family values, beliefs, and lifestyle include the following: (1) How does the family define health? (2) What health-promoting behaviors does the family engage in regularly? (3) What health-promoting behaviors are particularly enjoyable to family members? (4) Do all family members engage in these behaviors or are patterns of participation highly variable throughout the family system? (5) Is there consistency between family health values as stated and their health actions? (6) What are the explicit or implicit goals of the family in the area of health?

Variant family forms are common in today's society. Family units may be traditional two-parent families, one-parent families (most often mother only), blended families (parts of two preexisting families), extended families (nuclear plus a relative, often older), augmented families (additional members, not blood relations), married adult dyads, and unmarried adult dyads (blood and nonblood relations). Families are as diverse as individuals and need to be actively involved in planning their health promotion activities. The nurse working with families in the area of health promotion must be sensitive to both the commonalties and differences across varying family forms. Understanding the milieu for the promotion of health in families of varying types is essential to successful family health promotion counseling and behavioral interventions.

The family is a pivotal group to decrease risky behaviors and increase healthy behaviors among its members. For example, recent research has identified disruptive behavior early in childhood among children from alcoholic families as a possible risk factor for alcoholism in adulthood. A family-based program focused on the prevention of disruptive behavior among preschool sons of alcoholic fathers was designed to address this problem. A 10-month intervention was provided to 52 families with major alcohol misuse problems. The intervention focused on parent training and marital problem solving in attempting to influence child behavior and authoritative parenting. Parental expectations prior to the intervention influenced their investment in the program. Parental investment was positively related to an increase in authoritative parenting and a decrease in the disruptive behavior of their children.[1]

The effects of a home-based family intervention to decrease alcohol use and misuse among adolescents is described by Loveland-Cherry and colleagues.[2] Goals of the intervention were to (1) enhance parenting practices and family patterns proposed as protective of adolescents such as warmth, nurturance, monitoring, and parental self-efficacy in preventing alcohol use; and (2) minimize practices proposed to increase risk for alcohol use such as excessive permissiveness and parental drinking. A sample of 428 youths, 86% European American, from schools in an urban area and their families provided complete data for this intervention study. Youths entered the study in fourth grade. Each family was provided with materials to assist them in developing parent–family assets to build competence of teen members to prevent or decrease alcohol use and misuse. The intervention consisted of three one-hour in-home sessions with a family intervener, periodic family meetings organized by the parents, and follow-up telephone calls. During seventh grade, in-home booster sessions reviewed prior intervention components and addressed school transition and normal adolescent development. Following completion of the intervention, the lowest drinks per week were reported by adolescents who had no prior drinking history and were in the family intervention group. Reported alcohol use was higher in those who reported drinking prior to the intervention and in the control groups not receiving the intervention. This study illustrates the positive outcomes that can be achieved through family intervention and the importance of identifying those adolescents most responsive to the intervention.

Knutsen and Knutsen[3] used the family as the unit of intervention directed toward reducing coronary risk factors. Through an intervention delivered to families in the primary care setting, the goal was to reduce coronary risk by reducing sugar intake, dietary fat intake, and smoking, and increasing the amount of exercise. Families were randomly assigned to intervention and control groups. The intervention families were informed that they were at increased risk for coronary heart disease because of a shared family lifestyle. The intervention consisted of home visits and counseling, with special emphasis on diet. Smoking and exercise were also discussed, but in less detail. Based on dietary information from the family, the dietitian gave specific advice, using food models and other audiovisuals to reinforce her message regarding good nutrition. At rescreening approximately five years later, significantly lower risk factor levels were found in the men and their spouses in the intervention group compared with the control group. For children in the family, the difference in overall risk factors was minimal and generally nonsignificant. Families in the intervention group reported more positive health practices in relation to diet than in the control group. No differences were found between the two groups in smoking and exercise behavior. This study indicated that a family approach to risk reduction and health promotion is well accepted, moderately effective, and feasible in primary care. More powerful behavioral interventions for families need to be developed.

Families demonstrate a spectrum of abilities, insights, and strengths. The challenge for the nurse is to assist the family unit in identifying relevant health goals, planning for positive lifestyle changes, and capitalizing on their strengths to achieve desired family health outcomes. Nursing care directed at improving health behaviors in the family unit should include assessing current family lifestyle; planning collaboratively with the family for positive and enjoyable behavior change; promoting the knowledge, skills, and collective efficacy of family members to implement change; and evaluating family health behavior and health outcomes. Prenatal and postnatal visits with families offer windows of opportunity to initiate discussions of family health promotion. Motivation to create healthy family environments may be optimal during early infancy. Through health promotion counseling and strategic support, family members can be assisted to exert control over family health behaviors and health status.

Health Promotion in Schools

With a majority of the nation's children enrolled in elementary and secondary schools, school-based health promotion programs can exert a major influence on the acquisition of health-promoting behaviors among children and adolescents. Schools can be health-enhancing environments that build resilience and assist children to develop healthy behaviors such as positive nutrition and regular physical activity as well as avoid negative behaviors such as substance abuse and violence. Teachers and school health personnel need to set the normative expectations for healthy behaviors and serve as role models of health-enhancing lifestyles. Of critical importance is creating positive peer influences that foster health-promoting rather than health-damaging behaviors. Healthy schools need parents who are interested and involved in creating healthy school environments as well as carrying healthy lifestyles into the home environment.

Health promotion programs in school settings should be integral to the instructional program of the school. Critical functions of comprehensive school health promotion programs include:

1. Promote acquisition of knowledge and skills for competent self-care and informed decision making about health.
2. Reinforce positive health attitudes.
3. Structure environment and social influences to support health-promoting behaviors.
4. Facilitate growth and self-actualization.
5. Sensitize students to aspects of their environment and culture that are detrimental to health and well-being.
6. Foster positive life skills that enhance successful coping and supportive interpersonal relationships.
7. Include school–family partnership activities in health education courses and after school health promotion activities.

Health-promoting behaviors are acquired more readily in childhood, when routines and habits are being formed. Habits or behaviors developed in childhood and adolescence are more likely to persist as an integral part of lifestyle than changes made in health behaviors later in the adult years. Thus, development of healthy behaviors in very young children is critical to increasing the prevalence of healthy lifestyles in the population.

Increasing concern about the current and future health of our nation's children has resulted in new models of school health services. Schools are envisioned as the sites for health promotion education and primary care service delivery for children and families.[4]

Youth health promotion programs can address many of the pressing problems that today's youth face. Millstein and colleagues suggest the following guidelines for successful programs.[5] The programs should be:

1. Highly responsive to the population for whom they are developed, recognizing age-related differences
2. Sensitive to the diverse cultural and social contexts in which youth live
3. Inclusive of many individuals and institutions that affect the lives of youth
4. Responsive to the need for continuing education of parents, teachers, and health professionals to enable them to use "state of the science" strategies and interventions to meet the health promotion needs of youth

To address the pressing health problems of youth, Uphold and Graham propose that traditional school health services be restructured as family service centers to help families solve their interrelated educational, social, economic, and health care problems. The authors described the Family Services Center located at a middle school in Gainesville, Florida. The primary objective of the center is to empower families to make substantial life and health behavior changes and to escape the cycle of poverty. When a family seeks service at the center, a family liaison specialist completes a needs assessment and develops a contract that addresses issues such as parenting skills, literacy, substance abuse, and various aspects of health care. The specialist may conduct home visits as needed and referrals are made to other agencies for services not provided at the center. Adult education and job training are a central focus of the center. An education specialist works with parents to improve their ability to help their child succeed academically. Peer counseling, mental health counseling, social work, and health care services are available. Transportation is provided for families to the center and referral agencies. A school nurse specialist and health aides develop and implement health promotion and prevention care plans for families. Nurse practitioners and school nurses are an ideal team to provide leadership to health professionals and lay workers in developing family service centers that are school based or school linked.[6]

"Reach for Health" is an example of a school-based program for urban African American and Latino middle school students. Community involvement as a part of the program enhances orientation to caring for others, social skills, and related behaviors. The curriculum builds skills for avoiding risks such as drug and alcohol use, violence, sexual activity, and unintended pregnancy. After experiencing the program, students in the intervention group reported higher sexual abstinence and more frequent use of protection if sexually active in comparison to a control group. This program had a positive impact on the lives of the adolescent participants.[7]

The relative effectiveness of two school-based approaches to prevent substance use was tested among inner-city African American and Hispanic seventh and eighth graders. A culturally tailored intervention (CTI) was compared to a life skills training (LST) approach. Both focused on decision making, communication, resistance skills, stress management, self-esteem building, and help seeking. Intervention techniques included demonstration, behavioral rehearsal, and homework assignments. In addition, the CTI addressed specific risk factors for the targeted groups through a professional storyteller who related culturally relevant stories, through use of culturally appropriate videos and peer leaders, and by focusing attention on African American and Hispanic heroes and heroines as healthy role models.

Both interventions were shown to be effective in decreasing alcohol and substance use. However, the CTI was shown to have a more pronounced effect on increasing the hopefulness of youth that they could have a positive future.[8] Sensitivity to the many dimensions of race and culture in school-based interventions is essential to reach youth with effective interventions and programs.

In examining comprehensive school health and social programs for adolescents at risk, Dryfoos[9] identified several characteristics of programs that work. The programs that work (1) provide individual attention to children; (2) are multicomponent, multiagency, community-wide programs; (3) focus on intervention as early as preschool; (4) promote acquisition of basic academic skills; (5) create healthy school climates; (6) promote "real" parental involvement with paid or volunteer positions; (7) promote active peer involvement; (8) connect to the real world of work; (9) provide social and life skills training; and (10) attend to the needs of staff for training and supervision. These characteristics should be built into school health promotion programs to optimize their chances of success and meaningful impact on the youth they serve.

Health Promotion at the Work Site

With the escalating cost of health insurance benefits, employers are attracted to work site prevention and health promotion initiatives as a means of controlling costs and maintaining a healthy and productive workforce. Accumulating evidence suggests that such programs may increase productivity, decrease absenteeism, decrease use of expensive medical care, and lower disability claims resulting ultimately in a more productive and globally competitive workforce. Review of research suggests that comprehensive programs that address risk reduction counseling, modifications of workplace policies, and changes in the physical work environment are most likely to have successful long-term results.[10] Offering a variety of health promotion programs at the work site, using differing approaches, increases the appeal of the program to employees of varying cultural backgrounds and of differing ages.

A definite advantage of health promotion policies and activities at the work site is that they create a cultural milieu that supports health-promoting behaviors. For example, smoke-free workplaces have made major contributions to the recent declines in cigarette smoking in both the United States and Australia. In reviewing 19 studies of the impact of smoke-free workplace policies on workday cigarette consumption of employees, Chapman and colleagues found that 18 studies reported declines in daily smoking rates. They estimate that approximately 22.3% of the decrease in cigarette consumption in Australia and 12.7% of the decrease in the United States can be attributed to smoke-free workplaces. Policy changes also resulted in a major decrease in exposure of nonsmokers to environmental tobacco smoke at the work site.[11]

Workplace programs have many strengths including access to employees during the workday over an extended period of time, opportunities for health-promoting changes in policies and the environment to support behavior changes by employees, capabilities for modifying social norms and increasing interpersonal support of coworkers for change, and opportunities to put incentive programs in place to reward healthy behaviors. Change in workplace cultures is important to achieve broad-based support for health promotion programs. One study evaluated the effectiveness of management training in increasing health promotion programming. Twenty companies participated in the study that measured changes in health promotion programming over time. Seminar content for managers included organizational assessment, participation in analysis of health hazard appraisal data of employees, design of a plan to support employee health, miniconference for vendors with health promotion products and programs to display their wares, and evaluation and follow-up. Following intervention, the experimental group made greater strides than did the control group in changing the work milieu to support healthy living. Examples of changes at the work site included availability of an array of health materials, healthier foods in cafeteria and vending machines, healthier snacks at meetings, discounted rates at fitness centers for employees and families, periodic health screening, and on-site health fairs.[12]

Two work site programs are described here to inform the reader of the range of approaches that can be used to promote wellness at the work site. Lusk and colleagues[13] applied the Health Promotion Model to develop a tailored work site intervention for construction workers to promote use of hearing protection devices to decrease noise-induced hearing loss. Predictors of use of hearing protection from the HPM that were integrated into the intervention included the cognitive–perceptual influences of perceived self-efficacy, value of use, perceived barriers, and the modifying factors of peer modeling (interpersonal influence), availability of devices, and extent of noise exposure (situational influences). A tailored interactive video and print materials were used in the intervention.[13] Study results indicated that the intervention resulted in increased use of hearing protection among workers.

The impact of a work site behavioral skills intervention to increase physical activity was evaluated in a randomized control trial consisting of three months of intervention and six months of maintenance in which the intervention was gradually phased out. Employees were assigned to intervention and control groups. Both groups were given a free nine-month membership in a fitness center. In addition, employees in the intervention group were encouraged to exercise and taught behavioral skills to maintain exercise such as goal setting, time management, self-talk, social support building, relapse prevention, and environmental modification. Moderate physical activity was conducted during the group sessions. The intervention group also received four behavioral skills booster sessions spaced over the six-month maintenance period. Following the intervention, reported energy expenditure as measured by the Seven-Day Physical Activity Recall was significantly greater in the intervention group. Use of processes of change increased and television viewing decreased more in the intervention group than in the control group. The intervention group also reported considerable increase in enjoyment of exercise.[14] Thus, the intervention was effective in increasing exercise among employees and in decreasing the time spent in watching television and other sedentary pursuits.

Including families in work site health promotion programs is of interest to many employers because part of their outlay for health care costs is for family members. Studies have shown that smokers are more likely to have spouses who smoke and that individuals with physically active spouses are more likely to be active themselves, and their children are likely to be more active. Some companies have also invited teachers from local schools to participate in their training programs so that health promotion concepts in schools and work sites are consistent and integrated. This effort, if greatly expanded, could give rise to "seamless" health promotion programming in communities that would accelerate behavior change efforts across the life span.

Work site health promotion programs will expand in the future. Exciting possibilities exist for integrating these programs into a coordinated community effort. The effectiveness of work site programs will continue to be evaluated as more companies adopt this approach to promoting the health of employees and containing health-care costs.

Health Promotion in Nurse-Managed Community Health Centers

Nurse-managed community health centers represent an ideal setting for offering a spectrum of services including health promotion and prevention counseling, behavioral interventions to promote the adoption of healthy lifestyles, and screening for early detection of health risks. The focus on the "individual and family" rather than on "the presenting illness" has enhanced the appeal of nurse-managed centers for the delivery of care to a growing segment of the population. For example, many families prefer to obtain health care from nurse practitioners in a setting that is user friendly and respectful of both their unique assets and their needs. Nurse-managed centers provide family-oriented care that is culturally sensitive. With the diversity of populations today and the variation in composition of family units, most families need assistance with healthy parenting and with meeting the health promotion needs of all family members. Many centers include in their services not only direct care but education classes on highly relevant topics, small group support sessions, and family and individual counseling. Family-focused activities of nurse-managed centers serve as excellent health care-delivery models.

The University of Michigan School of Nursing and Health System founded the North Campus Nursing Center in 1991 to provide health care to international students living on campus. These students and their families may have a limited command of English, have minimal incomes, and feel alienated in a culture different from their home culture. The center, staffed by nurse practitioners and community health nurses, provides an array of services to international student families. Immunizations and well-baby checkups are available, as is health promotion counseling for family members. The center is located in an apartment in the campus housing area so it is maximally convenient to students and their families. The reception and examination rooms are welcoming and attractive. A living room and play area have been furnished to encourage informal conversations among clients and health care workers. The center is currently funded by a health maintenance organization (HMO), Medicaid, and various state and federal programs. Fee for service for the uninsured is on a sliding scale based on ability to pay.

Nurse-managed centers can be established in many different environments readily accessible to the people they are intended to serve. For example, some centers are set up at or near schools so that the pressing health needs of children and adolescents can be met in a confidential and developmentally appropriate manner. Locating nurse-managed centers in malls or storefronts where people congregate or spend time when not at school or work also provides easy accessibility. Nurse-managed centers offer new alternatives of care including family-focused care that enhances the health and well-being of all family members, interdisciplinary care that provides a range of health and social services, and integrated care that covers the life span of families and individuals.

With major national emphasis on cost containment in health care, nurse-managed centers are particularly appealing as integral components of the health care system. Health insurers, HMOs, and Medicare and Medicaid are increasingly interested in incorporating such centers into the cadre of health care providers. Particularly appealing are the opportunities to link schools of nursing in universities and nurse-managed centers so that the latest scientific developments can impact services through evidence-based practice. Computerized tracking systems of client outcomes are particularly critical to collect the data needed to evaluate the quality and cost effectiveness of health care delivered in nurse-managed centers.

Nurses need to address the legislative impediments that constrain the establishment of nurse-managed centers and the provision of reimbursed health promotion and prevention services to individuals and families. Nurse-managed centers are uniquely positioned in the health care system to negotiate with managed care organizations to be primary care providers to a growing segment of the population. The nursing profession and lay organizations should continue concerted efforts to bring nurse-managed community health centers into the mainstream in provision of health promotion and prevention services.

The Community at Large as a Setting for Health Promotion

The idea of changing the behavior of communities rather than of individuals or small groups is based on the efficiency gained by using community organizations, media, and information dissemination and support structures to mobilize large groups of individuals for environmental and behavioral change. Community-based health promotion and prevention programs encompass a range of activities such as community-wide health education, risk reduction intervention programs, environmental awareness and improvement programs, and initiatives to change laws or regulatory policies to be supportive of health.

Community activation, as a health promotion strategy, includes organized efforts to increase community awareness and consensus about health problems, coordinate planning of health promotion partnerships for environmental change, achieve interorganizational allocation of resources, and promote citizen involvement in these processes. Community activation is most closely associated with a social planning model that places emphasis on organizational change and the development of rational planning strategies to achieve goals.[15] A critical feature of community activation is matching programming to "real" community needs identified by those who reside in the community. It is critical to keep in mind that a community is a "living" organism with interactive webs among organizations, neighborhoods, families, and friends. The health of the community as an organism is directly related to the health of its members. The health of all is enhanced through effective social change.[16]

An excellent example of community health promotion programming is offered by The Well, a neighborhood-based wellness center for African American women in an urban setting. The mission of The Well is to promote health-enhancing change through mutual support, personal growth, community education, and collective action to foster personal and community empowerment for wellness initiatives. A nurse practitioner coordinates services offered at The Well, which is located in a low-income housing complex. Health promotion activities offered include sister circles that serve as self-help groups, exercise classes, weight-loss assistance, family planning, risk screening services, physical examination, substance abuse outreach, and health advocacy. Universities and community organizations provided support for activities at The Well. Four strengths of the program were identified: The empowerment process is integral to all services; there is shared ownership by community members; the center has a community-based location; and relationships with local universities were put in place to augment resources.[17]

Another community-based initiative, Project Salsa, was organized to promote heart healthy nutritional changes in a Latino community. A needs assessment was first conducted to determine the top-ranking community issues. The nutrition intervention was based on consideration of community input from varying sources. Using culturally appropriate materials, the intervention focused on nutrition for pregnant women, encouragement of breast-feeding, heart healthy nutrition cooking skills, nutritionally balanced diets for schoolchildren, risk screening, and instruction on positive dietary behaviors. After the five-year project ended, the school nutrition program and coronary heart disease risk factor screening program were institutionalized in the community, although other aspects of the program were not. Facilitators of institutionalization were a close fit between the activity and the mission of the adopting agency, a champion for the program within the agency, benefits for the agency, and economical cost of the institutionalized programs.[18]

The Black Churches United for Better Health Project, a community-based health promotion program, was aimed at increasing fruit and vegetable consumption among rural African Americans to address the greater incidence of cancer and chronic diseases in this population compared to European American counterparts. Fifty churches participated in the project, which consisted of a multicomponent intervention within an ecological framework targeted at individual, social, and community levels. Focus groups were used as a basis for constructing culturally sensitive messages. Concepts from the transtheoretical model, social cognitive theory, and social support models provided a basis for the intervention. Intervention components included printed materials and bulletin boards in churches, educational sessions on nutrition, cooking classes, gardening classes, and instruction in preparation of healthy meals to be served at church functions. Pastoral support and lay health advisers were also an important part of the intervention. Community grocers were also enlisted to provide healthy foods and nutrition information. Following the intervention, the proportion of the intervention group meeting the dietary guidelines of consuming five servings of fruits and vegetables a day increased from 23% to 33%, whereas the control group showed a decrease from 23% to 21%. More members of the intervention group were in the action and maintenance phases of dietary change than were members of the control group. This church-based intervention successfully modified the reported dietary behaviors of participants and has the potential for long-term institutionalization as an ongoing program.[19]

Community-based health promotion programs offer an excellent approach to reaching many communities, particularly impoverished communities, with limited resources. It is critical to provide health promotion services in the settings where people live, work, and play. Offering nutrition services in churches and mammography screening in malls exemplify bringing valuable services to people in real life settings. The synergy of bringing community strengths and resources together and the empowerment that subsequently results from early successes warrant continued attention in designing innovative and culturally sensitive health promotion programs for large aggregates.

Creating Health Partnerships

Various settings for health promotion have been discussed but, in reality, creative health partnerships across settings is critical in order to optimize the health of communities. Many economic, social, and health incentives for organizational partnerships exist in the current health care system. Partnerships promote continuity of care in health promotion and prevention and synergistic use of resources to achieve optimal effectiveness and efficiency. Partnerships may consist of any combination of work sites, schools, nursing centers, other health agencies and universities working together to improve the health of an entire community. In this section of the chapter, the advantages as well as the issues related to developing community health partnerships will be addressed.

A community partnership can be defined as a purposive relationship between collaborating parties committed to pursuing both individual partner and collective benefits.[20] Community partnerships recognize the value of community members and health care providers coming together to create new health care systems that are user friendly, accessible, and culture sensitive. Partnerships optimize the combined resources of all partners so that mutually valued goals are achieved. Braithwaite and colleagues[21] advocate for health partnerships as a way of using community organization to achieve health empowerment, to improve health in communities of color, and to eliminate health disparities. Significant advances in health for various racially and ethnically diverse populations will result from social-structural changes that remove constraints to good health and augment opportunities to pursue optimum health and well-being. Further, comprehensive health policies must be enacted that build a health-sustaining infrastructure within communities.[22]

To establish successful health partnerships, a relationship must be established with communities that clearly communicates respect for their right to identify problems and potential solutions to those problems. It is important to determine the community's norms for participation. Is community problem solving, at present, primarily an individual or collective effort? How in touch are citizens with each other? What are the units of interaction (e.g., neighborhoods, townships, housing complexes)? Do crime or other factors deter citizens from interacting on an ongoing basis? Some communities already have structures set up for community planning to address health concerns. Current patterns of citizen involvement, working relationships among community organizations already in existence, and organizations known for activating community involvement (e.g., churches, recreation centers, service clubs) should be analyzed to determine how partnerships for health promotion might be shaped in any given community. For some communities, flexible coalitions might be the appropriate organizing framework to address community health needs, whereas for others, a leadership board or council may be needed to combine the power of key community activists.

An important goal of community partnerships focused on health promotion is empowerment of the community. Community empowerment is defined as a social-action process in which individuals and groups act to gain mastery over their lives through changing their social and political environment.[23] Together the members of a partnership should create conditions that empower their joint efforts. Community partnerships for health promotion have the potential for bringing about institutional and policy changes that affect many people. It is to those broader goals of both positive social-structural and individual change that many community partnerships are committed.

The challenge of building partnerships requires substantial time and effort. It is important that the diverse interests of partners be acknowledged in the early stages of the partnership and efforts be made to address any cultural gaps that exist between partners. Issues that need to be addressed include:[24]

1. Finding the right mix of ownership and control among partners
2. Recognizing the assets of all partners
3. Valuing all partners at the table
4. Resolving ethnic, cultural, and ideological differences between partners

A shared vision among partners creates a common identity and a shared purpose. A vision is an image of what the partners see as the future product of their collaboration. Based on a shared vision, a shared mission can be crafted that identifies the primary reason(s) for the existence of the partnership. An example of a mission statements is:

> To assist individuals and families in the community to adopt healthy lifestyles, and to assist the community to develop culturally sensitive and cost-effective health promotion and prevention services.

Shared core values need to be identified among partners. Core values such as justice, creativity, and compassion guide the actions of the partnership in a manner consistent with its mission in pursuit of its vision.[25] The will to work together to accomplish highly cherished social and health goals will sustain a community partnership over time despite points of disagreement and difficulties.

The potential for fostering healthier lives for citizens of all ages lies in the power of partnerships that are multisectoral and reach well beyond the bounds of traditional medicine. Partnerships are critical to appropriately plan, implement, and evaluate community-based health promotion interventions. For example, if crime is a problem in a community, a wide array of youth activity programs can be offered to both foster greater cardiovascular fitness through physical activity as well as prevent crime. Partnerships can facilitate the safe transport of youth to programs and the assessment of the programs to determine if the desired outcomes were attained. Community partnerships can set priorities for use of health resources in ways that are likely to work in their community, whereas imported solutions may be unacceptable because they are neither culturally nor socioeconomically appropriate for a given community.

Action research involves community members and provides important information for community organizations. A community organization approach to health promotion partnering is based on the concepts of self-determination, shared decision making, bottom-up planning, community problem solving, and cultural relevance. The philosophy underlying this approach is that health promotion is likely to be more successful when the community at risk identifies its own health concerns, develops its own intervention programs, forms a decision board to make policy decisions, and identifies resources for program implementation. Communities that are empowered through organization and active participation in partnerships develop leadership skills and the ability to attack an array of conditions that compromise their health and well-being. The impact of individual behavior-change efforts is limited without efforts to bring about systematic change within the society and environment through health partnerships.[20]

Community health partnerships can bring greater "rationality" to health care expenditures by advocating that prevention and health promotion services be adequately funded by national, state, and private insurers. Politically active partnerships can redirect public and private health care dollars so that they are allocated as depicted in Figure 14–1 with major emphasis on population-based health care services and clinical preventive services. Environmental support, community education, and positive health policies are key elements for successful community health partnerships.

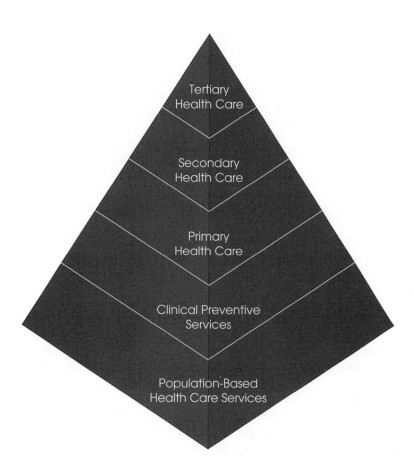

FIGURE 14-1 Health services pyramid (From U.S. Public Health Service. *A Time for Partnership: Report of State Consultations on the Role of Public Health, Prevention Report.* Washington, DC: U.S. Public Health Service; December 1994/January 1995.)

The Role of Partnerships in Education, Research, and Practice

Multidisciplinary education and collaborative work experience with community residents are critical to prepare health professions students for the diversity of health care roles that they will assume in the years to come. With the movement toward community-based care and away from traditional institutional care, except for the critically ill, knowledge of how to function in diverse community settings will be essential to meet the health needs of individuals and families from diverse backgrounds. Bartering student and faculty professional services for access to community educational experiences can be a win–win situation for both schools of nursing and communities. For example, students in the early stages of baccalaureate nursing education can experience various aspects of the role of community health worker by distributing health education materials in a community, participating in blood pressure screening programs, helping organize health fairs, collecting health data from communities, and surveying vending machines and fast-food stores in a community to determine the availability and cost of health-promoting options. More advanced baccalaureate students with a greater understanding of the impact of culture and socioeconomic class on health behaviors can provide nutrition classes at schools and work sites, assist community residents in identifying environmental risks to health, and provide self-care education to groups of individuals who have similar health-risk profiles.

Graduate students, faculty, and community representatives provide a superb team for training community health workers in underserved communities. In order to build a successful cohort of community health workers, schools of nursing must (1) establish rapport with the community; (2) collaborate with the community in the assessment of health needs; (3) hire workers from the community sufficiently language and culture fluent to gain the trust and participation of community residents; (4) share program ownership and decision making with community health care workers, empowering them to evaluate and refine program goals and redesign strategies for greater effectiveness; (5) facilitate program flexibility so workers can adapt it to changing needs; and (6) closely link workers with community health and social service agencies so that professional backup is available as necessary.[26]

The need has never been greater for schools of nursing to take an active role in developing enduring health promotion partnerships. The orientation of nursing to the whole person and the critical nature of the person–environment interaction in shaping health provides the professional background needed to work collaboratively with communities to accomplish health goals. With escalating reform in health care and the economic pressures to provide cost-effective, quality care with a mix of professionals different from that in the past, nurses are in an excellent position to make a difference in community health care systems as the twenty-first century commences. Incentives that have been identified to foster greater emphasis on partnering with communities for health improvement include:[27]

1. Increasing reimbursement for disease prevention and health promotion services
2. Federal grants to schools of medicine, public health, and nursing that are engaged in partnerships with underserved communities

3. Incentives in the form of grants, matching funds, and low-interest loans to communities that are engaged in partnerships with academic health centers

4. Tax benefits to businesses and financial institutions that provide direct support and low-interest loans to such community–academic health partnerships

Community–university health partnerships are valuable allies in research efforts. Assessment is a natural activity of community partnerships to enable them to understand the nature of the problems that they face and are trying to resolve. Assessment to obtain baseline data is also critical before implementing health promotion programs directed at large-scale social or environmental change. Partnering with universities throughout all stages of assessing, planning, and conducting health promotion interventions creates a sense of community ownership of the study and takes advantage of the expertise of university faculty. Partnerships foster more enthusiastic participation, greater attentiveness to subject recruitment, more thoughtful interpretation of findings in relation to a particular locality, and greater commitment to application of the findings to community programming.

Community partnerships can play a strategic role in creating the total community capacity to respond to health needs. In addition, they can set the expectation that the health care system will function as a copartner with other systems in the community to shape public policy and the environment to foster conditions for healthy living.

Directions for Research in Multi-Level Health Promotion Strategies

Nurse scientists need to explore both the content and the processes of successful and culturally appropriate prevention and health promotion services and health partnerships. Suggested directions for research include:

1. Explicating health promotion and disease prevention beliefs and practices in diverse families and communities as a basis for effective and culturally sensitive programming

2. Determining the synergistic effects of work site, school, family, and community health promotion efforts on population health outcomes

3. Identifying the interactive effects of unhealthy lifestyles and exposure to unhealthy environments

4. Identifying the short-term and long-term effects of poverty on the wellness potential of youth and their families

5. Testing community partnership strategies for optimizing health behavior and health outcomes for vulnerable populations

6. Developing valid and reliable community health outcome measures including quality-of-life indices

7. Developing uniform methods for assessing health outcomes and cost savings across a range of programs and communities

Although some anecdotal evidence suggests that community partnerships make a difference in health practices and the health of the community, few systematic studies have been conducted to determine the effectiveness and sustainability of community partnerships, particularly in communities with underserved populations.[20] Partnership intervention studies are critically needed. The intervention process should be carefully documented to facilitate identification of its most effective components and to allow replication. Numerous measures should be used to assess the behavioral, social, and environmental outcomes of partnership activities.

Directions for Practice to Promote Health in Diverse Settings

Multiple settings offer the opportunity for provision of health promotion services. Nurses, particularly nurses with an understanding of community health issues and problems, are ideally suited to provide leadership in the design, development, implementation, and evaluation of health promotion programs in schools, work sites, nursing centers, and other community settings. Financial support for such programs should be sought from a variety of public and private sources. The health problems of today can best be addressed by many sectors coming together in partnerships to impact the social and environmental conditions that compromise health. Partnerships offer a means of communication and collaboration and, thus, power to achieve solutions that single groups or organizations on their own do not have. Particularly exciting is the opportunity for schools of nursing to join with other health professions' schools, groups of health care providers, and communities in building health partnerships. These arrangements, if designed in a community-sensitive manner, can improve prevention and health promotion services provided to diverse populations.

SUMMARY

Health promotion services should be offered in multiple settings to optimize their reach to target populations. Development and maintenance of healthy lifestyles and healthy environments must be a central goal. Programs should be tailored to the needs of communities to enhance their cultural appropriateness and likelihood of success. Formation of community partnerships can create a network of community residents and health care providers that offer quality health promotion and prevention services to diverse populations.

SELECTED WEB SITES RELEVANT TO HEALTH PROMOTION IN COMMUNITY SETTINGS

Guide to Community Preventive Services—*www.thecommunityguide.org*

Centers for Disease Control and Prevention, National Center for Chronic Disease Prevention and Health Promotion—*http://www.cdc.gov/nccdphp/index.htm*

Centers for Disease Control and Prevention: The Planned Approach to Community Health (PATCH)—*http://www.cdc.gov/nccdphp/patch/*

Centers for Disease Control Prevention Guidelines Database—*http://aepo-xdv-www.epo.cdc.gov/wonder/PrevGuide/PrevGuid.htm*

References

1. Nye CL, Zucker RA, Fitzgerald HE. Early family-based intervention in the path to alcohol problems: Rationale and relationship between treatment process characteristics and child and parenting outcomes. *Journal of Studies on Alcohol.* 1999; (Suppl 13):94–102.

2. Loveland-Cherry CJ, Thompson Ross L, Kaufman SR. Effects of a home-based family intervention on adolescent alcohol use and misuse. *Journal of Studies of Alcohol.* 1999; (Suppl 13):94–102.

3. Knutsen SF, Knutsen R. The Tromso Survey: The family intervention study—The effect of intervention on some coronary risk factors and dietary habits, a 6-year follow-up. *Prev Med.* 1991;20:197–212.

4. Dryfoos JG. *Full Service Schools: A Revolution in Health and Social Services for Children, Youth and Families.* San Francisco: Jossey-Bass Publishers; 1994.

5. Millstein SG, Nightingale EO, Petersen AC, et al. Promoting the healthy development of adolescents. *JAMA.* 1993;269:1413–1415.

6. Uphold CR, Graham MV. Schools as centers for collaborative services for families: A vision for change. *Nurs Outlook.* 1993;41(5):204–211.

7. O'Donnell L, Stueve A, SanDoval A, Duran R, Haber D, et al. The effectiveness of the Reach for Health Community Youth Service Learning Program in reducing early and unprotected sex among urban middle school students. *Am J Public Health.* 1999;89(2):176–181.

8. Fogey MA, Schinke S, Cole K. School-based interventions to prevent substance use among inner-city minority adolescents. In Wilson DK, Rodrigue JR, Taylor WC, eds. *Health-promoting and health-compromising behaviors among minority adolescents.* Washington DC: American Psychological Association; 1997:251–267.

9. Dryfoos JG. Adolescents at risk: A summation of work in the field—Programs and policies. *J Adolesc Health.* 1991;12:630–637.

10. Heaney CA, Goetzel RZ. A review of health-related outcomes of multicomponent worksite health promotion programs. *Am J Health Prom.* 1997;11:290–308.

11. Chapman S, Borland R, Scollo M, Bownson RC, Dominello A, Woodward S. The impact of smoke-free workplaces on declining cigarette consumption in Australia and the United States. *Am J Public Health.* 1999;89:1018–1023.

12. Golaszewski T, Barr D, Cochran S. An organization-based intervention to improve support for employee heart health. *Am J Health Prom.* 1998;13(1):26–35.

13. Lusk SL, Hong OS, Ronis DL, Eakin BL, Kerr MJ, and Early MR. Effectiveness of an intervention to increase construction workers' use of hearing protection. *Human Factors* 1999;41(3);487–494.

14. Nichols JF, Wellman E, Caparosa S, Sallis JF, Calfas KJ, Rowe R. Impact of a worksite behavioral skills intervention. *Am J Health Prom.* 2000;14(4);218–221.

15. Wickizer TM, Von Korff M, Cheadle A, et al. Activating communities for health promotion: A process evaluation method. *Am J Public Health.* 1993;83:561–567.

16. Eng E, Salmon ME, Mullen F. Community empowerment: The critical base for primary care. *Fam Community Health*. 1992;15(1):1–12.

17. Elliott Brown KA, Jemmott FE, Mitchell HJ, Walton ML. The Well: A neighborhood-based health promotion model for black women. *Health and Social Work*. 1998;23(2):146–152.

18. Elder JP, Campbell NR, Candelaria JI, Talavera GA, Mayer JA, et al. Project Salsa: Development and institutionalization of a nutritional health promotion project in a Latino community. *Am J Health Prom*. 1998;12(6):391–401.

19. Campbell MK, Demark-Wahnefried W, Symons M, Kalsbeek WD, Dodds J, et al. Fruit and vegetable consumption and prevention of cancer: The Black Churches United for Better Health Project. *Am J Public Health*. 1999;89:1390–1396.

20 Cropper S. Collaborative working and the issue of sustainability. In: Huxham C, ed. *Creating Collaborative Advantage*. London: Sage; 1996:80–100.

21. Braithwaite RL, Bianchi C, Taylor SE. Ethnographic approach to community organization and health empowerment. *Health Educ Q*. 1994;21(3):407–416.

22. Neighbors HW, Braithwaite RL, Thompson E. Health promotion and African-Americans: from personal empowerment to community action. *Am J Health Prom*. 1995;9(4):281–287.

23. Wallerstein N, Bernstein E. Introduction to community empowerment, participatory education, and health. *Health Educ Q*. 1994;21(2):141–148.

24. Cheadle A, Beery W, Wagner E, Fawcett S, Green L, et al. Conference report: Community-based health promotion—State of the art and recommendations for the future. *Am J Prev Med*. 1997;13(4):240–243.

25. Nelson JC, Rashid H, Galvin VG, Essien JDK, Levine LM. Public/private partners: Key factors in creating a strategic alliance for community health. *Am J Prev Med*. 1999;16(3S):94–102.

26. Sherer JL. Neighbor to neighbor: Community health workers educate their own. *Hosp Health Net*. 1994 October 20;68(20):52–56.

27. Levine DM, Becker DM, Bone LR, et al. Community-academic health center partnerships for underserved minority populations. *JAMA*. 1994;272:309–311.

15

Protecting and Promoting Health Through Social and Environmental Change

- Health as a Social Goal
- Health in a Changing Social Environment
- Promoting Health Through Public Policy
- Promoting Health Through Environmental Control
  - A. Eliminating Health-Damaging Features of the Environment
  - B. Augmenting Health-Promoting Features of the Environment
- Voluntary Change versus Legislative Policy
- Economic Incentives for Disease Prevention and Health Promotion
- Directions for Research in Social and Environmental Change
- Directions for Practice to Promote Social and Environmental Change
- Summary

Recognition that health behavior is influenced by the social and physical environments in which people live has resulted in new ways to achieve behavior change.[1] New approaches argue that large-scale change is best accomplished by focusing on altering social and environmental structures that influence health as well as individual and group behaviors. Effective health promotion efforts, therefore, must take into consideration the dynamic relationships between individuals and families and changing social and environmental contexts. Health and social policies that fail to directly address harmful living conditions such as poverty, abuse, violence, hunger, and unemployment; environmental threats such as pollution in work sites and communities; and disparities in access and care will not be successful in promoting the health of individuals and communities. Individual and family efforts to adopt healthy behaviors are also likely to be ineffective as a result of environmental constraints and policies that do not promote healthy living. Any strategy for health promotion that focuses only on individual behavior change will fail without simultaneous efforts to alter the physical and social environment as well as the collective behavior of the community. In the Health Promotion Model described in Chapter 3, interpersonal influences and situational factors are proposed to affect decisions to engage in health-promoting behaviors. Creative initiatives to foster social and environmental conditions that actively promote health are addressed in this chapter.

Health as a Social Goal

Health needs to be identified as a social goal as well as an individual goal. The health of societies, communities, families, and individuals are integrated and inseparable. Health is influenced by social, cultural, economic, and political factors as well as biological and psychological factors.[2] Health promotion efforts involve working with communities to ameliorate conditions that contribute to poor health such as inadequate housing, an unsafe water supply, poor nutrition or interruptions in the food supply, chemical toxins, poor recreational facilities, inadequate access to care, and lack of economic opportunity, as these issues directly impinge on health. Therefore, behavior-change strategies need to be redirected beyond the individual to include community- and policy-level factors.[3]

Health as a social goal requires the integration of theories that address social change (e.g., critical social theory, ecologic framework, community organization, community empowerment) with theories that address individual behavior change (e.g., social cognitive theory, cognitive evaluation theory, theory of reasoned action) and family change (e.g., family stress theory, family development theory, family systems theory). The three theoretical perspectives are complementary. When nurses think only in terms of one-to-one relationships, the range and success of intervention possibilities are severely limited. Individual-level approaches are successful in patients with chronic diseases.[4] However, behavior change is more likely to be successful when the social context in which the individual acts is targeted as well. For example, smoking cessation programs must not only target the individual addictive properties of smoking. The social conditions in which smoking occurs must also be addressed, including the advertising and sale of cigarettes, the influence of the tobacco industry on certain sectors of the population, and the role of public policy in changing smoking behaviors. Tobacco public policy interventions have been successful in changing smoking behaviors through laws that reduce exposure to secondhand smoke in public facilities, excise taxes that increase the costs of cigarettes, limiting youth access to cigarettes, and regulating advertising and promotion of tobacco products.[5] Enduring, large-scale behavior change is best achieved by changing the standards of acceptable behavior in a community rather than by attempting to change the behavior of individuals against overwhelming social odds.

The pursuit of health as a social goal requires that people of a shared community engage together in the process of change to accommodate various social, political, and economic developments. Community models emphasize community strengths and the community's role in leading the change. Central concepts in these community-building models include participation, empowerment, critical consciousness, community competence, and issue selection.[6] Empowerment is a social action process through which individuals, and communities gain control over their lives and their environment to improve their health and quality of life. Community competence is closely related to the concept of empowerment, as it focuses on problem-solving ability as a central goal of the community. Competent communities can identify problems and needs of the community, achieve a working consensus on goals and priorities, agree on ways to implement agreed-upon goals, and collaborate effectively in the actions that need to be taken.[6] Health care providers can assist in the development of community competence by identifying natural leaders in a community who can undertake their own community assessments and actions necessary to strengthen the community. Leadership development is also a critical component in developing community competence. Leaders are needed who can stimulate people in the community to identify problems and solutions and act as facilitators to build group effectiveness. As a community gains competence in negotiating for resources to address a particular problem, the community becomes empowered, which enhances its problem-solving ability and capacity to cope with other problems as they arise. In addition, the community gains a sense of ownership in that it has a sense of responsibility for and control over the programs promoting change, as it has been involved in initiating and promoting them.[7]

Ecological models consider the relationships between individuals and their environments and explain how environments affect behavior as well as the interaction of behavior and environment.[8] Ecological models focus on changing the environmental context, including regulatory changes to support healthy behaviors. The *Healthy People 2010* objectives incorporate an ecological model of health promotion to address the social and physical context in which negative behaviors occur.[5] Social ecological models focus on the social context to produce large-scale social change. Social change refers to altering the social structures of a community.[1] Social change is generally followed by changes in the normative structures, or the shared rules and expectations (rules of conduct) that govern everyday life. When rules that govern behavior are modified, normative change takes place. Social change may occur through a functionalist view or conflict.[1] The functionalist view sees change as a gradual adaptive process oriented toward community reform and is based on cooperation and consensus. As the community changes, social norms change and new rules of conduct arise for the changed community. Social change focuses on the community's strengths and how these strengths can be used to best advantage in fostering continuing development of community competence. In the conflict view, social change occurs when a new community emerges. However, the system changes by coercive means or social control, in which those who control important parts of the community attempt to change social norms. A functionalist perspective is consistent with an expansive view of health. These two perspectives are contrasted in Figure 15–1. Social ecological models hold promise for successful health promotion. However, more research is needed on the environmental influences on behavior and evaluation of interventions that target the social context.

In summary, when health is considered a social goal as well as an individual goal, the most appropriate focus for health promotion is considered to be the community.[9] Individuals can govern their own behavior and should do so. Government can formulate broad policies and allocate funding. However, priority decisions and strategies for social change to control for more complex lifestyle issues can best be made collectively by members of the community. This strategy insures that the programs are relevant and appropriate for the people involved, and encourages greater involvement in the planning and implementation process.

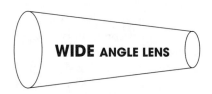

WIDE ANGLE LENS

Models for Intervention

Social change	*Social control*
Social analysis	Epidemiologic and demographic analysis
Focus on strengths	Focus on weaknesses
Goal is health outcome and increased community competence	Goal is health outcome
Organized around human categories	Organized around disease categories
Asks what are people's motives	Asks how can we motivate people

FIGURE 15-1 Comparison of social change with social control models (From Eng E, Salmon ME, Mullen F. Community Empowerment: the critical base for primary care. *Fam Community Health*, 1992; 15(1):1–2. Used with permission.)

Health in a Changing Social Environment

Despite the absence of comprehensive enabling legislation, health care reform in the United States continues to proceed at a rapid rate propelled by social, environmental, and economic forces. The rise of managed care and market competition has produced major changes in health care financing and delivery and has resulted in a shift in power from providers to purchasers.[10] Health care systems are beginning to take broader responsibility for the health of the communities they serve, as well as to support public policy to improve the forces that shape health.[11] New models of care are appearing that are based on various cost containment strategies, as national health care expenditures continue to be a major concern. Many of these models are based on a continuum of care, which is also known as an integrated system of care.[12] Integrated models of care focus on health promotion and maintenance across the life span as well as the provision of health care services.

Absence of guaranteed access to care has also been a major factor in the push for health care reform. Limitations in access to care include financial barriers, structural barriers, transportation barriers, and personal barriers such as cultural and language factors. As discussed in Chapter 5, disparities in access must be eliminated as access to health care increases (1) physical capacity, (2) personal resources to realize aspirations, and (3) ways to cope with the environment to improve one's health and quality of life.[13] Every community should be able to provide the services to monitor the health status of its members; inform, educate, and empower community members; and assist its members in accessing personal health services.[14] Successful reforms in health care systems will create new opportunities for communities, health care providers, and health systems to develop linkages to improve health.

In addition to health care reform, the communication revolution resulting from rapid technological advances, has changed our society to an information- and knowledge-based one. Information is available at the click of a mouse and the news media can now deliver health education and counseling to individuals as well as the public. Based on comprehensive, computerized health assessments, information systems can tailor health protection–promotion interventions to the knowledge, beliefs, motivations, and prior health-behavior histories of diverse individuals and families. Health promotion activities are beginning to take advantage of computer-based technologies such as CD-ROM and the World Wide Web to target audiences, tailor health promotion messages, and promote interactive ongoing exchanges about health.[5] Personal computers in the home offer informational resources, answer questions, and provide electronic access to support and discussion groups. One major issue will continue to be the scientific credibility of the information accessed on the Web in relation to the existing state of knowledge.[15] Information must be carefully screened and delivered with quality programs if it is to contribute to improving health promotion efforts.

Information systems are now enabling large segments of any community to be in touch with each other about the social problems that they face and their potential solutions. Furthermore, a composite plan for addressing health-related social and environmental conditions can be jointly developed by citizens without leaving their homes. Information technology offers the possibility of direct contact with policy makers in relation to health issues, formation of national networks to enhance local coalitions, and development of multiple communication links between health facilities and grassroots community groups.

The information era has also begun to bring about changes to empower families. Parents now often work at home as well as receive health information and health care at home through taking advantage of interactive computer technology.[16] Research results indicate that the Internet revolution is reshaping education, as individuals conduct health information searches and share information with their families and talk about it with their health care providers.[17] Computer-assisted health education is also being successfully implemented by means of the Internet.[18]

The information revolution is challenging health professionals to think creatively about the future of health care and new ways to educate health professionals in a multicultural society. Futurist perspectives need to be critically analyzed so that the nursing profession stays at the forefront in helping clients to enhance health amid conditions of rapid social and environmental change.

Promoting Health Through Public Policy

The importance of shaping healthy policies in the public and private sectors as the primary vehicle for achieving major improvements in health status for populations has been widely advocated. Policies set goals and limit and define choices; therefore, policy plays a vital role in achieving the goals of health promotion.[19] Personal, social, and political factors all influence the development and implementation of health policy. For example, at the personal level, changes in public sentiment have influenced the development of health policy related to smoking in public places in this country. At the political level, food lobbyists have been successful in maintaining the economic interests of the food and drug industries to prevent accurate labeling of foods and lower drug costs. On a more positive note, public policy has resulted in removal of cigarette commercials from television.

The idea of developing policies for healthier communities is not new. Historically, local governments have provided environmental safeguards against infectious diseases. However, the parameters of a healthy community have been expanded to include social and economic factors as well as environmental ones.[20] An underlying assumption of developing healthy communities is that local government plays a significant role through the development and implementation of policies to improve health, while community members actively participate in the decision making process. Thus policy formulation to promote health begins at the local level, through identification of problems and development of local ordinances to implement change.

The role of government in regulating health behavior remains undefined.[21] State and federal policies regulate a range of health behaviors, including alcohol, tobacco, seat belt use, food safety, and drug use. In addition, state and federal governments play a major role in the payment of health services. However, in many cases, a uniform health policy is missing, as in the case of immunization for measles or helmet use in motorcycle riding. One question that continues to be debated is how far should policy go in terms of individual behavior. The *Healthy People 2000* objectives emphasized individual responsibility, thus avoiding large-scale health policy mandates. However, an underlying premise of the *Healthy People 2010* objectives is that individual health is inseparable from the health of the larger community, which in turn determines the health status of the nation. The *Healthy People 2010* objectives and the national goal to eliminate health disparities challenge local, state, and federal governments, as well as policy makers, to be active participants in the development of policies that will improve the health of communities. For example, local governments can limit youth access to tobacco in local markets and vending machines. Local and state policies can also be developed to target economic development in communities with high unemployment or promote safe housing in poor neighborhoods.[22] Health policies have direct and indirect effects on health.[23] Long-term changes occur as a result of modifying the conditions under which people live.

Although policy making is usually thought to occur at the national and international level, local and regional policy making can be just as fruitful in health promotion efforts. Local and regional policy making can occur through social service agencies, local transportation authorities, public safety commissions, economic development zones, and professional organizations.[24] An advantage of beginning at the local level for policy making is that the policy will have an influence in the community almost immediately, as there is no trickle-down time. Community and political leaders, along with the local and state health departments, can advise and advocate large-scale changes to promote health.

Policy making is driven by the interplay of stakeholder interests and uses both science-based and nonscience-based information.[22] Policy making is value driven, dynamic, and often chaotic and is about social influence, as it involves persuasion, attitude change, decision making, and compromise. Facts, or science-based information, are usually used in the early phases of policy development to identify problems and solutions, including the economic costs. However, nonscience-based or less verifiable information presented by stakeholders who offer their informed judgments and personal experiences, is also used to promote the legitimacy of a proposed policy. Both types of knowledge are needed to gain support for successful policy making. Although the scientific knowledge is critical, stakeholders also need other information such as the political costs as well as the resources needed to implement the policies. This additional information assists in the development of consensus to achieve policy development.

Health policies are needed that encourage individuals and communities to place a higher value on health and provide them with the resources necessary to make healthy changes. This means that the necessary capacity and infrastructure relevant to health promotion must be developed and sustained in communities. Collaborative partnership models to develop health policy need to be implemented and tested to reduce disparities in access to information and resources. The value of individuals, communities, local and state government, as well as national government as active partners in this effort is critical.

Promoting Health Through Environmental Control

The quality of the physical environment in which people live is critical to the health of populations. Traditionally, environmental health practices have focused on controlling factors that are beyond the power of most people to control effectively. However, there are many external factors over which individuals have control, and today the goal is to help people change these factors in order to promote healthy environments.[25] Not only should health-damaging features of the environment be eliminated, but health-enhancing features should be augmented and actively used to promote improved health and well-being.

Eliminating Health-Damaging Features of the Environment

The harmful effects of toxic substances in the environment are vividly illustrated by the fact that 1 in 20 children have blood lead levels that exceed acceptable levels, and the risks are greatest for low-income racial and ethnic groups living in older housing.[26] Although there has been a dramatic reduction in the number of children with elevated lead levels due to screening and public education campaigns, much more remains to be done. Lead can be found in urban areas not only in paint but also in dust and soil. Exposure to high levels of lead can be fatal, but even low exposures can be toxic to the central nervous system, resulting in delayed learning, impaired hearing, and growth deficits. Such disorders severely limit the potential of children to compete successfully in school and make affected children prone to early dropout and compromised adult lives.

Leading indoor air hazards to which many thousands of people are exposed each year are tobacco smoke and radon. Environmental tobacco smoke is a cause of disease including lung cancer in nonsmokers. Children of parents who smoke are more likely to develop lower respiratory tract infections and middle ear infections than are children of parents who do not smoke. Asthma and other respiratory diseases are triggered or worsened by tobacco smoke and other substances in the air. Since the mid-1980s, asthma rates in the United States have risen to the level of an epidemic.[5]

The second leading cause of lung cancer, after smoking, is exposure to radon, a natural by-product of the breakdown of uranium that is found in many homes, offices, and schools.[27] Radon from soil gas is the main cause of radon problems. The Environmental Protection Agency reports that although inexpensive kits are available for radon testing, only 5% of homes have actually been tested. As many as 8 million homes may have radon at a level requiring correction.

Outdoor air quality continues to be a widespread environmental problem nationally as well as internationally. The effects are noted in premature deaths, cancer, and respiratory and cardiovascular diseases. Motor vehicles account for one-fourth of emissions that produce ground-level ozone, the largest problem in air pollution. The estimated annual costs of human exposure to outdoor air pollutants range from $40 billion to $50 billion, and an estimated 50,000 premature deaths.[5] Changes are beginning to occur by encouraging and rewarding individuals not to drive their cars, but to walk or use public transportation. Local and regional governments can devise public transportation systems that are amenable to communities and design streets that facilitate bicyclists and pedestrians. Nationally, support needs to be increased for the development and use of alternative fuels such as ethanol by commercial and private vehicles.

Water quality has once again become a major issue because of protozoa and chemical contaminants. Industry and agricultural runoff may contaminate water. For example, the development of intensive animal feeding operations has resulted in the discharge of improperly treated animal wastes into recreational and drinking water. The development of new molecular technologies to detect and monitor water contamination has eliminated the inability to detect parasitic contamination. These new technologies will greatly improve water monitoring and surveillance techniques.

Hazardous substances in the environment also pose significant health risks. For example, the Agency for Toxic Substances and Disease Registry (ATSDR) continues to publish a list of the most hazardous waste sites that need extensive cleanup.[5] Low-level radiation wastes deposited in landfills or carried from their source by air, groundwater, or surface runoff accumulate and have the capacity to affect surrounding populations. New job opportunities need to be made available to employees of hazardous waste sites to facilitate closure and cleanup of many of these sites. Second, the widespread use of pesticides continues to pose a threat, and children are at increased risk for pesticide poisoning.

Work-related injuries and illnesses result in billions of dollars in lost wages, lost productivity, and health care costs. In 1996, the National Institute for Occupational Safety and Health (NIOSH) developed a research agenda to guide occupational safety and research. Twenty-one priorities in three major categories were identified: disease and injury, work environment and workforce, and research tools and approaches. Areas not addressed by the research agenda that have been targeted by the *Health People 2010* objectives include preventive practices to reduce latex allergy, effective tuberculosis control programs, and rollover protective structures for agriculture tractors. In addition to occupational hazards in the work environment, as the economy continues to evolve from an industrial to a service-oriented one, the workforce is changing. Younger children (16 to 17 years), as well as women, minorities, and elderly, who are now in the workforce present new challenges for work safety and health.

Environmental variables have three functions important to health promotion.[7] First, environmental variables are part of a complex group of factors that lead to healthy and unhealthy behaviors as described above. Second, environmental variables moderate the effects of health promotion efforts. In other words, if the environment is not taken into account, the health promotion program may be ineffective. Last, environmental variables can be changed to achieve health promotion goals. Changing environmental variables requires targeting policy makers in private industry as well as government. Accomplishment of the *Healthy People 2010* objectives warrants attention to these factors.

Nursing as a health care profession must take responsibility for protecting and maintaining an environment that is health strengthening rather than health damaging. For example, noise is a feature of the environment that can be potentially stressful and health damaging. Hearing loss is a priority research area identified by NIOSH, as it ranks among the top 10 occupational hazards. Developing interventions to foster the use of hearing protection at work sites has been the target of ongoing research efforts by Lusk and her colleagues at the University of Michigan.[28,29,30] Based on her findings, Lusk, an occupational health nurse and clinical researcher, recommends that workers play a role in selection of hearing protection devices instead of basing choice exclusively on noise reduction, to increase use. In addition, training programs need to be tailored to level of education and trade group, as the percentage of workers who do not wear protective devices continues to be alarmingly high.

Risk assessment is the means by which currently available information about environmental public health problems can be organized and understood. The National Research Council has described four major steps in this risk assessment process: (1) hazard identification, (2) dose–response assessment, (3) exposure assessment (estimation of human exposure over time), and (4) risk characterization (determination of risk for human populations under various exposure scenarios).[19] In hazard identification, the range of toxic effects for a substance are identified from the literature. The second step, dose–response assessment, is used to describe as accurately as possible the relationship between magnitude, duration, frequency, and timing of chemical exposure and the frequency of manifestation of the chemical's adverse effects. Human exposure assessment identifies the range of exposures experienced by the target population of concern. In the fourth step, risk characterization, the particular risks that are likely to be experienced by the population of interest under actual expected exposure conditions are described. This four-step assessment framework can be applied to many types of health threats that arise within the environment, including potential threats arising from the introduction of new technologies. Comprehensive risk assessment directs attention to those sources of risk that, if reduced, will yield the greatest public health benefits.

Health professionals should note that the tolerance for risks on the part of individuals and families is based on the characteristics of the risk itself. For example:

1. Voluntarily assumed risks are tolerated better than those imposed by others.
2. Risks over which scientists debate and are uncertain are more feared than those in which scientific consensus endorses a risk.
3. Risks of natural origin are often considered to be less threatening than those created by humans.

Affective responses that differ according to the characteristics of the risk being considered can result in undue alarm or apathy. Individuals should be encouraged to consider objective information about the nature and extent of various environmental risks, rather than relying on feelings and emotions. Further, some societies base risk reduction priorities on the relative ease with which risk reduction can be achieved. Ease of resolution sometimes has a poor correspondence to the public health importance of the risks being attacked. Environmental risk reduction objectives should be based on the best available scientific knowledge about the relative risks of various pollutants to health rather than on what is emotionally appealing or politically attractive at a particular point in time.[31]

Many major environmental risks require intensive, multifaceted, and often long-term interventions to influence related attitudes and to reallocate resources for their control. By focusing on environmental change in the local community and its work sites, such as methods to reduce environmental pollutants; safe waste disposal; monitoring and surveillance to insure quality water; worker protection from toxic substances, diseases, and injuries, such as prevention of noise-induced hearing loss; nurses can play a proactive role in promoting health through environmental management.

Augmenting Health-Promoting Features of the Environment

Studies in environmental psychology have found that the environment can nurture, comfort, relax, strengthen, and add to a sense of well-being.[32] Important elements of a healing environment include color, lighting, furnishings, temperature, texture, nature, art, music, scents, and privacy. Restorative influences of viewing natural elements or nature scenes have been shown to promote a shift to a more positive emotional state and an increased attention span.[33] Understanding the uses of nature and its restorative properties may result in the development of innovative health promotion modalities for use by care providers in optimizing health and well-being.

Increasing evidence supports the importance of natural environments in assisting individuals to manage mental fatigue and, specifically, to regain directed attention capacities. Cimprich has developed nursing interventions that use the environment to assist cancer patients to cope with attentional fatigue created by the demands of their illness.[34,35,36] In a study of breast cancer patients, the intervention protocol consisted of explaining the restorative experience, choosing of restorative activities that would be performed for 20 to 30 minutes at least three times a week, contracting in writing to carry out the activities, and keeping track of restorative experiences. Examples of restorative activities selected were sitting or walking in the backyard, a garden, or a park; tending green living things; sitting by a pond, lake, or stream; and observing wildlife, birds, and animals. A comparison of intervention versus nonintervention groups on attentional performance across various tasks (e.g., Digit Span and Symbol Digit Modalities Test, Necker Cube Pattern Control, etc.) revealed that the intervention group showed a significant and steady improvement in attentional performance over time, whereas the nonintervention group showed inconsistent performance.

The research of Cimprich and her colleagues has important potential implications for creating health-strengthening environments for individuals of all ages in a wide array of contexts. Natural environments, as used in these studies, undoubtedly provide the best restorative milieus. However, simulated restorative environments that reduce environmental demands and promote rest are promising nursing interventions as well.

Supportive physical environments in health care settings have been implemented for patients undergoing bone marrow transplantation.[37] Nursing in collaboration with an interdisciplinary health care team created and implemented a quality-of-care model, of which one major component focused on changing the physical inpatient and outpatient environments to promote positive health outcomes, including quality of life.

Discovery of strategies to foster health and well-being through use of restorative environments in inner cities, at work sites, and in school settings will be a significant breakthrough in prevention and health promotion. Several important questions arising include What are the health-promoting aspects of the environment? How do features of the environment affect mental and physical health? What is the range of psychologic and biologic processes that can be affected positively by restorative environments?

Voluntary Change versus Legislative Policy

In a democratic society, it is widely assumed that matters of risk critical to survival and security are predominantly subject to regulatory decisions, whereas risks not clearly vital to general health and welfare are issues for personal decision and action. In a democracy, even vital risks may be left to individual decision, providing that they do not infringe on the rights of others. The role of government continues to be questioned in relation to legislating environmental and behavioral changes that promote good health and increase longevity. If the government uses the means at its disposal for regulating changes in behavior, it may be faced with problems of an ethical nature. On the other hand, educational approaches may fall short of achieving widespread change in self-damaging behaviors.

Government involvement in lifestyle reform is to some extent supported by the long-standing role of the federal government as a health care provider. In the face of high costs of health care, it may be cost-effective for the government to consider legislation that requires individuals to assume more self-care responsibility. Although such federal regulations might be cost effective if health promotion interventions are shown to reduce health care costs substantially, many individuals may resist legislation of preventive and health promotion measures as unethical or undue intrusion upon individual freedom. Ethical issues, including individual autonomy, must be thoughtfully considered in matters of health.

The two views are often labeled "individualism" and "paternalism."[38] Individualism is the American ideal, in which individuals are given maximum freedom in the area of health promotion. Health habits are considered personal, so outside interventions by governmental policy are not warranted. Poor health is attributed to individuals, thus society's responsibility is minimized. Paternalism, the philosophical counterpoint, holds that experts (professionals and policy makers) have a moral responsibility to solve health problems because individuals lack the ability to do so. Therefore, interventions, such as laws and public policies, are justified for the health of society. The role of the individual in this model is to adhere to the policies. Individuals are not blamed for their problems as they are viewed as the victims of circumstance. Both views have strengths that deserve mentioning. In the individualism model, control of health promotion is shared, as control is in the hands of the individuals, promoting a sense of efficacy and empowerment. Second, in the individualistic view, diversity of opinions is respected. The strength of the paternalistic view is that it is intended to reduce health disparities. Health policies are socially responsible as they apply to all segments of the population. In addition, problems greater than the individual, such as environmental issues, are recognized and addressed.

Both approaches have limitations as well. The overriding emphasis on individualism or personal responsibility for health results in victim blaming, which becomes problematic for poor people, because poverty is now widely accepted as a significant risk factor for illness and premature death.[39] However, overemphasis on paternalism or social responsibility ignores individual and group differences in human responses as well as the contributions of individuals to lifestyle change. The strengths of both approaches need to be combined to promote health in individuals and communities. Collaborative models of health promotion will promote community control, allow diversity, incorporate environmental issues, and reduce health disparities in different segments of the community.

Almost two decades ago, Pellegrino[40] suggested certain guidelines in considering trade-offs between individualism and social responsibility (paternalism) in relation to health. These guidelines remain timely.

1. Certain lifestyles result in disease, disability, and death, with economic consequences for the whole society. Thus, there is a social mandate to encourage healthier lifestyles in all citizens.

2. In a civilized and democratic society, individual freedom must be protected and is to be limited only when it violates the freedom of others. In an interdependent society, free acts are subject to justifiable restriction.

3. Coercive measures should be considered only when their effectiveness is unequivocal for large numbers of people and when control extends over a limited sector of life.

4. Even if a societal control measure meets all of the above criteria, it must accommodate as closely as possible the democratic principle of self-determination. Voluntary measures must be clearly inadequate at the outset or must have failed before coercive measures are contemplated.

While government regulation is sometimes deemed necessary for the public good, self-direction is valued by Americans because most individuals believe that they themselves are the best judge of what is good for them, and the process of choosing is considered a good in itself, even when the outcomes are health damaging. Some persons may voluntarily opt for a brief life span full of unhealthy practices. It can be argued that if the practices are not detrimental to others and are carried out in full awareness of the consequences, these people should be allowed to pursue the course they want. However, the role of the nurse is to make sure that individuals have as much information as possible on which to base informed decisions concerning lifestyle and health-related behavior.[25]

Deciding whether social changes to enhance health should be voluntary or mandatory presents society with a complex dilemma. Is coercion ever appropriate? If so, how and to what extent? Is it coercive to increase cigarette taxes in order to help defray the cost of smoking-induced disease? Should highly refined sugar products and high-cholesterol foods also be taxed more heavily to pay for the cost of health problems induced by obesity and atherosclerosis? Should taxes on large, high-speed automobiles be proportionately higher than taxes on smaller cars with limited speed and greater fuel economy? Which lifestyle, organizational, and social changes should be voluntary and which should be mandated through legislation? A balance of voluntary and mandatory action is needed, while continuing to pay close attention to the ethical dimensions of such health-related decisions.

Economic Incentives for Disease Prevention and Health Promotion

The dependence of the American people on diagnosis and treatment of disease to improve health and increase longevity is economically and socially rooted in our culture. Until recently, Americans have been willing to spend escalating proportions of both personal and public dollars on an increasing array of medical services, hoping for "magic bullets" to cure all ills. However, the availability of health care technology and medical interventions exceeds society's ability to afford them.[41] In addition, medical care is considered to account for only 10% to 15% of the declines in premature death in the Twentieth century, while factors that help to prevent illness have been responsible for the remaining decline. Health care systems are now undergoing restructuring and new health care policies are being implemented to attempt to achieve a balance among prevention, health promotion, and disease treatment services.

Health promotion programs continue to be at a competitive disadvantage for time and money, in spite of mounting evidence that health promotion and prevention efforts reduce morbidity and mortality for such conditions as heart disease, stroke, diabetes, injuries, and many cancers.[42] Those allocating resources continue to require evidence of potential for cost savings, indicating that health promotion programs will receive increased scrutiny as resources decline. If disease prevention and health promotion services are to be widely available to consumers in the twenty-first century, the public must be convinced of the value of staying well, the effectiveness of environmental and behavioral change in promoting health and preventing disease, and the economic and human advantage of shifting a portion of health care dollars from the treatment of illness to keeping people healthy. Nurse scientists and nurses in practice who develop health promotion interventions should be particularly sensitive to the need to evaluate costs as well as health outcomes.

Cost-effective analysis (CEA), cost–benefit analysis (CBA), and other economic evaluations discussed in Chapter 13 are increasingly assuming an important role in research and health care policy decisions.[43] These methods, particularly CEA, are useful for evaluating and comparing different health promotion strategies and providing health care professionals with important information related to patient preferences and priorities for prevention and health promotion.

Positive effects from any health promotion program require a chain of events: a structured program, participation continuing over time, and health enhancement or reduction of risk, measured by specified outcome criteria. For many disease prevention and health promotion programs, costs are incurred as the program is implemented while benefits may be obtained in the future. Although an extended time period between costs and benefits can be reconciled mathematically with cost-analysis procedures, consumers may not be willing to spend in order to protect themselves from a health problem with a 20-year latency to improve their health status when they feel well. Emphasizing short-term as well as long-term benefits may enhance consumer acceptance of disease prevention and health promotion interventions that require marked environmental and individual behavioral change.[43]

Current demands for medical services result in high rates of use of resource-intensive services and less emphasis on self-management, preventive, and health promotion services.[42] Insurance coverage offers little in the way of incentives to increase motivation for engaging in prevention and health promotion activities. For individuals and families who have insurance coverage for hospital care, few have coverage for disease prevention and health promotion services because such services cannot be related to a specific diagnosis or medical complaint. Even more distressing is the higher incidence of preventive screening in low-risk groups than in high-risk groups, when the latter group could benefit more from such services but does not have insurance to access them. This is referred to as reverse targeting. Unlike other countries, the United States does not assure that every person has health insurance. During the 1990s an increasing number of Americans found themselves uninsured or underinsured for health care costs, and this number continues to rise.[44] Those who are mainly affected include children and young adults, poor and middle-income families, blacks and Hispanics. States in the South and Southwest continue to have the highest rates of uninsurance. The disparities in disease and mortality rates among population groups will continue as long as this state of affairs persists, as lack of insurance has been associated with difficulties with access to the health care system, unmet medical needs, and less likelihood of obtaining preventive services such as mammograms.[44] It is obvious that the *Healthy People 2010* objectives cannot be achieved unless the financial barriers of receiving preventive and health promotion services are removed.

Managed care organizations have the potential to incorporate prevention and health promotion activities into the services provided. Rather than discouraging prevention and health promotion, as our present reimbursement system does, economic advantages for using such services need to be brought directly to consumers. The following suggestions for financial incentives are offered:

1. Expand insurance coverage to include primary health care services for prevention and health promotion.
2. Offer partial insurance premium refunds for maintaining good health or improving health status.
3. Develop a sliding scale for insurance premiums based on documented attendance at health education programs and use of early detection screening services.

Nurses are in a key position to work with consumer groups to shape health and social policies to offer more incentives for prevention and health promotion. Further, because of nursing's person–environment orientation, nurses can work in collaboration with other professionals and with target populations and communities to promote local, national, and global changes supportive of health and healthy lifestyles.

 # Directions for Research in Social and Environmental Change

Social and environmental change approaches to protect and promote health offer new vistas for nursing research. Social change approaches that realize human health potential will receive more attention in this century than ever before. New models that test public and organizational policy in managing risk and fostering health need rigorous evaluation. Suggested directions for nursing and interdisciplinary research efforts are as follows:

1. Test the effects of both family and community health promotion interventions on positively altering health-related social norms among children and adolescents.
2. Evaluate the effectiveness of interventions to decrease the exposure of children to passive smoke from parental smoking in their homes.
3. Develop and test models that proactively manage the environment to reduce health threats that are man-made or of natural origin.
4. Assess the targeted effects of various social and physical environmental interventions on behavior change
5. Test the effectiveness of various economic incentives in increasing health-promoting environmental and behavioral change.
6. Analyze the cost benefits and cost effectiveness of managed care plans that place major focus on health promotion and disease prevention services.
7. Test the effectiveness of eliminating environmental and financial barriers to healthy food choices and active lifestyles on the treatment and prevention of obesity.

The study of interactive effects of human and environmental factors in health and disease is complex and requires interdisciplinary research collaboration to address the many gaps in knowledge that now exist.

Directions for Practice to Promote Social and Environmental Change

Health promotion and prevention interventions can no longer focus exclusively on the individual if large-scale behavior change is to be achieved. It is now recognized that the social and physical environments, as well as individual behaviors, must be targeted. The comprehensive view of health promotion emphasizes the need for collaboration between health care professionals, health care organizations, and policy makers at the local, state, and national levels. Nurses will need to help build healthy communities by implementing interventions that focus on community development. Assessment skills are critical as the need to assess communities to identify resources, problems, and opportunities is necessary before prioritizing and planning interventions. Community development means that strategies are needed to involve the members of the community and provide them with training to develop the leadership necessary to play an active role in the change process. Because of the multiple factors involved in behavior change that go beyond the individual, nurses also need to become active in the promotion of health policy to decrease social and environmental risk factors present in many communities. This can be accomplished by working with local health departments and state legislatures to make change. Health promotion in the twenty-first century brings many challenges due to the rapid, ongoing changes in the population, workforce, technology, and health care environment. However, these challenges bring new opportunities for nursing.

SUMMARY

The focus of this chapter has been on society as a collective and the impact of public policy and social and physical environments on the health status of individuals, families, and communities. Attempts to change health behaviors without changes in the environments in which people live will result in frustration and failure of health promotion efforts. A balanced approach to disease prevention and health promotion within the United States requires attention to (1) the quality of the social and physical environments, (2) the disparities in health-promoting options available within the environment, and (3) the changes in health policy needed to create healthier communities. Because health is no longer viewed as an aim in itself, but as a resource for personal and social development, changes in public policies should become part of any effort to promote health.

WEB SITES OF CLEARINGHOUSES AND INFORMATION CENTERS OPERATED BY THE FEDERAL GOVERNMENT ON TOPICS COVERED IN THIS CHAPTER

Food and Drug Administration
www.fda.gov
Indoor Air Quality Information Clearing House
www.epa.gov/iaq

National Lead Information Center
epa.gov/lead/nlic.htm

Office on Smoking and Health
www.cdc.gov/tobacco

Clearinghouse for Occupational Safety and Health Information
www.cdc.gov/niosh/homepage.html

Drug Policy Information Clearinghouse
whitehousedrugpolicy.gov

REFERENCES

1. Thompson B, Kinne S. Social change theory: Applications to community health. In: Bracht N. *Health Promotion at the Community Level: New Advances.* 2nd ed. Thousand Oaks: Sage Publications; 1999:29–56

2. Hancock T. Future directions in population health. *Can J Public Health.* 1999;90(Suppl 1):S68–S70.

3. Reppucci ND, Woolard JL, Fried CS. Social, community, and preventive interventions. *Annual Reviews.* 1999; 50:387–418.

4. Steckler A, Allegrante JP, Altman D, Brown R, Burdine JN, et al. Health education intervention strategies: Recommendation for future research. *Health Educ Q.* 1995;22:307–328.

5. U.S. Department of Health and Human Services. *Healthy People 2010* (Conference Edition in Two Volumes). Washington DC: U.S. Government Printing Service; January 2000.

6. Minkler M, Wallerstein N. Improving health through community organization and community building. In: Glanz K, Lewis FM, Rimer BK, eds. *Health Behavior and Health Education.* San Francisco: Jossey-Bass Publishers; 1997:241–269.

7. Lichtenstein E, Thompson B, Nettekoven L, Corbett K. Durability of tobacco control activities in eleven North American communities: Life after the community intervention trial for smoking cessation (COMMIT). *Health Educ Res.* 1996;11:527–534.

8. Sallis JF, Owen N. Ecological models. In: Glanz K, Lewis FM, Rimer BK, eds. *Health Behavior and Health Education.* San Francisco: Jossey-Bass Publishers, 1997:403–424.

9. Green LW. Health education's contributions to public health in the twentieth century: A glimpse through health promotion's rear-view mirror. *Annual Reviews of Public Health.* 1999;20:67–88.

10. Oliver TR. Dynamics without change: The new generation. *Journal of Health Politics, Policy and Law.* 2000;25(1):225–232.

11. Olden PC. Well-being revisited: Improving the health of a population. *Journal of Healthcare Management.* 1998;43(1):36–48.

12. Kronenfeld JJ. Salient features of the U.S. health care infrastructure and delivery system. *In The Changing Role in U.S. Health Care Policy.* Westport, CT: Praeger; 1997:19–48.

13. Gulzar L. Access to health care. *J Nurs Schol.* 1999;31(1):13–19.

14. Speers MA, Lancaster B. Disease prevention and health promotion in urban areas: CDC's perspective. *Health Education and Behavior.* 1998;25(2):226–233.

15. Mechanic D. Issues in promoting health. *Social Science and Medicine.* 1999;48:711–718.

16. Goldstein D, Flory J. The Internet revolution: Transforming health care delivery. *Medical Interface.* 1997;10(2):56–58.

17. Leaffer T, Gonda B. The Internet: An underutilized tool in patient education. *Comput Nurs.* 2000;18(1):47–52.

18. Winzelberg AJ, Eppstein D, Eldredge KL, Wilfley D, Dasmahapatra R, Dev P, Taylor CB. Effectiveness of an Internet-based program for reducing risk factors for eating disorders. *J Consult Clin Psychol*. 2000;68(2):346–350.

19. Leeder SR. Health-promoting environments: The role of public policy. *Aust N Z J Public Health*. 1997;21(4 Spec No):413–414.

20. Harris E, Wills J. Developing healthy local communities at local government level: Lessons from the past decade. *Aust N Z J Public Health*. 1997;21(4 Spec No):403–412.

21. Buchanon DR. Relevance for professionals and issues for the future. In: Gochman DS. *Handbook of Health Behavior Research IV—Relevance for Professionals and Issues for the Future*. New York: Plenum Press; 1997:163–179.

22. Mileo N. Priorities and strategies for promoting community-based prevention policies. *Journal of Health Management Practice*. 1998;4(3):14–28.

23. Brownson RC, Newschaffer CJ, Ali-Abarghoui F. Policy research for disease prevention: Challenges and practice recommendations. *Am J Public Health*. 1997;87:735–739.

24. Mittlemark MB. The psychology of social influence and healthy public policy. *Prev Med*. 1999;29:S24–S29.

25. Armstrong B. Health-promoting environments: Prospects for national monitoring measures. *Aust and N Z J Public Health*. 1997;21(4 Spec No):415–416.

26. Salazar MK. Environmental health: Responding to the call. *Public Health Nurs*. 2000;17(2):73–74.

27. www.epa.gov/iaq/radon/pubs/citguide.html#risk.

28. Lusk SL, Kerr MJ, Kaufman SA. Use of hearing protective and perceptive of noise exposure and hearing lose among constructive workers. *American Industrial Hygiene Association Journal*. 1998;59:466–470.

29. Lusk SL, Ronis DL, Baer LM. Gender differences in blue-collar workers' use of hearing protection. *Human and Health*. 1997;25(4):69–89.

30. Lusk SL. Effects of hearing and protection of noise induced hearing loss. *AAOHN Journal*. 1997;45(8):397–405.

31. Rodricks JV. Risk assessment, the environment, and public health. *Environ Health Perspect*. 1994;102(3):258–264.

32. Neumann T, Mensik K. The healing power of design. *Innovator St. Luke's Episcopal Hospital*. Division of Nursing. 1993 spring.

33. Ulrich RS. How design impacts wellness. *Healthcare Forum Journal*. 1992 Sep–Oct;20–25.

34. Cimprich B. Development of an intervention to restore attention in cancer patients. *Cancer Nurs*. 1993;16(2):83–92.

35. Cimprich B. Symptom management: Loss of concentration. *Seminars in Oncology Nursing*. 1995;11(4):279–288.

36. Wintermeyer-Pingle S, Cimprich B, Marciniak K. Model allows nurses to prioritize patient teaching for chemotherapy. *Oncology Nursing Forum* 1997;24(3):456–457.

37. Murdaugh C, Parsons M, Gryb-Wysocki T, Palmer J, Glasby C, Bonner J, Tavakoli A. Implementing a quality of care model in a restructured hospital environment. *National Academies of Practice Forum*. 1996;1(3):219–226.

38. Ribisl KM, Humphries K. Collaboration between professionals and mediating structures in the community: Towards a "Third Way" in health promotion. In: Shumaker SA, Schron EB, Ockene JK, McBee WL. *The Handbook of Health Behavior Change*. 2nd ed. New York: Springer; 1998:535–554

39. Minkler M. Personal responsibility for health? A review of the arguments and the evidence at century's end. *Health Education and Behavior.* 1999;26(1):121–140.

40. Pellegrino ED. Health promotion as public policy: The need for moral grounding. *Prev Med.* 1981;10:371–378.

41. McGinnis, JM. Foreward. In: Gold MR, Siegel JE, Russell LB, Weinstein MC. *Cost-effectiveness in Health and Medicine.* New York: Oxford University Press; 1996, V–VII.

42. Fries JF, Koop CE, Sokolov J, Beadle CR, Wright D. Beyond health promotion: Reducing need and demand for medical care. *Health Affairs.* 1998;17(2):70–84.

43. Brown AD, Garber AM. A concise review of the cost-effectiveness of coronary heart disease prevention. *Medical Clinics of North America.* 2000;84(1):279–297.

44. Carrasquillo O, Himmelstein DU, Woolhandler S, and Bor DH. Going bare: trends in health insurance coverage, 1989 through 1996. *Am J Public Health.* 1999;89(1):36–42.

Index

Kluckhohn, FR, 110
Knutsen, R, 293
Knutsen, SF, 293
Koop, C. Everett, 211
Kreuter, MW, 51, 52

L

Latinos. *See* Hispanic Americans
Lazarus, RS, 218
LDL (low-density lipoprotein) cholesterol, 200, 204, 208
Lead, 316
Leahey, M, 136, 137
Legislative policy, 319–321
Leisure physical activity, 170
Lenz, ER, 44
Levine, LM, 19
Life-stress review, 127–132
Lifestyle, assessment of, 133–136
Lifestyle physical activity, 170
Lifestyle reform, government involvement in, 320
Literacy, 109
Loneliness, preventing, 251
Loveland-Cherry, CJ, 26, 88, 293
Low-density lipoprotein (LDL) cholesterol, 200, 204, 208
Lusk, SL, 67, 68, 297, 317

M

Mackenzie, Alec, 225
Maintenance stage, in transtheoretical model, 41
Malnutrition, 125
Mann, L, 41
Manual of Nursing Diagnoses: 1998-1999, 119
Manual of Nursing Diagnosis: 1998-1999 (Gordon), 205, 223
Marcus, BH, 42, 52, 179, 182
Marlatt, GA, 44, 45
Mass media, eating habits and, 199
McAuley, E, 71
McBride, JL, 132
McClowery, SG, 87
McDermott, RJ, 133
McKenzie, TL, 175
McKinlay, JB, 279
Measurement, of outcomes of interventions
  challenges in, 269–270
  deciding which outcomes to measure, 264–265

developing a plan to measure health outcomes, 268–269
  directions for nursing research in, 270
  timing of outcome measures, 266
Media campaigns, 280
Medications (drugs), foods and, 204
Menninger Foundation Biofeedback Center, 128
Mental health, 219. *See also* Stress
  concept of, 17
Mexican Americans, 37. *See also* Hispanic Americans
  children, 175
Middle-age adults, self-care for, 88–89
Midstream interventions, 279
Mischke-Berkey, K, 137
Motivation
  for health behavior, 34
  for learning, empowering competence and, 95
Muscular endurance, assessment of, 120–121
Mutual help groups, 241

N

National Cholesterol Education Program, 192–193
National Database of Nursing Quality Indicators (NDNQI), 264
National Institute for Occupational Safety and Health (NIOSH), 317
National Institutes of Health, 87
National Research Council, 317–318
Neuman, B, 19
Neuman Health-Care Systems Model, 137
Newman, MA, 21
Nichols, JF, 105
Nies, MA, 177
Nightingale, Florence, 260
Normality, definitions of health based on, 19, 20
North American Diagnosis Association (NANDA), 263
North American Nursing Diagnosis Association (NANDA), 118–119, 180
North Campus Nursing Center (University of Michigan), 298
Nurse-client contracts, 158, 162
Nurse-managed community health centers, 298–299
Nurses
  contribution to the prevention and health promotion team, 10
  empowering clients for self-care and, 84